AF833081

TUMORS OF THE CENTRAL NERVOUS SYSTEM – PRIMARY AND SECONDARY

Edited by **Lee Roy Morgan**

Tumors of the Central Nervous System – Primary and Secondary
http://dx.doi.org/10.5772/57014
Edited by Lee Roy Morgan

Contributors

Richard Michael Zuniga, Siddharth Joshi, Lee Roy Morgan, Igor Pessoa, Fabio Da Silva, Nilson Anselmo, Edivaldo Herculano Correa De Oliveira, Pinar Atukeren, Taner Tanriverdi, M.Ramazan Yigitoglu, Marc-Eric Halatsch, Georg Karpel-Massler, Adrianna Ranger, Navjot Chaudhary, Jonathan Lau, Hassan Mahmoud Fathallah-Shaykh, Paula Province, Davide Schiffer, Laura Annovazzi, Yasushi Shibata

Published by InTech

Janeza Trdine 9, 51000 Rijeka, Croatia

Copyright © 2014 InTech

Individual chapters are under their authors' copyright and distributed under the Creative Commons Attribution 3.0 license, which allows users to download, copy and build upon published chapters provided that the authors and publisher are properly credited, which ensures maximum dissemination and a wider impact of the authors' work. Any republication, referencing or personal use of the individual chapters or any of their contents must explicitly identify the original source.

Permission for commercial use of the book as a whole, such as (but not limited to) reprint rights, republication, distribution, sales, translation, and reproduction in any and all forms of media, must always be obtained from InTech.

Notice

Statements and opinions expressed in the chapters are these of the individual contributors and not necessarily those of the editors or publisher. No responsibility is accepted for the accuracy of information contained in the published chapters. The publisher assumes no responsibility for any damage or injury to persons or property arising out of the use of any materials, instructions, methods or ideas contained in the book.

Publishing Process Manager Iva Lipovic

Technical Editor InTech DTP team

Cover InTech Design team

First published June, 2014

Printed in Croatia

Additional hard copies can be obtained from orders@intechopen.com

Tumors of the Central Nervous System – Primary and Secondary, Edited by Lee Roy Morgan

p. cm.

ISBN 978-953-51-1576-2

We are IntechOpen, the world's leading publisher of Open Access books

Built by scientists, for scientists

4,200+
Open access books available

116,000+
International authors and editors

125M+
Downloads

151
Countries delivered to

Our authors are among the
Top 1%
most cited scientists

12.2%
Contributors from top 500 universities

WEB OF SCIENCE™

Selection of our books indexed in the Book Citation Index
in Web of Science™ Core Collection (BKCI)

Interested in publishing with us?
Contact book.department@intechopen.com

Numbers displayed above are based on latest data collected.
For more information visit www.intechopen.com

For EU product safety concerns:
IN TECH d.o.o., Prolaz Marije Krucifikse Kozulić 3, 51000 Rijeka, Croatia,
info@intechopen.com or visit our website at intechopen.com.

Meet the editor

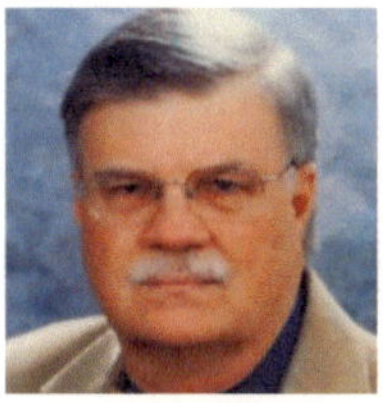

Dr. Morgan is a clinical pharmacologist and oncologist whose research interests are focused on developing new and novel agents that penetrate the CNS and are effective against both CNS primary and metastatic cancers. Dr. Morgan is currently CEO of DEKK-TEC, Inc. in New Orleans, Louisiana.

Contents

Preface IX

Section 1 CNS Cancer – Past, Present and Future 1

Chapter 1 **High Grade Glioma — Standard Approach, Obstacles and Future Directions 3**
Siddharth K. Joshi and Richard Zuniga

Chapter 2 **Paediatric Brainstem Cancers — Where We Have Been; Where We Are; Where We Are Going 31**
Adrianna Ranger, Navjot Chaudhary and Jonathan Lau

Section 2 New Diagnostic Approaches – CNS Tumors 61

Chapter 3 **Spatial Relationships of MR Imaging and Positron Emission Tomography with Phenotype, Genotype and Tumor Stem Cell Generation in Glioblastoma Multiforme 63**
Davide Schiffer, Consuelo Valentini, Antonio Melcarne, Marta Mellai, Elena Prodi, Giovanna Carrara, Tetyana Denysenko, Carola Junemann, Cristina Casalone, Cristiano Corona, Valentina Caldera, Laura Annovazzi, Angela Piazzi, Paola Cassoni, Rebecca Senetta, Piercarlo Fania and Angelina Cistaro

Chapter 4 **New Application of 123I-Iodoamphetamine SPECT for the Diagnosis of Primary Central Nervous System Lymphoma 95**
Yasushi Shibata

Section 3 Neurobiochemical – Considerations for the Future 103

Chapter 5 **Biochemical and Surgical Aspects of Epilepsy Related to Brain Tumors — Appraising Redox Biology and Treatments 105**
Pinar Atukeren, Taner Tanriverdi and M. Ramazan Yigitoglu

Chapter 6 **Alterations in TP53 gene – Implications in Tumorigenesis Process and Prognosis in Central Nervous System Cancer 127**
Igor Andrade Pessôa, Fabio P. Estumano da Silva, Nilson Praia Anselmo and Edivaldo Herculano C. de Oliveira

Section 4 Angiogenesis and Immune Therapy – New Therapeutical Approaches 175

Chapter 7 **Anti-Angiogenesis, Gene Therapy, and Immunotherapy in Malignant Gliomas 177**
Paula Province, Alexis Bashinski Shaefer, Benjamin McCullough and Hassan M Fathallah-Shaykh

Chapter 8 **Erlotinib in Glioblastoma – A Current Clinical Perspective 223**
Georg Karpel-Massler and Marc-Eric Halatsch

Section 5 New Drugs for CNS Tumors – The Hope for the Future 237

Chapter 9 **Comparative Preclinical Pharmacology and Toxicology for 4-demethyl-4-cholesteryloxycarbonylpenclomedine (DM-CHOC-PEN) — A Potential Neuro-Alkylating Agent for Glioblastoma (GBM) and Metastatic Cancers Involving the Central Nervous System 239**
Lee Roy Morgan, Andrew H. Rodgers, Gerard Bastian, Edmund Benes, William S. Waud, Christopher Papagiannis, Dan Krietlow, Branko S. Jursic, Robert F. Struck, Gerald LaHoste, Melissa Thornton, Melody Luttrell, Edward Stevens and Rodger Thompson

Preface

The treatment of malignancies involving the central nervous system – primary, as well as metastatic, has improved in recent years, however, the long term responses are still depressing.

The causes for the paucity of useful chemotherapeutic agents have been due to a reluctance to enroll patients with advanced CNS cancer in new clinical trials.

Thus, the knowledge of anti-cancer drug pharmacology in the brain is lagging. *Tumors of the Central Nervous System – Primary and Secondary* presents a concerted effort to appreciate the relationships between the pathophysiology of malignancies growing in the brain, the functions of the blood brain barrier (BBB), tolerance of the brain to potential new drugs, and new imaging techniques. Neurooncology has been a sleeping giant and finally the neurosurgeons, neuropharmacologists, neuro-oncologists, neuro-physiologists and the medicinal chemists are all working together to identify novel, safe and effective anticancer agents and procedures to treat CNS tumors. Plus the FDA's Orphan Designated Drug program has created an incentive for pharmaceutical industry involvement. Maybe we can *'catch up'* .

Every chapter in "*Tumors of the Central Nervous System – Primary and Secondary* " is an example of neuro-collaborations and contains new approaches, in-depth discussions and/or reviews of diagnostic and therapeutic concepts that will improve the management of key topics in neurooncology.

Neurooncology is still an *empirical subspecialty* when it comes to selecting treatment plans or cancer chemotherapy. We continue to face the *age old question* from patients and families during the treatment process – *will the patient respond, not when a response will occur* . This is often based on the fact that we lack the ability to predict whether or not a drug or drugs will:

Be absorbed

Be absorbed

Undergo the required activation or metabolism

Enter the cancer cell

Target a bio-sensitive site

and , if all the required pharmacological criteria are met, in fact *'will the cancer cell respond in the proper way to therapy – with death'!*

Tumors of the Central Nervous System – Primary and Secondary is designed to integrate concepts in surgery, diagnostic imaging, radiation and molecular pharmacology with results from empirical trials to promote our advancement on current neurooncology issues.

Perhaps the information presented in these chapters will help reverse the negative concept that *'Cancer of the Brain'* always has a fatal outcome.

I sincerely hope that all enjoy reading the book, as much as I have enjoyed writing a chapter and reviewing the book.

Lee Roy Morgan, MD, PhD
CEO
DEKK-TEC, Inc.
New Orleans, United States

Section 1

CNS Cancer – Past, Present and Future

Chapter 1

High Grade Glioma — Standard Approach, Obstacles and Future Directions

Siddharth K. Joshi and Richard Zuniga

Additional information is available at the end of the chapter

http://dx.doi.org/10.5772/58548

1. Introduction

Glioblastoma Multiforme is the most malignant of gliomas. These malignancies that arise from glial cells remain one of the pre-eminent and confounding therapeutic challenges in oncology and medicine at-large. Though uncommon, it continues to be responsible for disproportionate rates of morbidity and mortality the world over, as qualified by a median survival of only about 15 months despite optimal treatment [1, 2]. This is in large part due to its heterogeneous biology, exceedingly complex molecular pathogenesis, and the tumor's predilection for growth in the CNS. Ongoing research, particularly in the last decade, has provided the scientific and medical worlds with ever deeper insight into, and further elucidation of, the biology and molecular pathogenesis of Glioblastoma Multiforme (GBM). This in turn has led to compelling novel treatment modalities that range from rudimentarily conceptual to, excitingly, on the very cusp of implementation. This chapter aims to provide the reader with a comprehensive survey of Glioblastoma Multiforme contextualized within the broader realm of malignant gliomas.

GBM is the most common malignant primary brain cancer in adults, accounting for roughly 3 new cases per 100,000 people [3]. Underscoring its importance as a therapeutic target, GBM accounts for nearly 16% of all brain tumors and, furthermore, nearly 46% of malignant gliomas [3]. The average age at diagnosis of GBM is 64 years of age, and, for reasons yet unclear, it has demonstrated a clear male predilection, being about 1.6 times more common in males than females [3].

Running in tandem with the quest for more effective therapies for GBM has been a long and intensive search for clear risk factors positively associated with the development of GBM. This search, however, has been fraught with many dead ends. Indeed, no clear inciting cause has been identified for the vast majority of cases of GBM and the only bona-fide established risk factor is exposure to ionizing radiation. The cause-effect relationship between ionizing

INTECH
open science | open minds

© 2014 The Author(s). Licensee InTech. This chapter is distributed under the terms of the Creative Commons Attribution License (http://creativecommons.org/licenses/by/3.0), which permits unrestricted use, distribution, and reproduction in any medium, provided the original work is properly cited.

radiation and the development of GBM was established with studies that demonstrated that children treated with radiotherapy for malignancies like leukemia have a markedly increased risk for developing GBM [4]. Family history of cancer of any type also has a suggested association, being found in the family members of roughly 19% of patients diagnosed with GBM in one small study [5]. In a small minority, approximately 5%, of diagnosed primary brain tumors, there is the presence of genetically inherited syndromes (e.g. Neurofibromatosis Types I and II, Li-Fraumeni Syndrome, von Hippel-Lindau Syndrome, Turcot Syndrome, Tuberous Sclerosis), which suggests a putative genetic relationship [6]. As with other malignancies, it has also been suggested that viral infections, specifically by SV40, HHV-6, and CMV, may be associated with the development of GBM by tumorigenesis through integration of viral genetic material into normal DNA [7-10]. Another putative association that has garnered much in the way of publicity is the relationship between cell phone use and development of primary brain tumors. This is a weakly-supported association based on the aggregate epidemiological data on hand that deserves further study and follow-up in the years to come as cell phone use becomes more ubiquitous the world over [11,12].

2. Histopathology

GBM is, in a manner of speaking, the pathological culmination of and histological end point on the broader continuum of gliomas/astrocytomas. The word Glioma literally translates in Greek into the English equivalent of "glue" [13]. This connotates the functional conception of the cells that beget gliomas, i.e. gliomas arise from those cells in the CNS that form the support framework for neurons. It merits a side note here that though this has been the traditional conception of glial cells, new studies have shown them to possess a more autonomous role than previously supposed [15]. The WHO has classified gliomas/astrocytomas into 4 grades that, successively, convey graver prognostic significance (See Table 1); this is the 4th iteration of this classification system published in 2007 and originally conceived in 1979 [15]. This method of classification, based on histopathological features, is one that has built a certain assumed relevance for clinical decision making. The neuro-oncologist uses it as a template to guide whether a patient may qualify for a conservative strategy of watchful waiting, as with Grades I and sometimes with Grade II, or aggressive radiotherapy with chemotherapy, as with Grades III and IV. Indeed, only Grades III (Anaplastic astrocytoma/oligodendroglioma) and IV (GBM) are considered malignant gliomas. There are discrete histological features that qualify Grade III and IV astrocytomas as malignant. Grade III gliomas when compared to lower grades, is distinguished by a significant increase in cellularity, mitotic activity, and nuclear atypia [16] (See Figure 3). Grade IV gliomas, in addition to these telltale harbingers of malignant transformation, is embodied, uniquely, by areas of microvascular proliferation and/or neoplastic tissue necrosis [16] (See Figure 4). Indeed, it is worthy of emphatic mention that one of the overarching and typifying characteristics of malignant gliomas is their histological heterogeneity, i.e. consisting of both neoplastic and stromal tissue [16]

http://dx.doi.org/10.5772/58548

Localized Astrocytoma
WHO Grade I
Pilocytic Astrocytoma
Pleomorphic Xanthoastrocytoma
Subependymal Giant Cell Astrocytoma
Diffuse Astrocytomas/Oligodendrogliomas
WHO Grade II (Astrocytoma)
Fibrillary
Protoplasmic
Gemistocytic
WHO Grade II (Oligodendroglioma_
WHO Grade III (Anaplastic Astrocytoma) WHO Grade III (Anaplastic Oligodendroglioma)
WHO Grade IV (Glioblastoma Multiforme)
Giant Cell Glioblastoma
Gliosarcoma

Table 1. WHO Classification of Gliomas

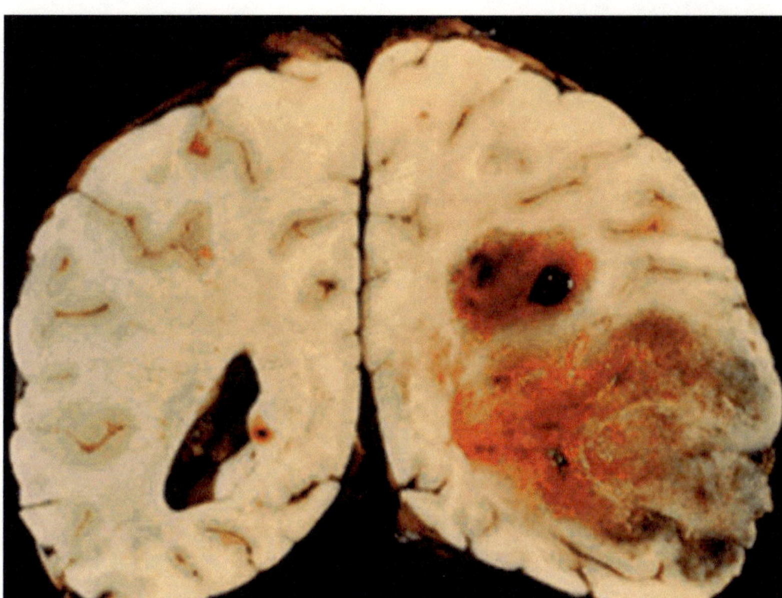

Figure 1. Gross Appearance of GBM

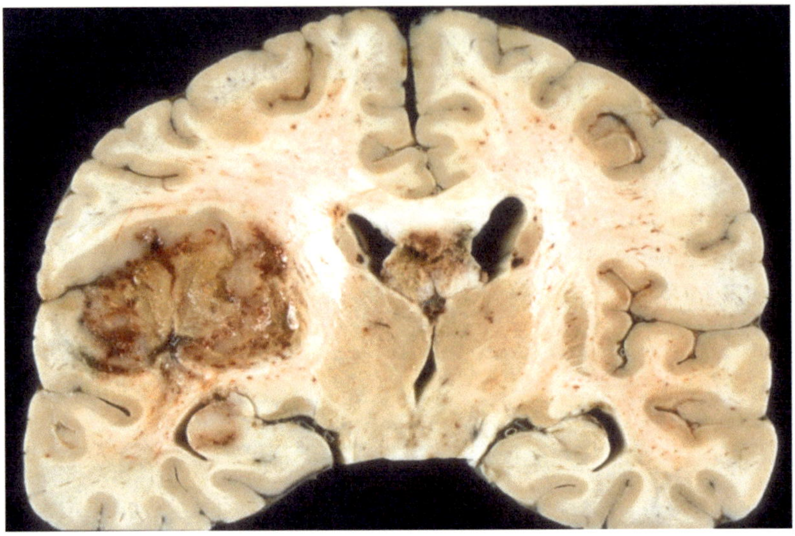

Figure 2. Gross Appearance of GBM

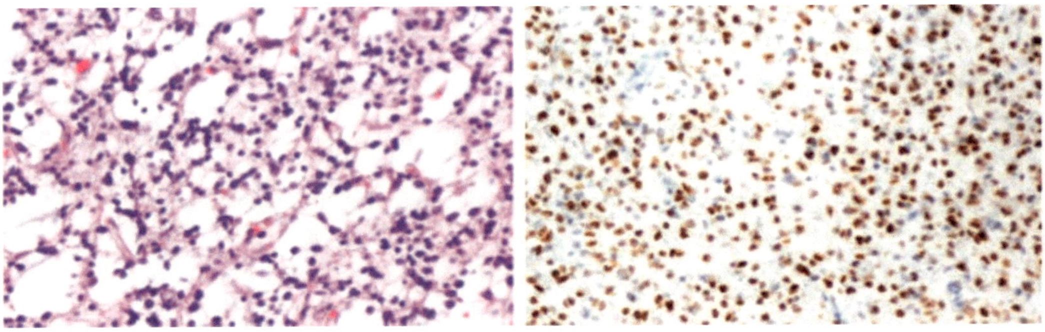

Figure 3. Histological Appearance of Grade III Anaplastic Oligodendroglioma. [16]

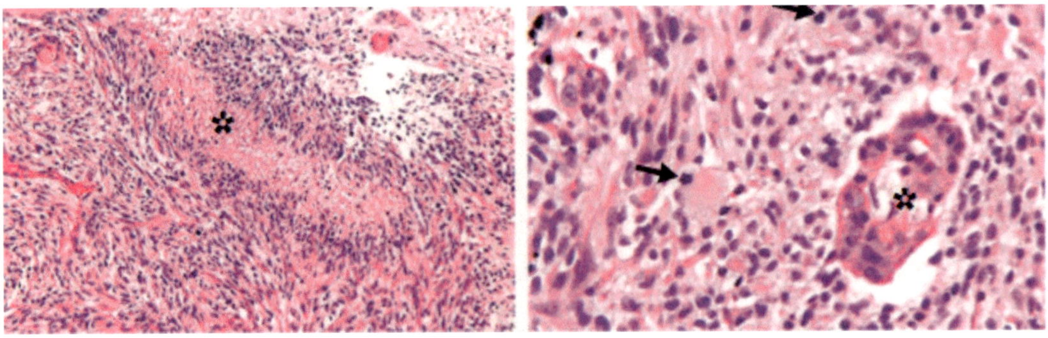

Figure 4. Histological Appearance of GBM. First Panel shows Pseudopalisading Nuclei at area of asterisk; second panel shows mitotic figures at arrows and endothelial proliferation at asterisk. [16]

The pathology of GBM, quite simply, is summated by foci of necrotic tissue surrounded by anaplastic cells and microvascular hyperplasia. The anaplastic cells surrounding the foci of necrosis are unique for malignant gliomas and are known as "pseudopalisading cells" due to their configuration around the necrotic foci (Refer to asterisk in Figure 4, which shows a necrotic center surrounded by pseudopalisading cells). It is interesting to note that the pseudopalisades, hyperplastic vasculature and necrotic centers are all inextricably linked to one another. The pseudopalisading cells are found to be severely hypoxic which causes over-expression of hypoxia-inducible factor (HIF-1) and secretion of pro-angiogenic factors VEGF and IL-8. It is thought that the telltale hypoxia and necrosis that distinguish malignant gliomas arise as a result of vascular occlusion and intravascular thrombosis that are inevitable consequences of tumor outgrowing blood supply. By this model, then, the pseudopalisading nuclei are seen as waves allowing for tumor cells to extend outwards from necrotic foci into normal surrounding parenchyma [33]. Another tumor type of neuroepithelial tissue with malignant capacity is oligodendroglioma. This type of tumor usually presents in younger patients within the white matter of the frontal and temporal lobes. Histologically, oligodendrogliomas are characterized by round nuclei and perinuclear halos dispersed in a monotonous pattern. The perinuclear halos are a preparation artifact that is characteristic of oligodendrogliomas and are frequently described as having a "fried-egg appearance". This type of tumor can be classified as WHO grade II or III (diffuse oligodendroglioma and anaplastic oligodendroglioma respectively) and the presence of a high mitotic rate (most 5-10%), vascular endothelial hyperplasia and nuclear pleomorphism categorizes the tumor as Grade III anaplastic oligodendroglioma.

When one considers the origin of malignant gliomas, i.e. the inciting events that herald transformation of normal glial tissue/parenchyma into malignant tissue, they conform to the general oncological orthodoxy. That is, they are basically the end-result of stepwise mutations in genes responsible for essential biological processes, most notably cell growth, proliferation and controlled cell death. Oncogenesis of GBM is essentially representative of that basic canon in oncology--activation of oncogenes and silencing of tumor suppressor genes. In other words, stepwise acquisition of new biological properties/characteristics by oncogenesis confers phenotypic characteristics that allow the malignant cells to outcompete their wild-type counterparts in their micro-mileu.

3. Primary vs. secondary GBM

Upon diagnosis, GBM is customarily delineated into one of two broad categories--Primary GBM, which arises *de novo* in brain tissue, or Secondary, which develops from lower grade astrocytomas (Refer to Table 2 for salient respective features and differences). In addition to the fundamental etiological difference, primary GBM possesses categorically different genetic and epigenetic differences from Secondary GBM. (Epigenetics refers to those meiotically or mitotically heritable traits resulting in phenotypic/gene expression patterns not related to changes in the underlying actual DNA code.) The vast majority of cases are GBM are primary, i.e. *de novo,* and comprise upwards of 90% of diagnosed cases. Epidemiologically, Primary

GBMs are almost always found in the elderly population with a mean age of diagnosis of 62 years and is characterized by a rapidly inexorable course till death [27]. The genetic/epigenetic features that beget the malignant transformation in primary GBM and encompass its difference from secondary GBM include: mutations in and amplification of EGFR, loss of heterozygosity of Chromosome 10q, deletion of the phosphatase and tensin homologue (PTEN) on Chromosome 10, and p16 deletion [16,23]. Secondary GBM, on the other hand, predominantly affects younger patients with a mean age at diagnosis of 45 years, and is characterized by a much slower, more smoldering course than Primary GBM [23]. Secondary GBM evolves from Grade II (Low Grade Well-Differentiated) and Grade III (Anaplastic) astrocytomas, has a predilection for the frontal lobes, and develops from its precursors over the course of years. An epidemiological study from 2005 showed that the time of progression from low-grade astrocytoma to GBM was approximately 5.3 years whereas the time of progression from anaplastic astrocytoma to GBM was approximately 1.4 years [28]. This stands in stark contrast to the rapidity of Primary GBM progression, with roughly two-thirds of patients having a clinical history from time of diagnosis to death of less than 3 months [27]. As stated, secondary glioblastoma has a genetic/epigenetic footprint that differs from Primary GBM, the exception being the commonality of loss of heterozygosity of Chromosome 10q. The differences in this epigenetic footprint include: mutations in p53, over expression of Platelet-Derived Growth Factor Receptor (PDGFR), aberrancies in p16/Retinoblastoma pathways, and global differences in transcription patterns and DNA copy numbers [16]. It is worthy of emphatic mention here that primary and secondary GBM, though developing through distinct genetic and molecular pathways, are grossly and histologically indistinguishable from one another.

	Primary GBM	**Secondary GBM**
Mean Age at Diagnosis	~ 62 years of age	~45 years of age
Percentage of Cases	> 90%	< 10%
Clinical Course	Rapid	Smoldering
Genetic Hallmarks	EGFR, etc.	PDGFR, etc.

Table 2. Primary vs. Secondary GBM

4. Clinical characteristics

The clinical presentation of GBM is, as intuited, dependent in large part on the location of the tumor. Continuing to bode ill for both treatment and prognosis is the sobering fact that malignant gliomas, and GBM in particular, grow insidiously and largely asymptomatically until they are big enough to elicit symptoms by sheer mass effect. By that time, tellingly, the options for surgical resection are relatively limited given extension into vital CNS parenchyma. Common presenting symptoms include recalcitrant headaches, unprovoked new-onset seizures, unprecedented memory loss, unaccountable changes in personality or consciousness, cognitive/language impairments, and other miscellaneous symptoms, i.e. nausea/vomiting.

http://dx.doi.org/10.5772/58548

Though there are no pathognomonic symptoms that may help the clinician to reliably distinguish between the two WHO Grades of malignant gliomas, there have been cohort studies done that have shown some nuances in symptomatology between Anaplastic

Astrocytoma and Glioblastoma Multiforme (See Table 3). Prognostic factors boding favorably for patients diagnosed with malignant gliomas include a lower tumor grade, resection of tumor mass, younger age (less than 50 years) at time of diagnosis, higher performance status (e.g. ECOG) score and intact neurological function [35].

Symptom	Grade III, %	Grade IV, %
Headache	53	57
Seizure	56	23
Memory Loss	26	39
Motor Weakness	25	36
Visual Symptoms	23	21
Language Deficits	22	36
Cognitive Changes	22	39
Personality Changes	11	27
Change in Consciousness	11	18
Nausea and Vomiting	8	15
Sensory Deficit	5	12
Papilledema	5	5

Table 3. Initial Symptoms in 565 Patients with Grade III or Grade IV Malignant Glioma (Data from Glioma Outcomes Project [29])

5. Diagnosis

The diagnostic modalities for suspected GBM in the appropriate clinical setting are, broadly, twofold: imaging and biopsy. The cornerstone of imaging is MRI with and without Gadolinium contrast enhancement. Prior to administration of contrast, malignant gliomas are hypo-intense on T1-weighted images (See Figure 5). Upon administration of Gadolinium, it is found that tumor enhances heterogeneously; this allows it to be distinguished from surrounding edema that remains hypo-intense on T-1 weighted images (See Figure 5). Another ancillary MRI sub-modality is FLAIR (Fluid Attenuated Inverse Reconstruction) MRI (See Figure 5) [30]. The utility of FLAIR MRI is that, as an inversion recovery MRI technique, it can essentially nullify or subtract the effects of fluid, thereby suppressing CSF in brain imaging. This can be especially useful in planning radiation therapy (to be discussed in more detail below) when it is of vital importance to delineate malignancy from native vital brain parenchyma [31].

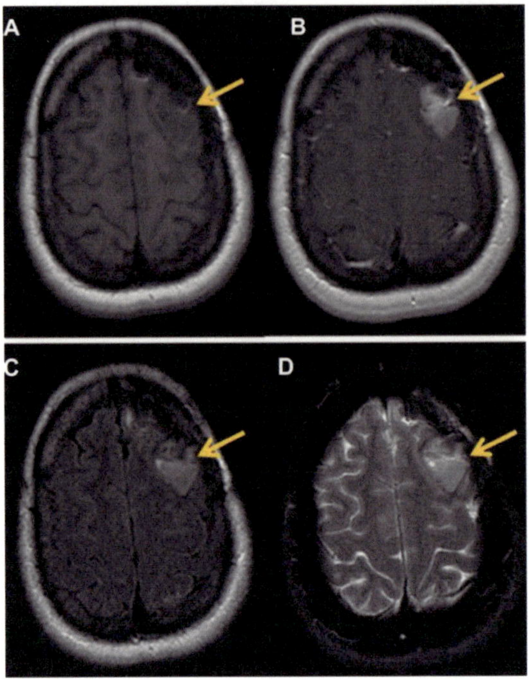

Figure 5. (A) T1 pre-contrast images exhibit a hypointense lesion in the left frontal lobe region (arrow). (B) Axial T1 post-contrast images, after injection of 20 cc of intravenous MultiHance®, demonstrate a focus of enhancement in left frontal lobe. (C) Axial T2 FLAIR images show increase in FLAIR signal in the left frontal lobe, which demonstrates enhancement. (D) T2 FSE images also demonstrate increase in signal in the region of the left frontal lobe.[30]

The gold standard for diagnosis, of course, remains procurement of tissue for histological confirmation that can either be accomplished either diagnostically through stereotactic biopsy or, more commonly, diagnostically and therapeutically with tissue samples obtained during craniotomy for the purposes of tumor resection or debulking.

6. Role of surgical resection

The standard treatment for newly-diagnosed GBM has remained relatively staid as evinced by the relatively abysmal prognosis over the aggregate of decades. However, caveat emptor must once again be invoked as there is a sea change in elucidation of the molecular features of GBM that promises much in the way of therapeutic potential on the horizon. This will be discussed in detail in content to follow.

The first modality in treatment is maximally safe surgical resection. This, it needs bearing in mind, is not curative. At the time of diagnosis, newly-found GBM has invariably infiltrated extensively into normal brain parenchyma. GBM is almost always diagnosed after it has grown large enough to elicit symptoms due to mass effect and parenchymal disruption. However, the benefits of maximally-safe surgical resection of tumor are manifold: sampling of tissue for pathological diagnosis, palliation of mass effect, and some indication of improvement in survival [16]. Though rote surgical resection has remained somewhat limited due to the intricate insinuation of the tumor into brain tissue, new surgical technologies have allowed for more elegant and discriminating extrication of malignant tissue. One example is neuroendoscopy, use of an endoscope deployed through the ventricles for a minimally-invasive approach to allow for biopsy, resection and alleviation of lesions causing obstructive hydrocephalus [13]. Another surgical technology is fluorescence-guided resection. This involves the administration of a non-fluorescent prodrug 5-aminolevulinic acid (ALA) that, when taken up by tumor tissue, is converted to fluorescent metabolite protoporyphyrin IX (PpIX) and accumulates to a marked degree in Grade III and IV gliomas. The neurosurgeon intra-operatively deploys "blue light" which allows tumor tissue to be visualized as "red" due to the fluorescent biomarker. This, in turn, has been shown to allow for more optimal and extensive tumor resection [13] (See Figure 6).

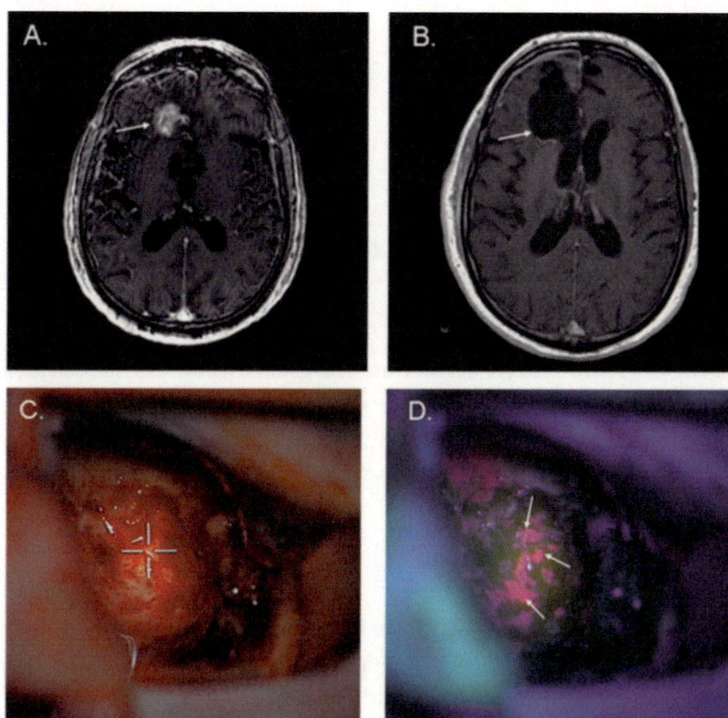

Figure 6. Flourescence/ALA-Guided Surgical Resection of GBM [13]

An important concept to invoke here in the discussion of surgical treatment is Extent Of Resection (EOR), i.e. the extent of tumor tissue that can be safely resected. There is, as would be intuited, a likely positive association between (EOR) and patient survival/patient outcome. Data from the ALA-glioma Study Group out of Germany provided the highest level of evidence--2b--for a positive association between patient outcome, i.e. progression free

Survival	RT	RT + TMZ
Median, mos	12.1	14.6
2 yr, %	10.9	27.2
3 yr, %	4.4	16.0
4 yr, %	3.0	12.1%
5 yr, %	1.9	9.8

Figure 7. EORTC/NCIC Trial 5-Yr Follow-up [35]

survival, and EOR [34]. There are, however, some retrospective studies (volumetric and non-volumetric) that have shown no survival benefit with increased EOR. However, the aggregate of evidence does support the thesis that patients with high-grade gliomas do show survival benefit with increased EOR.

7. Standard adjuvant therapy

After maximally-safe surgical resection, the standard of care for GBM is a 6 week course of External Beam Focused Radiation Therapy with concurrent chemotherapy followed by 6 months of adjuvant chemotherapy.

With the support of Level IA evidence, fractionated focal radiotherapy (60 Gy, 30-33 fractions of 1.8-2 Gy) is the established radiation regimen after resection or biopsy of malignant gliomas [37]. The fundamental nature of the ionizing radiation utilized has, needless to say, not changed; however, leaps and bounds have been made in efforts to focus the beam, tailor it to the highly-serrated and convoluted contours of tumor, and limit the dose to nearby critical structures/tissue by the use of intensity-attenuated and image-guided technologies, all with positive effect.

The single first-line chemotherapeutic agent for GBM is temozolomide, an oral alkylating agent that exerts its anti-tumorigenic effect by methylating/alkylating DNA at the N-7/O-6 positions of guanine residues, thereby causing irreparable damage to (tumor) DNA and instigating the process of tumor cell death. The benefits of the addition of concurrent with adjuvant chemo-therapy to the foundation of radiation therapy were demonstrated by a seminal landmark study by Stupp *et al* that showed a 14.6 to 12.1 month median overall survival benefit and showed a sustained survival advantage of 9.8% vs 1.9% at 5 year analysis (Figure 7) [35].

High-dose corticosteroids have a role to play in reduction of tumor-associated edema and associated symptoms but are not indicated for long periods of time [37]. There is an established role for anti-seizure therapy in patients who present with seizures, but the role for seizure prophylaxis after surgery is only indicated in symptomatic patients. It ought to be kept in mind that many anti-epileptics, particularly of the first generation (e.g. phenytoin, carbamazepine), may decrease the serum concentration of certain chemotherapy agents by dint of inducing increased hepatic metabolism [37].

As evinced by the yet-sobering statistics on overall GBM survival/patient outcome, there are many-a-challenge and obstacle that remain in treatment, especially regarding the development of resistance to both radiation therapy and, more so, to temozolomide chemotherapy.

8. Signaling pathways in high grade glioma

To understand the fundamentals of GBM oncogenesis, it is essential to understand that that there are certain cellular signal transduction pathways responsible for cell proliferation that are normally highly regulated. However, in malignant gliomas, these pathways aberrantly lose regulatory control and end up constitutively activated to disastrous consequence. This occurs mainly through anomalies in the receptors that initiate the signal transduction cascades for growth factors. In one common mechanism, epigenetic mutations result in overexpression or amplification of the genes that encode growth factor receptors. Increased expression of these growth factor receptors results in increased activation of signal transduction cascades. This ultimately yields exponentially increased expression of growth factors which begets malignant cellular proliferation [16].

Some of the best-characterized growth factor mutations in GBM oncogenesis are, as previously introduced, EGFR in primary GBM and PDGFR in secondary GBM. In upwards of 40% of cases of primary GBM, EGFR is amplified to significant pathologic effect (27). Most cases have a genetic lesion of EGFR from deletion of exons 2-7 that results in the anomalous gene *EGFR-vIII*. The normal gene product of the wild-type *EGFR* gene is the EGFR receptor. This receptor, by default, is phosphorylated at the intracellular domain which sets in motion a cascade of signal transduction events that culminates in cell proliferation and survival. In normal cells, the EGFR receptor is regulated by binding of extracellular ligands to the extracellular domain which acts to antagonize phosphorylation at the intracellular domain and thereby down-regulate the mitogenic function of the growth factor cascade. The mutant gene *EGFRvIII* generates the aberrant gene product EGFRvIII that is constitutively phosphorylated/activated due to lacking a down-regulating extracellular ligand-binding domain that would otherwise have been coded by the missing exons 2-7 [16].

There is an ever-burgeoning body of information with the molecular features of malignant gliomas that casts the WHO system in a stark light for the limitations it makes apparent. This molecular information has allowed for determination of discrete subtypes of gliomas within each WHO grade that, through the rigors of clinical trials, have borne out true clinical utility for diagnosis, prognostication and treatment [13]. Within one grade, molecular signatures have identified subtypes that respectively take demonstrably different clinical courses and have discrete treatment responses. Another aspect illuminated by molecular markers is that, when placing a new specimen into one of the 4 WHO grades, there still remains, considerable variability between pathologists/centers. This is particularly so for Grades III and IV [17].

9. Predictive and prognostic molecular markers: Clinical implications

Before embarking further on the discussion of molecular profiling of malignant gliomas, it is imperative to make the distinction that, on the face of it, appears but a matter of simple semantics. Within the context of this discussion, there exists a fundamental difference between Prognostic and Predictive. Prognostic connotes the effect a certain marker gives an outcome that is independent of the therapeutic intervention(s) employed. On the other hand, when a marker is said to have predictive utility, this indicates that it foretells benefit specifically from one type of treatment over others [17].

This discussion will first consider 1p/19q codeletion, a molecular profile that comes from unbalanced translocation between chromosomes 1p and 19q, leading to net loss of genetic material which ultimately leads to loss of one hybrid chromosome, and ultimately, loss of heterozygosity [17]. Mutations have been found in genes that correspond to this translocation; however, the biological underpinnings of these mutations have yet to be understood. The 1p/19q Codeletion has been reliably found in oligodendroglial tumor subtypes that are interspersed between the WHO Grades [17]. Three randomized clinical trials (RTOG 9402, EORTC 26951, NOA-04) have shown that anaplastic oligodendroglioma patients with 1p/19q codeletions have a survival benefit over those without the codeletion when receiving radiation therapy (RT), alkylating chemotherapy, or both [18-20].

First, the RTOG 9402 trial randomly assigned 289 patients with anaplastic oligodendroglioma or anaplastic oligoastrocytoma to receive either adjuvant RT alone or four cycles of Procarbazine/CCNU/Vincristine (PCV) chemotherapy followed by RT (PCV-> RT). Of 201 patients tested by FISH, 93 (46%) were found to have the codeletion. The first initial analysis of results at 3 years out found a median progression free survival (PFS) of 1.7 years for the RT alone contingent vs. 2.6 years for the PCV-> RT contingent; however, no overall survival benefit of either study arm was found at this time, with a median overall survival (OS) of 4.9 years in the PCV-> RT group vs. 4.7 years with RT alone. The 1p/19q codeletion was found to confer an overall survival benefit, with a median OS of > 7 years vs. 2.8 years in those patients without the codeletion. The type of treatment (RT vs. PCV-> RT) was not found to have statistically significant bearing on this increase in OS in patients with tumors possessing the codeletion at this interim analysis of study results. Extended follow up of patients in 2012 continued to show an OS benefit of the 1p/19q codeletion but also found, interestingly, that PCV-> RT did improve survival. At the 2012 reevaluation, those patients without the codeletion had median OS of 2.6 years for PCV-> RT vs. 2.7 years for RT alone, corresponding to earlier results. Those patients with the codeletion who received PCV-> RT were found to have a median OS of 14.7 years vs. 7.3 years with RT alone, yielding a hazard ratio of 0.59 (95% CI, 0.37-0.95; P=0.03).

Very analogous to the RTOG trial was the EORTC 26951 trial, which randomized 368 patients with anaplastic oligodendroglioma or anaplastic oligoastrocytoma to receiving either RT or RT followed by six cycles of PCV (RT-> PCV). In this study, there were 78 patients (21%) whose tumors were found to have the 1p/19q codeletion by FISH. When taken as a whole, the results were similar to the RTOG study, finding that addition of PCV to RT increased PFS to 23 months vs. 13.2 months but not finding a statistically significant difference in OS between the RT alone group (30.6 months) and the RT-> PCV group (40.3 months) at a median follow-up of 60 months. On stratification of patients based upon co-deletion status, a discernible survival benefit was once again found, with no median OS reached for patients possessing the co-deletion (irrespective of RT-> PCV vs. RT alone) vs. median OS of 25.2 and 21.4 months for RT->PCV and RT alone, respectively, in patients with partial or no deletion. Updated results from 2012, reflecting a median follow up of close to 12 years, went further to demonstrate that receipt of adjuvant chemotherapy in patients possessing the co-deletion conferred an additional survival benefit, the median OS for the subgroup of 42 patients with co-deleted tumors and receiving RT-> PCV having not been reached vs. median OS for the subgroup of 38 patients with co-deleted tumors receiving RT alone being 9.3 years. With respect to patients without the co-deletion, this study's results were in accord with the RTOG trial, with a median OS of 25 months for the RT-> PCV subgroup vs. median OS of 21 months for the RT alone subgroup.

The third trial, NOA-04, by the German Neuro-Oncology Group, randomized 318 patients with anaplastic astrocytoma, anaplastic oligodendroglioma, and mixed anaplastic oligoastrocytoma into three single modality treatment groups--RT, PCV, or TMZ--by the ratio of 2:1:1, respectively. This study had crossover design built into it, with patients experiencing unacceptable toxicity or progression from RT being further randomized to receive either PCV or TMZ, or patients experiencing unacceptable toxicity or progression from chemotherapy further randomized to RT. In this study, FISH analysis revealed 74 patients (23%) to possess 1p/19q co-deletion. The first analysis of results was undertaken at 54 months of follow-up at which time 43% of patients had met the criteria for treatment failure, the primary endpoint of the study. This analysis revealed that across all groups there was similar PFS and similar OS. As with the RTOG and EORTC studies discussed above, the 1p/19q co-deletion was found to bode well for prognosis, conferring a risk reduction of nearly 50% irrespective of treatment arm.

Thusly, the molecular signature of 1p/19q codeletion has a predictive and prognostic utility as it shows increased overall survival in patients who receive alkylating chemotherapy, radiotherapy or both as compared to those who do not possess it. However, this benefit was not demonstratedin the group comprised of anaplastic astrocytoma which included 53% of the patient population in this study. There was no statistical difference in outcome, time to progression, nor overall survival whether patients were first treated with RT or alkylating chemotherapy. However, given the worse overall prognosis in patients with anaplastic astrocytoma the generally accepted approach to therapy is combined adjuvant chemotherapy-radiation. This approach is extrapolated from data obtained in trials including patients with glioblastoma.

MGMT is a DNA repair protein that canonically exemplifies the concept of chemotherapeutic resistance. It does so by removing the alkylation of the O6 position of Guanine, which represents the seminal mechanism of action of alkylating chemotherapeutic agents. The beneficial epigenetic profile associated with MGMT is methylation of the MGMT promoter, which silences the MGMT gene and thereby reduces the repair of chemotherapy induced alkylation of DNA. This molecular marker was first suggested to have predictive utility by Stupp *et al* in 2005 [21] in a post-hoc analysis of 203 (out of 573 patients treated in that study) assessable tumors. In that analysis, MGMT methylation status had significant bearing on progression free survival (PFS) in patients from the experimental arm receiving TMZ in addition to RT whereas it showed minimal benefit in PFS in those patients from the control arm receiving RT alone. It was then shown to have prognostic, but not predictive, utility by the results of the RTOG 0525 study, which showed an overall survival benefit of 23.2 months in patients with MGMT methylated tumors vs. 16 months in patients with unmethylated tumors irrespective of whether in the experimental arm (3 weeks on-one week off adjuvant dose-intensified TMZ) or the control arm (standard TMZ) [22]. Based on these results, MGMT methylation status is only accepted as a prognostic factor without predictive value in the population studied. It is also very intriguing to note herein the results of studies aimed at studying single vs. combined modality treatments in elderly patients greater than 70 years of age in whom combined modality treatments are less tolerable and perhaps less effective. These studies showed that in this subset of patients, MGMT methylation status has a predictive utility. Patients with MGMT methylation had longer PFS when receiving chemotherapy plus RT or chemotherapy alone as opposed to RT alone whereas patients without MGMT methylation accrued no comparable survival benefit from chemotherapy [17]. This supposition--that MGMT status is useful as a predictive tool in stratifying elderly patients to receipt of either chemo or RT--was further corroborated by two trials--the NOA-08 trial and the Nordic Trial. The NOA-08 trial, in brief, set out to prove non-inferiority of TMZ alone (one week on one week off) with RT alone in patients 66 years of age and older. While there was no OS or PFS difference between the two arms, it was noteworthy that patients with MGMT methylation showed PFS of 8.4 months vs. PFS of 4.6 in the TMZ arm whereas in the RT arm, MGMT methylation status had the opposite effect, conferring a PFS of 4.6 months in those without MGMT methylation vs. 3.3 months in those with [23]. It is important to note that the temozolomide regimen used in this study varies significantly from the standard schedule used today for patients with glioblastoma. In the Nordic Trial, patients were randomized into one of three groups--standard RT (60 Gy) vs. hypofractionated RT (34 Gy over 2 weeks) vs. standard TMZ schedule. Between the three groups, OS was found to be inferior in the standard RT group when compared to TMZ and hypo fractionated RT. However, MGMT methylation did show better OS in TMZ-treated patients whereas no such benefit was found in RT treated patients [24]. In addition, a recently published meta-analysis performed by Yin et al [25], also supports the predictive value of MGMT methylation status in the elderly population. These results make it reasonable that MGMT status be brought to bear when considering single modality treatment with RT or TMZ in elderly glioblastoma patients.

A third example of genetic/molecular markers that has proven prognostic is the genes IDH1 and IDH2 which encode the ubiquitous metabolic enzyme Isocitrate Dehydrogenase in the cytoplasm and mitochondria, respectively. The native function of wild-type IDH protein is to produce alpha-ketoglutarate. IDH Mutants catalyze a reaction that converts the native metabolic intermediary alpha-ketoglutarate into D-2-hydroxyglutarate, an onco-metabolite (this can be reliably measured by magnetic spectroscopy in situ and mediates the oncogenic activity of the provoking IDH mutations [26]. The classification of gliomas based on IDH is to categorize them based on IDH-wild-type vs. IDH-mutant gliomas. IDH-wild-type tumors are inclusive of Grade I Pilocytic Astrocytomas and Primary Glioblastomas; these, of course, acquire their tumorigenesis independently of IDH-mutating pathways. IDH-mutant gliomas are inclusive of most Grade II and Grade III Gliomas along with a few Secondary GBMs. It is exceedingly interesting to note that IDH mutants tend to carry a better prognosis than IDH-wild-type gliomas of the same histological grade (e.g. Secondary GBM carries a better prognosis than Primary GBM). Indeed, an insightful pooled analysis of 382 WHO Grade III and IV gliomas by Hartmann et al in 2010 corroborated this--that IDH status bears more valuable prognostic information than simple histological grade [27]. So revelatory has the delineation of gliomas been based on IDH status that, despite unequivocal similarities in histological grade and morphology between tumors that would otherwise have classified them together, it is now considered insufficient that they be grouped together if one were to be IDH-wild-type and the other IDH mutant.

10. Angiogenesis: Vascular Endothelial Growth Factor (VEGF) and Glioblastoma stem-like cells (GSC)

As alluded to earlier in the chapter, angiogenesis is an essential part of the pathogenesis of malignant gliomas which, as a rule, are among the most vascularized of tumors [40, 41]. This is due to: (1) upregulation of genes encoding proangiogenic factors, which include VEGF, fibroblast growth factor (FGF), IL-8 and-6, hypoxia-inducible factor 1 alpha (HIF-1alpha) and angiopoietins, and (2) downregulation of angiogenesis inhibitors, including thrombospodins, angiostatin, endostatin and interferons. Indeed, the lynchpin that begets the transformation from low grade to high grade gliomas is induction of expression of the above-cited proangiogenic factors [40]. The most prominent and well-characterized of the proangiogenic factors is VEGF-A, commonly denoted simply as VEGF, which is directly secreted by tumor cells. VEGF exerts its function by binding the receptor VEGFR2 on endothelial cells nearby the tumor. This action initiates a paracrine signaling loop that results in the proliferation of endothelial cells and, as a result, neo-vasculature. Interestingly, the level of VEGF produced by a tumor is proportional to the degree of malignancy, the aggressiveness and poor outcome; high-grade tumors are found to have orders of magnitude more VEGF than low grade tumors [13, 42]. There has thusly been a significant amount of clinical research focus on anti-angiogenic therapy for malignant gliomas. Anti-angiogenic therapy has multiple hypothesized mechanisms of action for the treatment of malignant gliomas. The primary mechanism of action is direct cytotoxicity to endothelial cells, inducing apoptosis. This, by merit of the resultant attenuated blood supply, decreases oxygen and nutrient delivery to tumor cells which preempts further growth for a short period of time. A second hypothesized mechanism of action based upon the results of select clinical studies is that, when used alongside cytotoxic chemotherapeutic agents, anti-VEGF agents are thought to synergistically sensitize endothelial cells to penetration by these cytotoxic agents. Intriguingly, it is also very likely that anti-VEGF agents work to counteract an upsurge of VEGF expression and endothelial cell recruitment observed with the tumoral insult caused by chemotherapy and radiation. Another hypothesis is that, during a discrete window of time after administration, anti-VEGF agents elicit a phenomenon known as "vascular normalization" during which there is reduced vessel diameter/permeability, improved vessel perfusion, a reduction in tumor interstitial pressure, and improved tumor oxygenation. Summarily, these changes all translate into an observed improvement in the delivery and efficacy of cytotoxic chemotherapy. A newer and exceedingly compelling hypothesis is that antiangiogenic agents appear to exercise antagonism to Glioblastoma stem-like cells (GSCs). GSCs play an inextricable part in the angiogenic potentiation of malignant gliomas. They appear to contribute to the resistance that glioblastoma is known to have to cytotoxic chemotherapy treatment by augmenting the repair of DNA damaged by cytotoxic agents and activating the DNA damage checkpoint response system. Antiangiogenic therapy appears to antagonize the functionality of GSCs by merit of GSCs embodying a categorically structural and functional vascular niche in the tumoral micro-milieu. GSCs have been found to upregulate VEGF expression, instigate formation of very angiogenic tumors in animal models, and bear a predilection for stem cell hot beds in areas around endothelial cells. In the self-same animal models, antiangiogenic agents appear to fundamentally disrupt the structural framework of the hot beds in which GSCs reside and resultantly provoke GSC death.

The canonical agent that has garnered the most investigation and use is the humanized anti-VEGF monoclonal antibody bevacizumab, originally used for treating colorectal cancer and also used routinely for metastatic lung adenocarcinoma. Its use for CNS tumors, recurrent gliomas in particular, was conceived of after improved outcomes were noted when it was used in conjunction with chemotherapy for colorectal and lung cancers. Recurrent gliomas have historically had a low radiographic response rate after re-exposure to temozolomide after failing initial therapy, ranging from only 5-8%. However, in the very first published study of the use of bevacizumab with irinotecan, a radiographic response rate of 66% (19 of 29 patients) was found [40]. This was followed by a number of retrospective studies on recurrent gliomas which showed progression free survival at 6 months (PF6) of 32-64% with bevacizumab vs. 21% PF6 rate for temozolomide [13]. The aggregate of these very positive results prompted two phase 2 trials designed for the purposes of fast track FDA approval of bevacizumab for the indication of recurrent gliomas. These two trials corroborated the prior results--a significant radiographic response rate and increase in PF6. The largest bevacizumab trial to date, designated the BRAIN trial and conducted by Freidman et al in 2009, randomized patientswith glioblastoma either after first or second recurrence to be treated with bevacizumab alone(n=85) or bevacizumab plus irinotecan (n=82). Both response rates (using MacDonald response criteria) and six month progression free survival were markedly higher when compared to historical controls in both groups (higher response rate in bevacizumab plus irinotecan group). However, overall survival was not statistically significant between the two groups at 9.2 months for bevacizumab alone and 8.7 months for the combination regimen. Bevacizumab was well tolerated. The most common or significant adverse events included thromboembolicevents, hypertension and proteinuria.

It is important to remind the reader here of the interdependence between angiogenesis and the propagation of peritumoral edema in malignant gliomas. In fact, the original name for VEGF was vascular permeability factor due to its increasing the permeability of tumor vessels, which leads to the phenomenon of vasogenic brain edema. Vasogenic brain edema is a telltale hallmark of malignant gliomas and qualifies much of the morbidity associated with them. It

http://dx.doi.org/10.5772/58548

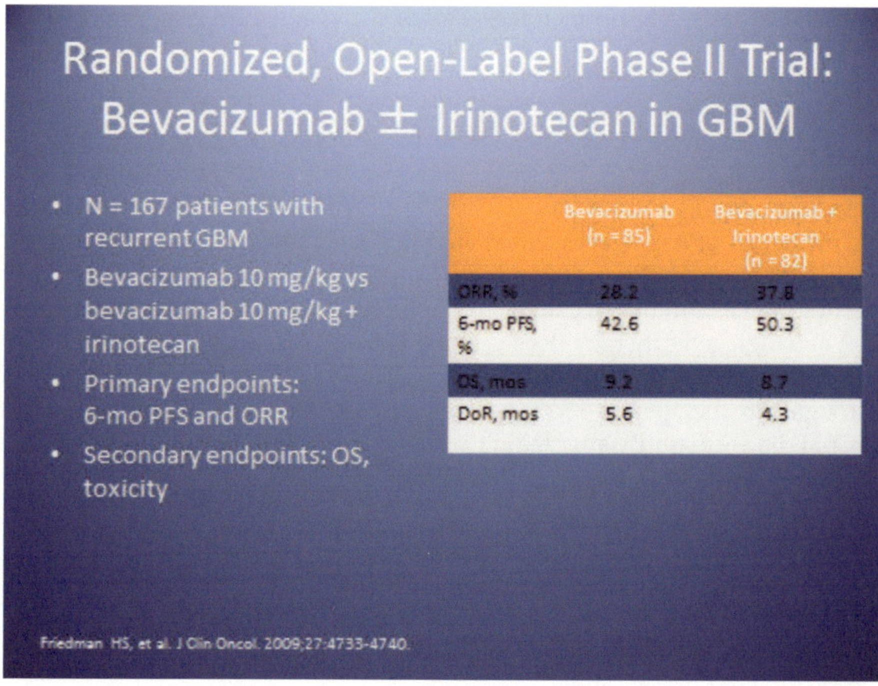

is for this reason that many patients with brain tumors are maintained over long periods of time on high doses of corticosteroids, not without insubstantial side effects. Both clinical and radiographic studies have found reductions in peritumoral edema with the administration of anti-VEGF agents. This in turn allowed for reduction in corticosteroid use by as much as 50%, a significant benefit for many of the patients experiencing the multifarious ill effects of chronic corticosteroid use [41].

11. Hypoxia as means of resistance and poor outcome

Despite the many promising aspects of antiangiogenic therapy outlined above, there have recently come to the fore many challenges that remain to the use of antiangiogenic agents for the treatment of malignant gliomas. One challenge that has become evident is based upon, in a matter of speaking, "tipping the balance" too far towards antiangiogenesis by significant use of antiangiogenesis agents. Animal and human biopsy results have showed that when used overzealously, antiangiogenic therapy actually works to promote a hypoxic environment within the tumor bed. Tumor hypoxia has been well established as a formidable means of resistance to chemotherapy and radiation [38]. Pre-clinical data obtained from xenograft models suggests that hypoxia and the hypoxia-inducible factors (HIFs) play a central role in maintaining the stem-like fraction in gliomas. This is achieved by providing the essential cellular interactions and signals needed to arrest differentiation of these stem-like cells. These interactions lead to stem-like cell survival and self-propagation. Upregulation of HIF-1alpha also activates autophagy, a lysosomal degradation pathway which may promote tumor cell survival.

Though clinical trials have largely focused on VEGF-A antagonism through bevacuzimab, there are a multitude of other pro-angiogenic factors/cytokines that contribute to glioma angiogenesis, including basic FGF (bFGF), angiopoietins, PDGF, interleukin-8 (IL-8), and hepatocyte growth factor/scatter factor (HGF/SF). It is thought that the contribution of these alternative mediators of angiogenesis mediate the phenomenon of antioangiogenic therapy resistance. In other words, these alternative proangiogenic factors are thought to allow for continuing angiogenesis in the face of VEGFR inhibition. Quite sobering is the harsh reality that though antiangiogenic therapy does prolong PFS and response rates are high in patients with recurrent GBM/gliomas, progression of disease inevitably occurs and once tumor burden breaks through, no therapeutic recourse presently exists. Confoundingly, patients with recurrent GBM die very shortly after failing antiangiogenic therapy (figure 8) [44].

Author	N	Treatment	Median PFS, Wks	6-Mo OS, %	Median OS, mos
Norden[1]	23	Bevacizumab + a different chemo (most often carboplatin)	7	2	NS
Kreisl[2]	19	Bevacizumab + irinotecan	4	0	NS
Quant[3]	35	Bevacizumab + carboplatin	5	3	3.0
Iwamoto[4]	19	Bevacizumab + chemo	8	0	5.2

Figure 8. Post-Bevacizumab Salvage Therapy [44]

12. Response criteria and pseudoprogression

Anti-angiogenic agents also have made assessing response and progression a nebulous task. Prior to the era of anti-angiogenic agents, response assessment was performed via the MacDonald criteria which only utilized post-gadolinium MRI sequences. It was previously accepted that a decrease in enhancement represents eradication of tumor but this has proven not to be entirely valid with the use of anti-angiogenic agents. The development of a post-treatment hypoxic microenvironment favors a metabolic change in the tumor cells toward glycolysis, which leads to enhanced tumor cell invasion into the normal brain that is not represented by MRI contrast enhancement. Pre-clinical data suggests that Anti-VEGF treatment reduces vessel contrast leakage, reduces vessel density and promotes invasiveness of tumor cells which can be observed by an incongruent decrease in contrast enhancement along with hyper-intense T2 FLAIR MRI signal. Due to this new understanding, a revised response criteria was developed that, in addition to post-gadolinium sequences, incorporates FLAIR MRI sequences, steroid dependence and clinical stability. This new set of criteria is known as the RANO criteria (Response Assessment in Neuro-Oncology) and now is standard in clinical practice.

Response	Criteria	
	Macdonald criteria	RANO criteria
Complete response	All: complete disappearance of all enhancing measurable and nonmeasurable diseases sustained for at least 4 weeks, no new lesions, no corticosteroids, and being stable or improved clinically.	All: T1 gadolinium enhancing disease, none; T2/FLAIR, stable or decreasing; new lesion, none; corticosteroids, none; clinical status: stable or improving.
Partial response	All: ≥50% decrease in sum of products of perpendicular diameters of all measurable enhancing lesions sustained for at least 4 weeks, no new lesions, stable or reduced corticosteroid dose, and being stable or improved clinically.	All: T1 gadolinium enhancing disease, ≥50% decrease; T2/FLAIR, stable or decreasing; new lesion, none; corticosteroids, stable or decreasing; clinical status: stable or improving.
Stable disease	All: being not qualified for complete response, partial response, or progression; being stable clinically.	All: T1 gadolinium enhancing disease: <50% decrease but <25% increase; T2/FLAIR: stable or decreasing; new lesion: none; corticosteroids: stable or decreasing; clinical status: stable or improving.
Progression	Any: ≥25% increase in sum of the products of perpendicular diameters of enhancing lesions, any new lesion, or clinical deterioration.	Any: T1 gadolinium enhancing disease: ≥25% increase; T2/FLAIR: increasing; new lesion: none; corticosteroids: not applicable; clinical status: deteriorating.

RANO: Response Assessment in Neuro-Oncology; FLAIR: fluid-attenuated inversion recovery.

An important concept to invoke at this juncture, and one unique to the treatment of Glioblastoma with chemotherapy and radiation, is that of Pseudoprogression. A few months after completion of concurrent temozolomide with radiation, many patients show increased contrast enhancement and T2/FLAIR hyperintensity in the radiation treatment field. This generally occurs about 3 months after completion of chemo-radiation and sometimes persists for about 6 months. The MacDonald criterion does not take this phenomenon into account when defining disease progression. The more contemporary RANO criteria defines progression at less than 12 weeks after chemoradiotherapy as the development of a new area of enhancement outside of the prior radiation field, confirmed tumor via biopsy, or clinical decline. Pseudoprogression, as the name implies, denotes these changes that are not due to tumor progression, but rather due to unique cytotoxic effects on the tumor and its microenvironment. Approximately ⅓ of patients with pseudoprogression are found to be symptomatic due to associated inflammation and edema and require treatment with corticosteroids. There is preliminary evidence at hand that indicates that administration of an anti-VEGF agent with standard of care concurrent temozolomide and radiation may reduce the incidence of pseudoprogression [45]. As in the case of vasogenic cerebral edema, this may spare, if not limit, the ill effects of heavy corticosteroid use in many patients. Distinguishing pseudoprogression and true disease progression is very challenging and new imaging techniques (i.e. MR spectroscopy, MR perfusion study) are being developed to help with this dilemma and guide treatment approach. Accumulating data shows promise using these new techniques but have yet to be validated in large clinical studies.

13. Bevacizumab as first line therapy

Two large phase III double-blinded randomized studies published in NEJM in February, 2014 evaluated the use of bevacizumab in the first line setting in patients with glioblastoma. Gilbert et al, led a study that randomized 637 patients with newly diagnosed glioblastoma to standard six weeks of chemo-radiotherapy (adjuvant temozolomide and concurrent radiotherapy) followed by up to twelve months or until disease progression of maintenance temozolomide, with or without bevacizumab starting at week four of chemo-radiotherapy [46]. The results were disappointing in that no survival benefit was determined between the two groups. The bevacizumab group reported a median overall survival (OS) of 15.7 months and the placebo group had an OS of 16.1 months. Progression-free survival favored the bevacizumab group at 10.7 months vs. 7.3 months in the placebo group. Interestingly, over time the patients who received bevacizumab did not benefit from a quality of life standpoint despite better response rates. These points further reinforce the question as to whether PFS is an appropriate surrogate maker for overall survival.

A second published in the same issue of NEJM performed by Chinot et al, studied the use of bevacizumab in the front line setting as well [49]. Similar conclusions were reported in this study compared to the performed by Gilbert et al. The treatment regimen used in the study differed in that after 6 months of maintenance temozolomide with or without bevacizumab were continued with bevacizumab alone or placebo until disease progression or until suffering from intolerable side effects. The results were again disappointing in that the addition of bevacizumab to standard chemo-radiation and maintenance therapy with this anti-angiogenic agent did not provide a survival benefit (72% and 33.9% one and two year survival rate respectively in the bevacizumab group versus 66.3% and 30.1%) despite a significantly better PFS (10.6 months in bevacizumab group vs. 6.2 months in placebo group). Baseline quality of life was maintained for a longer period of time in the bevacizumab group.

These results, in particular the study by Gilbert et al, appears to possibly support the use of maintenance temozolomide for twelve months instead of traditional standard therapy with six months as conducted in the landmark study by Stupp et al now considered standard of care. This is a question that every neuro-oncologist has to address when treating patients with newly diagnosed glioblastoma. Although difficult to extrapolate data from two separate studies, no large scale study has been performed making a direct comparison of twelve months versus six months of maintenance temozolomide. However, this data suggests that twelve months of maintenance temozolomide leads to an improvement in OS reporting 16.1 months versus14.6 months reported in the EORTC trial led by Stupp et al.

14. Patterns of recurrence

As we gain more experience using anti-angiogenic agents in high grade gliomas, we also learn more about what occurs after treatment failure. Mancuso et al. conducted a pre-clinical study using a mouse xengraft model to address the reversibility of VEGF inhibition after cessation of anti-VEGF therapy. It was noted that even after a 50–60% reduction of tumour vascularity, "empty sleeves of basement membrane were left behind." By day 7 after drug cessation, tumours were fully re-vascularized, suggesting that these remaining empty sleeves of basement membrane and pericytes are responsible for this tumor revascularization. These basement membranes also serve as storage sites for angiogenic growth factors as well as "tracks" for tumor vascular regrowth. This "rebound" phenomenon has also been observed in clinical studies (figure 9) [46]. This phenomenon appears to be associated with rapid clinical demise and dismal prognosis.

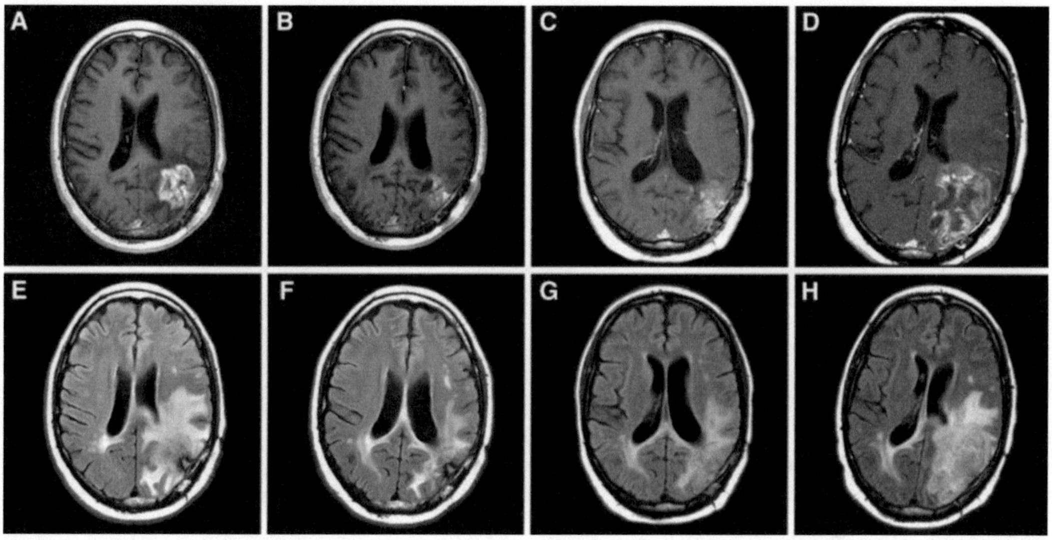

Figure 9. Rebound progression after discontinuation of bevacizumab: Original tumor area seen on post-Gd T1 weighted (a) and FLAIR MRI (e) sequences prior to initiating therapy with bevacizumab in a patient with recurrent high-grade glioma. Post-Gd T1 weighted (b) and FLAIR MRI (f) sequences that demonstrate partial response after 1 six-week cycle of treatment with bevacizumab. Post-Gd T1 weighted (c) and FLAIR MRI (g) sequences at the time of bevacizumab failure and subsequent cessation of bevacizumab therapy. Post-Gd T1 weighted (d) and FLAIR MRI (h) sequences at the time of "rebound" progression demonstrating a dramatic increase in area of enhancement and abnormal FLAIR signal 6 weeks after cessation of therapy with bevacizumab. [44]

15. MicroRNA – Potential target

MicroRNAs (miRNAs) are molecules of RNA numbering 20-23 nucleotides that function to interfere with messenger RNA (mRNA) translation into protein, the final step in gene expression. Through a complex and elegantly-characterized molecular sequence of steps, miRNAs function to "flag" mRNAs for decay, translational inhibition, or cleavage prior to the process of translation. This, in turn, results in a decreased level of encoded proteins, which in turn affects a myriad of essential cell functions, i.e. growth, proliferation, metabolism, apoptosis, etc. [43] Interestingly, though miRNA constitutes roughly 1-3% of the human genome, it is postulated that these molecules have influence on as much as ~30% of all gene expression [44]. The expression of one mRNA may be affected by numerous miRNAs; on the same token, one miRNA may affect the expression of multiple mRNAs [44]. The deregulation of miRNA has been pivotally implicated in tumorigenesis; a positive association has been found between those sites in the human genome associated with cancer and areas of miRNA expression [44]. Furthermore, miRNAs have been found to exemplify both oncogenic and tumor suppressor functions in the tumorigenesis of pancreatic cancer, prostate cancer, thyroid cancer, ovarian cancer, colon cancer, breast cancer, and melanoma. Of recent, the same has also been found in GBM wherein a multitude of miRNAs have been reported to have roles in tumor suppression or oncogenesis. Therapeutic strategies with respect to miRNA aim to augment tumor suppression or antagonize oncogenesis, respectively. In the former case, it is postulated that viral vectors may be utilized to deliver gene therapy to increase the *in situ* expression of tumor suppressive miRNAs. In the latter case, studies pursuing anti-miRNA therapies, e.g. the use of anti-miRNA oligonucleotides, are underway for downregulation of oncogenic miRNAs [44].

16. Promising treatment approaches: Convection enhanced nanoparticle delivery

An utterly novel modality of treatment actively under investigation is the utilization of nanoparticles for the directed delivery of radionuclides into tumor bed. The premise behind this modality is to maximize delivery of radiation therapy to tumor tissue while limiting damage to surrounding normal tissue; external beam radiation is limited to 60 Gy due to toxicity to normal tissue and lack of clinical benefit with higher dose of EBRT. Recently, studies have been published in which radionuclide particles, e.g. 186-Rhenium, are encased in liposomal nanoparticles and injected straight into the GBM tumor bed. In a study published in 2012, Brenner *et al* injected 186-Rhenium liposomes directly into GBM Xenografts transplanted into the brains of rat models. It was found that up to 1850 Gy could be delivered by this method without overt clinical or microscopic evidence of toxicity. Those animals in the experimental arm treated with 186-Rhenium liposomes were found to have a median survival of 126 days vs. a median survival of 49 days for those animals in the control group. Compellingly, it was found that a large number of the animal subjects that were treated 21 days after tumor grafting were found to have multiple objective indicators of tumor cure (See Figure 10). This included lack of detecting contrast-enhancing tumor on MRI, lack of detecting luminescence by the luminescent molecule embedded in tumor cells, and no tumor cells found on histopathology of resected animal brain tissue. These results suggest that nanoparticle delivery of radioisotopes to the cavities of resected GBM either intra-or postoperatively may have limitless therapeutic potential, particularly when used alongside adjuvant cytotoxic chemotherapy [45].

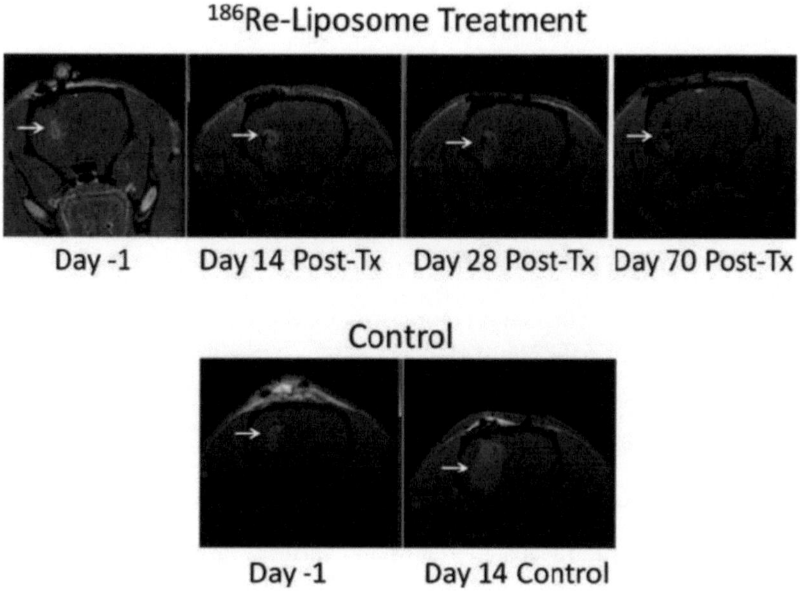

Figure 10. [45]

17. Conclusion

Glioblastoma is a deadly and devastating disease that is, as this chapter has made abundantly clear, in need of the development of effective new agents to treat this aggressive tumor. Our understanding of the intrinsic molecular and genetic make of this tumor, although still lacking, has improved rapidly over the past decade and has shed light on current obstacles and is leading to an array of promising agents on the horizon.

Author details

Siddharth K. Joshi[1] and Richard Zuniga[2*]

*Address all correspondence to: rickzunigaperu@hotmail.com

1 Department of Medicine, New York Methodist Hospital, Brooklyn, New York, USA

2 Department of Medicine-Division of Hematology-Oncology, New York Methodist Hospital, Brooklyn, New York, USA

References

[1] Bleeker, FE et al. Recent Advances in the Molecular Understanding of Glioblastoma. J Neurooncol 2012;108:11-27.

[2] Krex, D. et al. Long-term survival with glioblastoma multiforme. Brain 2007;130:2596-2606.

[3] Ostrom Q.T. et al. CBTRUS Statistical Report. Neuro-Oncology 2013;15:ii1-ii56.

[4] Neglia J.P. et al. New Primary Neoplasms of the CNS in Survivors of Childhood Cancer 2006. JNCI 2006;98(21):1528-37.

[5] Grossman SA, et al. CNS Cancers in First-Degree Relatives and Spouses. Cancer Invest 1999;17:299-308.

[6] Alentorn, A. et al. [Genetics and Brain Gliomas] Presse Med 2013;42(5): 806-13.

[7] Vilchez, RA et al. Simian virus 40 in human cancers. Am J Med 2003;114(8): 675-84.

[8] Crawford JR et al. Detection of human herpesvirus-6 variants in pediatric brain tumors: association of viral antigen in low grade gliomas. J Clin Virol 2009;46(1):37-42.

[9] Chi, J et al. Human herpesvirus 6 latent infection in patients with glioma. J Infect Dis 2012;206(9):1394-8.

[10] Cobbs, CS et al. Human Cytomegalovirus Infection and Expression in Human Malignant Glioma. Cancer Research 2002;62:3347-3350.

[11] Kan, P et al. Cellular phone use and brain tumor: a meta-analysis. J Neurooncol 2008;86(1):71-8.

[12] Hardell, L et al. Epidemiological evidence for an association between use of wireless phones and tumor diseases. Pathophysiology 2009;16(2-3):113-22.

[13] Van Meir, EG et al. Exciting New Advances in Neuro-Oncology: The Avenue to a Cure for Malignant Glioma. CA Cancer J Clin 2010;60(3):166-193.

[14] Smith, SL et al. Dendritic spikes enhance stimulus selectivity in cortical neurons in vivo. Nature 2013;503(7474):115-120.

[15] Louis, DL et al. The 2007 WHO Classication of Tumours of the Central Nervous System. Acta Neuropathol 2007;114:97–109.

[16] Wen, PY and Kesari, S. Malignant Gliomas in Adults. NEJM 2008;359:492-507.

[17] Weller, M et al. Personalized care in neuro-oncology coming of age: why we need MGMT and 1p/19q testing for malignant glioma patients in clinical practice. Neuro-Oncology 2012;14:iv100-iv108.

[18] Cairncross JG et al. Chemotherapy plus radiotherapy (CT-RT) versus RT alone for patients with anaplastic oligodendro-glioma: long-term results of the RTOG 9402 phase III study. J Clin Oncol 30:2008b.

[19] Van den Bent MJ et al. Adjuvant procarba-zine, lomustine, and vincristine improves progression-free survival but not overall survival in newly diagnosed anaplastic oligodendrogliomas and oligoastrocytomas: a randomized European Organisation for Research and Treatment of Cancer phase III trial. J Clin Oncol 2006;24:2715-2722.

[20] Wick W et al. NOA-04 randomized phase III trial of sequential radiochemotherapy of anaplastic glioma with PCV or temozolomide. J Clin Oncol 2009;27:5874-5880.

[21] Stupp, R et al. MGMT Gene Silencing and Benefit from Temozolomide in Glioblastoma. NEJM 2005;352:997-1003.

[22] Gilbert MR, et al RTOG 0525: A randomized phase III trial comparing standard adjuvant temozolomide (TMZ) with a dose-dense (dd) schedule in newly diagnosed glioblastoma (GBM). [Abstract] J Clin Oncol 2011; 29:2006.

[23] The NOA-08 Study Group of the Neuro-oncology Working Group (NOA) of the German Cancer Society. Temozolomide chemotherapy alone versus radiotherapy alone for malignant astrocytoma in the elderly: the NOA-08 randomised, phase 3 trial. Lancet Oncol 2012;13:707-715.

[24] Malmstrom A et al. Temozolomide versus standard 6-week radiotherapy versus hypofractionated radiotherapy for patients aged over 60 years with glioblastoma: the Nordic randomized phase 3 trial. Lancet Oncol 2012;13(9):916-26.

[25] Yin A-a, Zhang L-h, Cheng J-x, Dong Y, Liu B-l, et al. The Predictive but Not Prognostic Value of MGMT Promoter Methylation Status in Elderly blastoma Patients: A Meta-Analysis. PLoS ONE 2014;9(1):e85102.

[26] Stupp R et al. Molecular neuro-oncology in clinical practice: a new horizon. Lancet Oncol 2013;14:e370-79.

[27] Hartmann C et al. Patients with IDH1 wild type anaplastic astroctytomas exhibit worse prognosis than IDH1-mutated glioblastomas, and IDH1 mutation status accounts for the unfavorable prognostic effect of higher age: implications for classification of gliomas. Acta Neuropathol 2010;120:707–18.

[28] Ohgaki, H and Kleihues, P. Genetic alterations and signaling pathways in the evolution of gliomas. Cancer Sci 2009;100(12):2235-2241.

[29] Ohgaki, H and Kleihues, P. Population-based studies on incidence, survival rates, and genetic alterations in astrocytic and oligodendroglial gliomas. J Neuropathol Exp Neurol 2005;64:479–89.

[30] Chang, SM et al. Patterns of care for adults with newly diagnosed malignant glioma. JAMA 2005;293(5):557-64.

[31] Stall, B et al. Comparison of T2 and FLAIR imaging for target delineation in high grade gliomas. Radiation Oncology 2010;5:5.

[32] Stummer W et al. Extent of resection and survival in glioblastoma multiforme: identification of and adjustment for bias. Neurosurgery 2008;62:564-76.

[33] Stupp R. et al. Radiotherapy plus Concomitant and Adjuvant Temozolomide for Glioblastoma. NEJM 2005;352(10):987-96.

[34] Rong Y et al. 'Pseudopalisading' necrosis in glioblastoma: a familiar morphologic feature that links vascular pathology, hypoxia, and angiogenesis. J Neuropathol Exp Neurol 2006;65(6):529-39.

[35] Smirniotopoulos, JG et al. Patterns of Contrast Enhancement in the Brain and Meninges. Radiographics 2007;27:525-551.

[36] Stupp, R. and Roila, F. Malignant glioma: ESMO Clinical Recommendations for diagnosis, treatment and follow-up. Annals of Oncology 20 (Supplement 4) 2009; iv126-iv128.

[37] Stark VV. Bevacizumab and CPT-11 in the treatment of relapsed malignant glioma. Neurooncol 2005;7:369.

[38] Reardon, DA and Wen, PY. Therapeutic Advances in the Treatment of Glioblastoma: Rationale and Potential Role of Targeted Agents. The Oncologist 2006; 11:152-164.

[39] Reardon, DA et al. Glioblastoma multiforme: an emerging paradigm of anti-VEGF therapy. Expert Opin Biol Ther 2008;8(4):541-553.

[40] Leon, SP et al. Microvessel density is a prognostic indicator for patients with astroglial brain tumors. Cancer 1996;77(2):362-72.

[41] Moller, HG, Rasmussen AP et al. A Systematic Review of MicroRNA in Glioblastoma Multiforme: Micro-modulators in the Mesenchymal Mode of Migration and Invasion. Mol Neurobiol 1996;47:131-144.

[42] LeBrun, DL and Li, M. MicroRNAs in Glioblastoma Multiforme: Profiling Studies and Therapeutic Impacts. Mol Cell Pharmacol 2011;3(3):93-105.

[43] Phillips WT, Zuniga, RM, Brenner, AJ *et al*. Rhenium-186 liposomes as convection-enhanced nanoparticle brachytherapy for treatment of glioblastoma. Neuro-Oncology 2012;14(4):416–428.

[44] Zuniga, RM, Torcuator R et al. Rebound tumour progression after the cessation of bevacizumab therapy in patients with recurrent high-grade glioma. J Neurooncol 2010;99(2):237-42.

[45] Pinho M, Polaskova P, Jennings D, et al. Impact of adjuvant anti-VEGF therapy on treatment-related pseudoprogression in patients with newly diagnosed glioblastoma

receiving chemoradiation with or without anti-VEGF therapy. J Clin Oncol 2012;30(suppl;abstr 2025).

[46] Gilbert, M et al. A Randomized Trial of Bevacizumab for Newly Diagnosed Glioblastoma. N Engl J Med 2014;370:699-708.

[47] Chinot, O et al. Bevacizumab plus Radiotherapy–Temozolomide for Newly Diagnosed Glioblastoma. N Engl J Med 2014;370:709-722.

Chapter 2

Paediatric Brainstem Cancers — Where We Have Been; Where We Are; Where We Are Going

Adrianna Ranger, Navjot Chaudhary and Jonathan Lau

Additional information is available at the end of the chapter

http://dx.doi.org/10.5772/58297

1. Introduction

In North America and Europe, cancer involving the central nervous system (CNS) ranks second as the most common malignancy seen in infancy through adolescence, second only to leukaemia [1-7]. Consistent with this are figures on cancer-related mortality. In the year 2004, for example, there were 566 confirmed cases of leukemia-related death among children in the United States, followed by 555 CNS cancer-related deaths; these numbers accounted for 25.5% and 25.0% of the total number of cancer deaths in individuals less than 20 years old, respectively [4].

In general, survival from cancer has improved dramatically over the past forty years, presumably due to a combination of improved treatments and earlier detection. This is especially true in the paediatric population, among whom the overall long-term survival rate across all cancers has risen from under 50% to roughly 70% [4;8;9]. Even with brain cancer, the prognosis in children has improved, such that long-term survival is now achieved in more than half of patients [10]. This being said, the neoplasm originates in the brainstem in roughly 10-20% of children with CNS cancer [7;11-13], accounting for 150 to 300 new cases per year in the U.S. [11;13] and thus rendering it more common in children and adolescents than in adults [14;15]. And in this subset of children, the prognosis generally is considered extremely bleak, akin to that of glioblastoma multiforme [1;4;14;16-19].

Despite a continued poor prognosis, much has changed over the past several decades — like how paediatric brainstem tumours are diagnosed and classified, if and when surgery is considered, approaches to surgery, the use of adjunct therapies like radiation and chemotherapy, and the evolution of several new therapeutic options. Once lumped together as a single

INTECH
open science | open minds

© 2014 The Author(s). Licensee InTech. This chapter is distributed under the terms of the Creative Commons Attribution License (http://creativecommons.org/licenses/by/3.0), which permits unrestricted use, distribution, and reproduction in any medium, provided the original work is properly cited.

entity that was considered inoperable and, hence, completely incurable, recent developments in imaging and surgical techniques have led to the classification of several different types of brainstem tumour; and, for some of these, surgical resection is considered the treatment of choice [16;18;20].

This chapter reviews the historical progression of understanding of paediatric brainstem tumours, including evolving beliefs regarding their classification, diagnosis, management, prognosis and prognosticators, dating from the 1970s to current times. It then describes current diagnostic and management protocols for these tumours, ending with a glance forwards towards potentially promising treatments and technologies and how they might, hopefully within the near future, favourably alter outcomes in these patients, both in terms of their survival and quality of life.

2. Where we have been

2.1. Definitions, diagnosis and classification

The brainstem has been defined as extending from the midbrain (tectal plate) to the medullary cervical junction [7]. Brain stem tumours are, by definition, tumours that involve the brainstem. However, they include tumours not just in the brainstem *per se*, but also in the upper cervical spine [16]. In the paediatric population, posterior fossa tumours significantly outnumber those that are supratentorial [10;21;22], and brainstem tumours account for roughly 25% of all tumours found within the posterior fossa [16;23]. The vast majority of these are primary lesions, since just 3 to 5% of all brain metastases are found in the brainstem [24]. The most common paediatric posterior fossa tumours are cerebellar astrocytomas, medulloblastomas, ependymomas and brainstem gliomas [25].

Traditionally, the term *brainstem glioma* has been used to incorporate all brainstem tumours, largely because biopsies often were not performed and the majority of brainstem tumours in childhood are, in fact, of glial cell origin [26;27]. However, other histological forms of tumours do exist, though they comprise but a small percentage of brainstem tumours, and generally tend to be exophytic, growing either external to the brainstem or on its surface. Even among such exophytic tumours, gliomas form the clear majority. In their series of 75 paediatric patients with exophytic tumours seen between 1970 and 1990, Pierre-Kahn et al. [28] noted 69 glial tumours (92% of the total), of which 58 were astrocytomas and 11 oligodendrogliomas. The remaining six non-glial tumours were two ependymomas; two primitive neuroectodermal tumours (PNET); one ganglioglioma; and one of unknown histology [28]. In a much more recent review of non-glial brainstem tumours, other brainstem lesions noted to occur anecdotally included medulloblastomas invading the brainstem, cavernomas, lymphomas, haemangioblastomas, and other ganglionic and mixed tumors [29]. Nonetheless, many continue to use the term *brainstem glioma* generically, given that the vast majority of brainstem tumours are glial cell based.

Up until the development of advanced imaging techniques — like computed tomography (CT) and, to an even greater extent, magnetic resonance imaging (MRI) — brainstem tumours tended to be lumped together as a single clinical entity and considered uniformly inoperable [30]. Since they were presumed gliomas and surgery was deemed contraindicated, there was no call even to biopsy them, except in certain instances in which the diagnosis was in doubt. For example, in 1969, Matson wrote: "brainstem gliomas must be classified as malignant tumors since their location in itself renders them inoperable" [21]. And as late as 1984, Tomita et al. [31] wrote: "Since biopsy specimens often misrepresent the true pathology... surgery undertaken to obtain precise histological verification of brain stem gliomas is futile." Instead, these latter authors recommended computed tomography (CT) with high-resolution metrizamide CT cisternography to distinguish surgically resectable extra-axial tumors adjacent to the brain stem from non-resectable intrinsic brain stem gliomas. Such sentiments — that tumours only were worth a biopsy if they were either completely exterior to brainstem tissue or, at worst, on the surface — were echoed by others [32]. Consequently, early classification of brainstem tumours often subdivided lesions into those that were exclusively or primarily intra-axial, and those that were exclusively or primarily extra-axial. Meanwhile, brainstem tumours were collectively contrasted against those involving the midbrain or thalamus, both of which exhibited considerably superior prognoses [33].

This being said, there were early reports of certain patients with brainstem tumours who survived long-term. For example, in 1971, Lassiter et al. reported on 37 patients with presumed brainstem gliomas (22 of them children), among whom there were four children with large, surgically-drained neoplastic cysts who achieved long-term survival: two of these children died 7½ and 13 years later, and two still were alive 8½ and 9 years post diagnosis, one of them going on to graduate from college and the other with residual hemiparesis and mental retardation [34]. In 1975, Hara et al. reviewed the cases of 24 brainstem gliomas, and found that the median survival was 9 months, except for one patient who survived beyond 4½ years and another who lived for 14 years and 10 months before succumbing to the disease [35]. Similar isolated cases of long-term survival with brainstem gliomas, especially cystic lesions, were reported as far back as 1937 and 1940 through the mid nineteen seventies and early eighties [36-42]. And, contrary to conventional wisdom, even then, some neurosurgeons were routinely performing biopsies and surgery on select patients with brainstem gliomas [27;40;41;43-46].

In the nineteen sixties and early nineteen seventies, angiography and pneumoencephalograms were largely used to identify brain and brainstem tumours [47-50]. These imaging modalities were replaced in the mid nineteen seventies as computed tomography (CT) emerged as the imaging tool of choice for the detection and diagnosis of both supra-and infra-tentorial lesions, including brainstem tumours [51-54]. By this point, some surgeons were starting to distinguish outcomes between different subsets of patient who were able to undergo either partial or radical resection of brainstem cancers [27;40;41;43-45]. The first to propose what he termed a staging system for brainstem gliomas was Epstein, in 1985, who first categorized tumours as intrinsic, exophytic and disseminated; and then subcategorized intrinsic (actual brainstem) tumours as either diffuse, focal or cervico-medullary [43]. In 1986 and again in 1988, Epstein et al. published series of paediatric patients undergoing surgery for brainstem cancer, again classifying patients as focal, diffuse or cervico-medullary; in the latter report, they added a category for cystic lesions [27;44]. What these authors noted was uniformly dismal outcomes in children with diffuse lesions, but often favourable outcomes in those patients with any one of the three other classifications. In the 1988 report, co-authored by Wisoff [27], among 66 children with intrinsic brainstem gliomas diagnosed between 1980 and 1986 who underwent radical surgical resection and either CT, MRI or both pre-operatively, 27 (41%) were found to have diffuse tumors, all of whom died within 12 to 18 months of surgery with malignant neoplasms that had not benefitted from surgery. However, five of nine children with cystic tumors, three of five with focal tumors, and twenty of twenty-four with cervicomedullary tumors were discovered to have a histopathologically low-grade lesion, and these 28 children all remained alive between one and six years post-operatively. The authors proposed criteria combining clinical and neuroradiological findings to predict which patients with brainstem tumors were likely to benefit from radical surgical intervention [27].

Since that time, several additional and very different classification systems have been proposed for brainstem tumours, including those by Stroink et al., Barkovich et al., Albright, Fischbein et al., Choux et al., Fisher et al., Mehta et al. and, most recently, Ramos et al. [45;55-61]. (See Table 1) The system proposed by Stroink et al., published in 1987, was born out of a study of 16 children (9 girls, 7 boys; age range 1½-12 years) with dorsally exophytic transependymal benign brainstem gliomas diagnosed between 1962 and 1985 at Sick Kids Hospital in Toronto, Canada [45]. Of these, 13 were low-grade (grade I-II) astrocytomas, one a grade III astrocytoma, and two gangliogliomas. All 16 patients underwent subtotal resection of their tumours, and seven had post-operative radiation therapy. One died 18 months after surgery, but the remaining 15 remained alive an average of eight years post-operatively (median=7 years; range=8 months to 23 years). Based upon these results, Stroink et al. proposed dorsal exophytic gliomas (Type I) as a distinct clinical entity, to differentiate them from hypo-dense, non-enhancing intrinsic tumours (Type IIa); hyper-dense, contrast-enhancing exophytic intrinsic tumours (Type IIb); focal, enhancing cystic intrinsic tumours (Type III); and focal iso-dense and contrast-enhancing intrinsic tumours (Type IV) [45].

Author(s)	Year Published	Imaging	Classification System
Epstein [43]	1985	CT, MRI	Intrinsic - diffuse; focal, cervicomedullary
			Exophytic - anterolateral; posterolateral
			Disseminated - positive cytology; positive myelography
Epstein et al. [44]	1986	CT, MRI	Diffuse
			Focal
			Cervicomedullary
Epstein et al. [27]	1988	CT, MRI	Diffuse
			Focal
			Cervicomedullary
			Cystic

Author(s)	Year Published	Imaging	Classification System
Stroink et al. [45]	1987	CT with contrast	Type I: dorsal exophytic glioma
			Type II intrinsic brainstem tumour
			* IIa - hypodense with no contrast enhancement
			IIb - hyperdense with contrast enhancement, exophytic
			Type III: focal cystic tumour with contrast enhancement
			Type IV: focal isodense tumour with contrast enhancement
Barkovich et al. [55]	1990	MRI	Tumours characterized by -
			(1) Location - midbrain, pons, medulla
			(2) Focality - focal or diffuse
			(3) Direction & extent of tumour growth
			(4) Degree of brainstem enlargement
			(5) Presence/absence of exophytic growth
			(6) Presence/absence of haemorrhage or necrosis
			(7) Evidence of hydrocephalus
Albright [58]	1996	MRI	Focal - midbrain; pons; medulla
			Diffuse
Fischbein et al. [56]	1996	MRI	Midbrain - diffuse; focal; tectal
			Pons - diffuse; focal
			Medulla - diffuse; focal; dorsal and exophytic
Choux et al. [57]	2000	MRI	Type I - diffuse
			Type II - intrinsic and focal
			Type III - intrinsic and exophytic
			Type IV - cervicomedullary
Fisher et al. [59]	2000	MRI	Pilocytic astrocytomas
			Fibrillary astrocytomas
			Other tumors
Mehta et al. [60]	2009	MRI	Intrinsic tumours - expanding; diffuse infiltrative; purely ventral
			Extrinsic tumours
Ramos et al. [61]	2013	MRI	Diffuse intrinsic/diffusely infiltrative
			Posterior exophytic/cervicomedullary gliomas; other focal tumours
			Dorsal exophytic tumours
			Cervicomedullary tumours
			Focal tectal tumours

Table 1. Classification Systems for Brain Stem Tumours-1985 to Present

It was in the mid to late nineteen-eighties that magnetic resonance imaging (MRI) started to replace CT as the imaging modality of choice for the diagnosis and classification of brainstem tumours [62]. As such, it was based upon MRI studies that Barkovich et al. proposed their criteria for brainstem tumours in 1990 [55]. Their criteria were derived from the results of retrospectively-reviewed MRI studies for 87 paediatric patients with brainstem gliomas. T2-weighted images were deemed most appropriate for use, given that they were the most accurate at demonstrating the extent of tumour. In this much more elaborate classification scheme, tumours were characterized in terms of (1) their location of origin, into midbrain, pons and medulla; (2) their degree of 'focality' (whether diffuse of focal); (3) the direction and extent of tumour growth; (4) the degree of brainstem enlargement; (5) the degree of exophytic growth; (6) the presence or absence of cysts, necrosis or hemorrhage; and (7) the presence or absence of hydrocephalus. This classification scheme was never scientifically validated to determine its ability to predict outcomes, however, and failed to achieve widespread acceptance. Likely reasons for this failure were how cumbersome the system was, and the lack of any firm guidelines as to its use.

As such, subsequent classification schemes have been much simpler, starting with those proposed by Albright, in 1996, who returned to the very simple categorization of lesions as being either focal (further distinguished by location, into midbrain, pons or medulla) or diffuse [58]; and Fischbein et al., also in 1996, who again categorized lesions as focal or diffuse, but categorized both forms of lesion by location — again into midbrain, pons or medulla [56]. Harkening back to the four-category system initially proposed by Epstein in 1985 [43], Freeman et al., in 1998, and Choux et al., in 2000, adopted the four relatively straight-forward categories largely in use today: diffuse intrinsic; focal intrinsic; focal exophytic, and cervicomedullary [18;57]. In 2009, Mehta et al. proposed a modified sub-categorization of intrinsic tumours, into expanding, diffuse infiltrative, and pure ventral varieties, achieving good surgical results and reasonable survival with the first of the three subtypes [60]. Then, most recently, Ramos et al. adopted yet another classification system that included 'diffuse intrinsic and diffusely infiltrative' as a single category, followed by four additional categories of various focal lesions [61]. The authors' conclusion was that "brainstem tumors are a heterogeneous group of tumors." Clearly then, in terms of how brainstem tumours are now perceived, there has been a 180 degree reversal from early statements [21;30;31] about their homogeneity and the inappropriateness of biopsies for brainstem tumours. The questions remain, however: Who warrants such biopsies? And how could biopsies and surgery influence outcomes?

2.2. Outcome predictors and indications for surgery

Early universal pessimism regarding the fate of children with brainstem tumours has also clearly changed in recent years, with reports of better than 90% five-and ten-year survival rates in children with certain types of tumour [23;63]. The primary objective of all the classification schemes proposed to date has been to identify which patients warrant surgical treatment and how aggressive such treatment should be. Contrary to early years, when all brainstem tumours were considered inoperable [21;30;31], for the past thirty years neurosurgeons have been operating to either de-bulk or completely excise lesions when doing so was felt to be of clinical benefit, potentially positively influencing quality of life and/or survival. As stated earlier, that a subset of patients existed for whom long-term survival was possible has been suspected for almost eighty years [36;37]. Once again, it was Epstein et al. who first identified diffuse lesions as being the most rapidly fatal, and focal and cystic lesions as being more amenable to treatment and long-term survival [27;43;44]. Since then, other prognostic factors have been identified that can influence the decision to operate (See Table 2).

Factor	Studies	Year Published	Imaging	Comments
Focal (vs. diffuse intrinsic) tumour	Sandri et al. [77]	2006	MRI	87.4% 4-year vs. 12.3% 2-year survival
	Mauffrey [20]	2006	MRI	90% vs. 22% 2-year survival
	Fried et al.	2012	MRI	89% vs. 3% 5-year survival
Cystic appearance	Lassiter et al. [34]	1971	not identified	All 4 children with cystic lesions
Prolonged pre-diagnosis symptoms	Fisher et al. [59]	2000	MRI	Cox regression→ survival ↓w/ symptoms > 6 mo (p = .004)
	Shuper et al. [17]	1998	MRI	Mean survival 19.5 vs. 12.9 mo with >1 mo symptoms
Other than pons location	Fisher et al. [59]	2000	MRI	Cox regression→ survival ↓w/ pons involvement (p=.0002)
No presenting eye symptoms/eye palsies	Fisher et al. [59]	2000	MRI	Cox regression→survival ↓w/ abducens palsy (p<.0001)
	Shuper et al. [17]	1998	MRI	Mean survival 17.5 vs. 12.3 mo with no eye symptoms
Basilar artery engulfment	Fisher et al. [59]	2000	MRI	Cox regression→survival ↓w/ basilar artery engulfed (p=.006)
Tectal location	Poussaint et al. [65]	1998	MRI	All 32 children with tectal tumours alive
				after a mean 5 years follow-up
Non-enhancing on gadolinium MRI	Poussaint et al. [65]	1998	MRI	Gadolinium enhancement of tectal lesions
				increased odds of disease progression x15
Contrast enhancement on MRI	Dellaretti et al. [64]	2012	MRI	Mean survival with contrast enhancing lesions = 21.7 mo.;
				with non-enhancing lesions 54.2 months (p < .001)
Maximum diameter < 0.5 cm	Poussaint et al. [65]	1998	MRI	Each 1 cm increase in maximum diameter
				increased odds of disease progression x5
Neurofibromatosis type 1	Fried et al. [72]	2012	MRI	All 7 children with NF-1 had non-focal
				lesions & long-term survival
	Other papers			Numerous isolated anecdotal reports in other papers

Table 2. Factors Predicting Favourable Outcomes in Paediatric Brainstem Tumour Patients

One of the earliest attempts to empirically look at prognostic factors beyond imaging results was published by Fisher et al. in 2000 [59]. They reported on the results of a study of 77 patients, 21-years old or younger, seen between 1980 and 1997. In this study, they sought to identify characteristics statistically associated with poor survival. The factors that they identified were (a) symptom duration less than six months before diagnosis (p=0.004); (b) abducens palsy at presentation (p < 0.0001); (c) a pontine location (p=0.0002); and (d) engulfment of the basilar artery (p=0.006). Twenty of their patients were found to have pilocytic astrocytomas, which were associated with a very favorable 5-year overall survival rate of 95%, as well as with location outside the ventral pons (p=0.001) and dorsal exophytic growth (p=0.013). Another histological type they could predict based upon clinic-radiographic findings was fibrillary astrocytoma, of which they had 14 cases. These lesions were associated with symptoms < 6 months (p=0. 006), abducens palsy (p < 0.001), engulfment of the basilar artery (p=0.002), and a one-year survival rate of just 23% (p < 0.0001). Shuper et al. also found, in their analysis of 24 children operated upon between 1981 and 1997, that a shorter duration of symptoms (< 4 weeks) and visual symptoms at presentation were associated with shorter survival and lower survival rates [17]. Meanwhile, Dellaretti et al. found that contrast-enhancing lesions on MRI were associated with a significantly shorter mean duration of survival versus non-enhancing lesions (21.7 vs. 55.2 months, p < 0.001); however, on Cox proportional hazards regression analysis, tumour grade was the only significant predictor of survival, suggesting that contrast enhancement in that sample was an indicator of higher tumour grade [64].

Poussaint et al. specifically sought to determine which clinical and imaging findings best correlated with outcomes in children with tumours involving the midbrain tectum, via a retrospective review of the medical records and imaging studies of 32 children (16 boys and 16 girls; mean age, 8 years) with tectal tumours [65]. Of this number, eight children had undergone CT, 11 MRI, and 13 both CT and MRI studies. Over a mean follow-up period of five years (range, 3.6 months to 17 years), all patients experienced hydrocephalus, for which all but one required cerebrospinal fluid (CSF) diversion. The tectum was the centre of the tumour in all cases; and the majority of the tumours appeared iso-dense on CT scans, iso-intense on T1-weighted MR images, and hyper-intense on T2-weighted images. Twenty patients required no further treatment. In this group, the mean maximum tumour diameter was 1.8 cm, and enhancement occurred in only two cases (10%). At follow-up, 18 tumours were the same size as at baseline, one was larger due to cyst formation in the setting of stable symptoms, and one was smaller. The remaining 12 patients required further treatment (excision and/or radiotherapy) because of disease progression, indicated either by increased tumour size or by worsening symptoms. In this group, the mean maximum tumour diameter was 2.5 cm and contrast enhancement occurred in nine (75%). Further follow-up in this group showed decreased tumour size in eight and stable residual tumor in three. The authors then used regression analysis to calculate and compare the likelihood of a patient requiring further treatment with various-size enhancing versus non-enhancing tumours and identified two trends: larger tumours were more likely to require further treatment; and the same was true for enhancing lesions. Combining these two factors was especially predictive. For example, whereas 31% of lesions with a maximum diameter of 0.5 cm required further treatment, same-sized non-enhancing lesions warranted such treatment less than one percent of the time.

http://dx.doi.org/10.5772/58297

Corresponding percentages for lesions of maximum diameter 1.0, 1.5, 2.0, 2.5, 3.0, 3.5 and 4.0 cm were 48 and 1%, 67 and 3%, 80 and 6%, 90 and 11%, 95 and 21%, 97 and 36%, and 98 and 54%. By the time a lesion reached 4.5 cm in maximum diameter, virtually all (99 and 70%) required further treatment, irrespective of whether they did or did not enhance. Overall, the odds of surgical or radiation treatment were almost five times greater for each 1 cm increase in maximum tumor diameter (odds ratio, 4.9; 95% confidence interval, 1.3-19.3; p=0.015); and 15 times greater when the tumor enhanced versus when it did not (15.0; 2.2-106.5; $p < 0.003$). The investigators thereby concluded that, though paediatric tectal tumors exhibit somewhat variable behavior, patients generally do well, and that larger tumours, and especially those that that enhance with contrast on MRI, are highly likely to be more aggressive [65]. Whether size and contrast-based enhancement on MRI or CT predict the need for treatment or ultimate outcomes with other non-diffuse intrinsic or exophytic brainstem tumours has not yet been demonstrated.

Another factor long believed to place individuals at increased risk of brainstem and other CNS malignancies, but also to confer a relatively favorable prognosis, is the presence of type 1 neurofibromatosis (NF-1), though this belief is largely based upon anecdotal reports [66-72]. In the large study of 223 children with brainstem tumours reported by Fried et al., however, there were seven children with concomitant NF-1; and all had low-grade brainstem tumours [72]; the statistical likelihood that this occurred merely by chance, assuming a fifty-fifty split of low-to high-grade lesions (which is roughly what they observed across the sample), is less than one percent.

Overall in NF-1 patients, brainstem gliomas comprise a heterogeneous group of lesions, consisting of three main subtypes: (1) diffuse brainstem enlargement; (2) focal enhancing nodules with or without cystic areas; and (3) peri-aqueductal gliomas. All of these subtypes, including diffuse brainstem enlargement, generally exhibit a very indolent course and do not require treatment, though MRI monitoring is indicated until their indolent course is confirmed. Some lesions even regress on their own [73]. The diffuse brainstem enlargement is somewhat similar in appearance to the unidentified bright objects (UBOs) that are the most commonly observed CNS lesions on MRI in patients with NF-1 [74]. Like UBOs, they exhibit abnormal signals on T1-weighted images. The major differences are that, as opposed to UBOs, there usually is a mass effect, and these lesions also tend to be considerably larger than most UBOs. What the diffuse enlargement represents remains controversial. Many presume them to be gliomas, but they exhibit a much more indolent course than brainstem gliomas seen outside of NF-1, such that adjuvant treatment is only required in the minority of patients whose lesions progress. However, ongoing monitoring is required to detect the few who do progress, before neurological deficits ensue, which often are irreversible. Rarely, these gliomas progress to more malignant forms of astrocytoma, including glioblastoma [73;75].

The focal enhancing nodules seen in the brainstem of NF-1 patients, which may occur with or without cystic areas, generally are thought to represent pilocytic astrocytomas, given their imaging characteristics. Like pilocytic astrocytomas elsewhere, they generally are indolent; but their course is unpredictable and the brainstem so susceptible to major deficits, relative to the cerebral hemispheres, that ongoing monitoring is required. Small, focal intrinsic lesions may enlarge and then regress spontaneously. Exophytic tumours often are more aggressive and require treatment.

Periaqueductal gliomas occur adjacent to the aqueduct of Sylvius between the 3rd and 4th ventricles in the midbrain. They typically manifest with late-onset aqueductal stenosis, leading to hydrocephalus. Presumably, they represent low-grade gliomas or glial hamartomas, and typically are indolent. However, because of their location, CSF shunting often is necessary. But, as with the other two forms of brainstem tumour seen in NF-1 patients, resection usually is unnecessary [73;75].

Table 3 summarizes currently published research on tumour characteristics that predict a favourable outcome. What is most evident is the dearth of confirmatory studies. These findings aside, the brainstem tumour characteristic that is unquestionably the one most likely to dissuade surgeons from operating is evidence that the tumour is intrinsic and diffuse, due both to the known high risks of surgery and to the lack of evidence suggesting any benefit, in terms of either quality of life or survival time [16-18;20]. The corollary to this is that, contrary to thirty years ago when most surgeons preferred to leave all brainstem tumours alone, focal, exophytic and cystic tumours are increasingly being accessed and resected, often with good results [16-18;20;23;60].

	Year	**Study**	**Study subjects**	**5-year survival**	
Author(s)	**Published**	**Type**	**N =**	**N =**	**% =**
Lesniak et al. [76]	2003	Retrospective	57	26	45.6%
Sandri et al. [77]	2006	Retrospective	17	15	88.2%
Mauffrey [20]	2006	Retrospective	14	8	57.1%
Teo et al. [63]	208	Retrospective	34	27	79.4%
Fried et al. [72]	2012	Retrospective	108	96	88.9%
Klimo et al. [23]	2013	Retrospective	52	51	98.1%
OVERALL			**282**	**223**	**79.1%**

Table 3. Survival in Paediatric Patients with Non-Diffuse Intrinsic Brainstem Tumours

2.3. Treatment and outcomes

In 1984, Tomita [31] wrote that "radiation therapy is the choice of treatment, should CT indicate clear evidence of intrinsic brain stem tumor... posterior fossa craniotomy should be undertaken only for aspiration of cystic intrinsic stem tumors, resection of extra-axial juxtastem tumors and, although rare, in instances when CT is unable to definitively distinguish extra-axial from intra-axial mass for verification of lesion location." Clearly, sentiments have changed; but has the increase in surgical interventions altered outcomes?

In 1998, Shuper et al. published the results of their study of 24 children with brainstem tumours operated upon between 1981 and 1997 [17]. The main question they asked was: are we improving outcomes? A tissue diagnosis was achieved in only six of the children. Although the investigators did not perform inferential statistical analysis, average survival in five patients seen before 1990 was 8.6 months, versus 19.4 months in the five patients seen in 1990 through 1994, and 20.0 months in those seen in 1995 and 1996. Moreover, raw data were provided, allowing the current author to perform a statistical comparison of months of survival pre (8.6) versus post (19.7) January 1st 1990. This difference, despite the low numbers, is significant (t=2.379, df 13, p=0.03). However, these patients generally were offered radiation +/-chemotherapy, and not surgery. In addition, other biases might have erroneously generated these results, like alterations in referral patterns or the earlier recognition of tumours as a result of major technological advances in imaging.

More recently, several authors have reported survival rates in paediatric patients treated surgically for non-diffuse tumours (Table 3). In 2003, Lesniak et al. [76] retrospectively reviewed the charts of all pediatric patients admitted to Johns Hopkins University Hospital with a diagnosis of a brainstem tumor between January 1985 and December 2000: 89 patients met the inclusion criteria, among whom 57 (64.0%) underwent surgical resection, while 32 (36%) were treated with radiation and/or chemotherapy. Of the surgical candidates, 57 (100%) had an accompanying MRI scan significant for an enhancing lesion in the midbrain, pons or the medulla. The pathology was consistent with juvenile pilocytic astrocytoma in 30 patients (52.6%) and glioblastoma multiforme in 12 patients (21.1%). The remaining cases consisted of ten patients (17.5%) with fibrillary astrocytomas, three (5.3%) with gangliogliomas, one (1.8%) with an oligodendroglioma and one (1.8%) with a primitive neuroectodermal tumor. Total surgical resection was attained in 29 patients, near total resection (>90%) in eight, subtotal resection (50-90%) in 15, and partial resection (<50%) in five. The progression-free survival of all patients, which included the twelve with glioblastomas, was 71.9% at 3 years and 45.6% at 5 years. Excluding the 12 patients with known glioblastomas, all of whom died prior to three years, these survival rates rise to 83 and 53%, comparable to rates observed in a subsequent study by Sandri et al. [77].

In 2006, Sandri et al. [77] published their series of 31 children admitted to their institution from 1995 to 2003, 14 of whom were classified on MRI as having diffuse and 17 as having focal brainstem tumours. Patients with diffuse lesions were treated with locoregional radiotherapy (1.8 Gy/day for 54 Gy) and weekly vincristine for radiosensitization (1.5 mg/sm for six total doses). Meanwhile, patients with focal tumours underwent surgical resection, with adjunct chemotherapy and/or radiotherapy considered on a case-by-case basis. Among the 14 with diffuse tumours, ten experienced a partial response, three exhibited stabilization of their disease, and one progressed. General and/or neurological symptoms improved in more than 80% of these patients. However, the median time from diagnosis to progression and from diagnosis to death were just 8 (range of 3-13) and 13 (range of 4-25) months, respectively, with a 2-year overall survival rate of just 12.3%. Conversely, among the 17 children with focal lesions, gross total removal was achieved in 4/17 cases, subtotal removal in 7/17, and partial removal in 6/17. There was one surgery-related death. Eight out of 17 patients had adjuvant chemo-and/or radiotherapy after progression, among whom six remained free of neurological symptoms and two died secondary to tumor progression. The 4-year overall and disease-free survival rates were 87.4 (SE 8.4) and 58.8% (SE 11.9), respectively, with the extent of resection identified as the best predictor of survival (p=0.012) [77].

Also in 2006, Mauffrey reported on his retrospectively reviewed series of 27 paediatric patients admitted to hospital in Turin, Italy with a diagnosis of brainstem glioma [20]. Thirteen patients had a diffuse pontine tumour on MRI scan, while fourteen had other brainstem gliomas. Those in the first group had a shorter mean duration of symptoms prior to diagnosis (2.6 vs. 10.6 months), never demonstrated gadolinium enhancement of their tumour on MRI (vs. 78.6% in the other group), and were much more likely to have symptoms or findings indicating cranial nerve involvement (77.0 vs. 28.5%). None of the 13 with diffuse gliomas underwent radical surgery, whereas it was the treatment of choice in the remaining 14. Two-year survival rates were 25% and 90%, respectively, and 60% of the latter remained alive at five years [20].

In 2008, Teo and Siu [63] reported on their results with 34 consecutive patients between 3 and 16 years of age who underwent endoscope-assisted microsurgery for focal brainstem gliomas with the intent of radial resection between 1999 and 2005. More than 90% tumour resection was achieved in 31patients, while >50% was attained in the remainder. There was no peri-operative mortality and the average follow-up was 46 months. Twenty-three patients (74%) harboured low-grade and 11 (26%) high-grade gliomas. Kaplan-Meier survival analysis revealed marked differences in the 5-year survival rates between the two groups (100% vs. 33%). Multivariate analysis demonstrated that the degree of tumour resection was not associated with poor outcome at 6 months.

Two papers published over the past couple of years are those by Fried et al. [72], based at The Hospital for Sick Children in Toronto Canada, and Klimo et al., based at George Washington University in Washington, DC [23]. The latter study, like all those described previously, was relatively small, with just 52 patients (32 boys), all with radiographically-confirmed, low-grade focal brainstem gliomas seen from 1986 to 2010. The median duration of follow-up was 10.0 years, and the median age at diagnosis 6.5 years (range 1-17 years). Tumors were located in the midbrain (n=22, 42%), pons (n=15, 29%), and medulla (n=15, 29%). Surgical extirpation was the primary treatment in 25 patients (48%). Five-and 10-year event-free survival and overall survival rates were 59% and 98%, and 52% and 90%, respectively. Surprisingly, children with intrinsic tumors trended towards slightly higher event-free survival at 5 years than those with exophytic tumors (p=0.054), but not at 10 years (p=0.147). No other variables were predictive of event-free survival [23].

The retrospective study by Fried et al. is by far the largest to date, assessing a total of 223 children with brainstem tumours (12% of all CNS tumours seen) followed at The Hospital for Sick Children in Toronto over the preceding 25 years [72]. Ninety-five of these tumours were diffuse and an additional 17 were high-grade astrocytomas (grade III or IV). The investigators made several novel observations. First, whereas 75% of tumors involving the pons were high-grade, 98% of tumours lacking pontine involvement were low-grade (p = 0.0001). Second, residual tumour after surgery, even when visualized, did not adversely alter either progression-free survival or overall survival. And, among those requiring further treatment, 5-year progression-free and overall survival were comparable between those receiving chemotherapy (53 and 93%) and those administered radiotherapy (66 and 83%) (p = 0.26 and 0.30, respectively). Among those with focal lesions, five-year progression-free survival (PFS) and overall survival (OS) were 57% and 89%.

Combining the results of these last seven studies (Table 3), in which children with non-focal brainstem tumours were identified and treated, either surgically or non-surgically, there were 282 such children, of whom 223 (79.1%) survived long-term (beyond 4 years and most beyond 5 years). In the largest study, which had 108 such children [72], 90% remained alive 10 years post diagnosis. Several comments are warranted. First, every one of the above-mentioned studies had significant methodological issues, not the least being that they all were retrospective. Moreover, because patients were selected for surgery, it is not possible to rule out the possibility that the characteristics that made them surgical candidates in the first place (e.g., a focal vs. diffuse tumour) were responsible for their survival, rather than the surgery itself. Nonetheless, what is clear is that long-term survival among children with non-diffuse tumours clearly is not at all uncommon. In fact, it seems likely for four out of five such children, making it the rule and not the exception, which is radically distant from both the beliefs and outcomes of thirty and forty years ago, and considerably improved from survival rates in at least one older study in which those with non-diffuse tumours were identified but not offered surgery [78]. Fried et al. concluded that children with non-diffuse brainstem tumours do well even with conservative management; but their conservative management appears to have consisted of surgical resection in most cases, with adjuvant chemotherapy or radiation considered more aggressive [72]. Ideally, from a purely methodological standpoint, future studies would randomize surgery-eligible patients to surgery versus non-surgery groups. Practically, however, this author considers it unlikely that most parents would consent to allow their children to be randomly assigned to one group or the other when surgery offers at least the potential of cure.

The good news, then, irrespective of methodological questions regarding the true effectiveness of surgery, is that children with several types of brainstem tumour appear to do well. The bad news is that the majority of brainstem tumours in children continue to be either diffuse intrinsic lesions or high-grade astrocytomas [72], and the prognosis for either remains dismal, with only about 10% of children alive two years after diagnosis [79;80]. One major challenge currently facing researchers and clinicians is to identify non-surgical ways to better target these otherwise poorly responsive tumours.

3. Where we are and where we are going

Clearly, the past forty years have brought about substantial changes in the way brainstem tumours are both perceived and managed. No longer is the term 'brainstem glioma' used to lump all brainstem lesions together as homogenous, untreatable and ultimately fatal. Now, either three or four heterogeneous classes of tumour are described, and all but one is considered to be an indication for aggressive, often surgical treatment. Some investigators sub-classify lesions further, related to their anatomical location (e.g., midbrain, pons, medulla). In essence, though, irrespective of the number of tumour types proposed, all categorization systems ultimately separate diffuse intrinsic lesions from all others.

Current diagnosis largely depends on the use of patient histories and physical findings, especially paying attention to the duration of symptoms prior to diagnosis and the type(s) of neurological deficits identified (e.g., ocular palsies), followed by magnetic resonance imaging, both with and without contrast. Lesions that are intrinsic and diffuse, and lesions that involve the pons are generally considered to be a contraindication to surgery, though many clinicians are now biopsying them to determine if they are high-or low-grade to estimate course and likely survival time [81]. Conversely, lesions that are focal, cystic, and extraphytic are usually considered treatable, with surgery to remove as much of the tumour as possible often considered the treatment of choice. Table 4, utilizing the most recently proposed classification system of Ramos et al. [61], summarizes current general practices. Following the 2013 publication of guidelines promoting the biopsy of diffuse intrinsic brainstem lesions to aid in the development of targeted therapies [82], stereotactic biopsies must now be at least considered standard of care for these patients. Radiation therapy, sometimes combined with chemotherapy, appears to induce brief clinical remissions in patients with diffuse tumours for whom surgery is not indicated, and may prolong survival slightly [83]. With other tumours, surgery often plays the major role; though some patients merely require monitoring and others respond well to radiation or conservative measures like CSF shunting alone.

Tumour type	Typical location	Usual histology	Biopsy	Surgery	Radiation	Chemotherapy	2-year survival
Diffuse Intrinsic or	Pons	grade III-IV gliomas	Yes	No	Yes	+/-	10%
Diffusely Infiltrative		fibrillary astrocytomas					
Focal	Medulla	pilocystic astrocytomas	Yes	Complete resection	+/-	+/-	≥ 90%
	Brainstem	gangliocytomas		often possible			
Dorsal Exophytic	Mostly in 4th	pilocystic astrocytomas	Yes	Usually only partial	+/-	+/-	≥ 90%
	ventricle	other low-grade glioma		resection is possible			
Cervicomedullary	Epicentre either	pilocystic astrocytomas	Yes	Complete resection	+/-	+/-	~ 100%
	in medulla or	gangliocytomas		possible in ~75% of pts			
	cervical spine						
Focal Tectal	Tectum	low-grade gliomas	Yes	Shunt placement	Yes	Usually not	~ 100%
				Resection often			
				unnecessary			

Table 4. Current Management of Paediatric Brainstem Tumours

There remains no consensus, however, as to how to best categorize lesions; and the lion's share of brainstem tumours continue to be considered untreatable and to have a dismal prognosis. Consequently, three major challenges that remain are (1) coming to some consensus as to classifying lesions, so as to best predict their course, likely response to treatment and, hence, when and how best to treat them; (2) developing more effective non-surgical treatments to treat the intrinsic diffuse tumours for which all current treatments, including surgery, have been ineffective and the prognosis remains abysmal; and (3) optimizing quality of life in these children and their families, irrespective of long-term prognosis. With a view to these three main objectives, we now briefly explore current and future directions in the detection, diagnosis and classification of brainstem tumours, and in their non-operative and operative management.

3.1. Enhanced diagnostics and classification

In few fields have there been as many and as dramatic advances as in the field of diagnostic imaging, and this appears to be having a significant impact upon how brain and brainstem tumours are now detected and diagnosed. Increasing recognition that not all brainstem tumours are a diverse collection of pathological entities with distinct courses and responses to treatment, has led to attempts to distinguish between them using advanced imaging. Typically, for example, diffuse intrinsic fibrillary astrocytomas appear hypo-intense on T1-weighted images, while heterogeneously hyper-intense on T2-weighted images; they also exhibit indistinct margins that reflect the tumour's highly infiltrative nature [61]. Beyond distinctions made using different MR sequences, various contrasts are now being used to try to detect lesions that otherwise might be missed [84] and to delineate low-from high-grade lesions [19; 45;56;64;76]. For example, dorsal exophytic tumours often are low-grade pilocytic astrocytomas that, like high-grade fibrillary astrocytomas, may be hypo-intense on T1-weighted images and hyper-intense on T2-weighted images; however, they classically appear well-demarcated. Moreover, after gadolinium infusion, a cystic component often is identified, as only the solid portion of the tumour is enhanced, revealing a hypo-intense centre [61;85;86]. More recent advances in MR scanning — like MR spectroscopy, MR perfusion, and diffusion tensor imaging (DTI) — are also being utilized to further establish the histopathologic diagnosis of brainstem lesions [18;61]. An additional advantage of these newer MR technologies is that they are better at monitoring for disease recurrence or progression after treatment, since radiation-induced necrosis may be mistaken for tumour re-growth with traditional MRI [87-90]. In addition, functional scans — like functional MRI (fMRI), positron emission tomography (PET), and single-photon emission computed tomography (SPECT) — are emerging as additional imaging tools to identify and characterize lesions in the brain, brainstem and spinal cord [19;91-95]. Further development of these tools may aid in further delineating the various brainstem tumours, even obviating the need for tissue in those patients for whom biopsies pose undue risk.

This being said, among the most major imaging advances related to brainstem tumours relates to stereotactic biopsies. A *stereotactic biopsy* utilizes a computer and images performed in at least two planes, first to localize a target lesion, like a tumour, in three-dimensional space; then to determine its depth; and finally to guide the removal of tissue for pathological examination. Stereotactic biopsies rely on the underlying principle of *parallax*, a process that initially was used in astrology to estimate distances between stars [96]. *Parallax* is the concept of using multiple site lines to visualize the same object relative to objects of known position in front of and behind it. Since objects closer to the observer tend to move more than objects that are more distant when the point of observation changes, measuring the degree of movement of the target lesion relative to reference points, combined with recording the change in viewing angle, permits one to estimate the depth or "Z-dimension" of the target lesion [97]. Long used to aid in the biopsy of breast lesions [98], CT-guided stereotactic biopsies have been used for the diagnosis of brain lesions since the nineteen seventies [99;100], but not with brainstem lesions until more recently. Just this year, Cage et al. reported on their results specifically biopsying diffuse brainstem tumours; they also extensively reviewed the literature [81]. In their own series, nine children with pontine lesions were biopsied, with successful tissue collection achieved in all cases. Among these lesions, four were found to be low-grade (grade I or II) astrocytomas, and five high-grade (grade III or IV) gliomas, demonstrating heterogeneity even among diffuse pontine lesions. Moreover, only one patient experienced any post-operative complication – transient seizures and hydrocephalus. In their review of the literature, the same authors identified twenty case series besides their own, ranging in size from a single paediatric patient [101] to 52 children [102]. In this latter series, among 52 paediatric brainstem biopsies, only five patients experienced any post-operative morbidity, in four instances transient; and there were no deaths. Biopsy was felt to alter management in 18% of the cases. In another one of the larger series, Kondziolka and Lunsford reported on their use of CT-guided stereotactic biopsies in 40 consecutive patients seen over a 13-year interval [103]. Of this number, 20 patients had midbrain lesions (n=20), 18 pontine lesions, and two medullary lesions. Midline lesions were approached via a coronal, trans-thalamic trajectory; lateral brain stem lesions usually were approached via a trans-cerebellar route. A histologic diagnosis was achieved in 38 patients (95%), and no post-biopsy haemorrhages were noted on CT performed immediately after the procedure. Only one patient (2.5%) experienced a complication, which was transient diplopia. Altogether across the twenty-one papers Cage et al. reviewed, there were 294 documented brainstem biopsies in paediatric patients, among whom there were 16 cases of an intra-operative complication (5.4%); 42 cases of increased post-operative morbidity (14.3%) that was transient in the vast majority of cases; 29 inconclusive biopsies (9.9%); and two procedure-related deaths (0.7%) [102]. The authors concluded that brainstem biopsies are safer than widely perceived and that, when used judiciously, might be both safe and of advantage in terms of determining treatment. Stereotactic biopsies have been demonstrated to be superior to MRI alone in accurately diagnosing brainstem lesions [104].

3.2. Enhanced non-operative management

Many have argued against biopsying diffuse intrinsic brainstem lesions, since they cannot be surgically removed or even de-bulked without causing unacceptable neurological deficits because of their location and infiltrating nature, and given the lack of enduring response that the vast majority of patients demonstrate to traditional chemotherapy and radiation. But this pessimistic outlook may be changing, given emerging knowledge about potential therapeutic targets and optimized ways to cross the blood-brain barrier. In fact, one key rationale behind obtaining tissue in patients with diffuse pontine lesions stems from recent work to further classify lesions based upon a number of identifiable genetic and molecular alterations that may render these tumors susceptible to targeted therapies [79-81].

Until the last couple of years, the biology of diffuse intrinsic brainstem tumours was entirely unknown. However, tissue analysis has now identified a number of identifiable genetic and molecular alterations — like amplification of receptor tyrosine kinases and cell-cycle regulatory genes, and alterations in membrane proteins and the Hedgehog (Hh) signaling pathway [79;105-109] — that could serve as therapeutic targets. Much of this research is being aided by the development of human glioma cell lines that can be studied in the lab [110]. One particular membrane protein that has garnered considerable recent interest is B7-H3 (also called CD276), a type I trans-membrane glycoprotein that is part of the B7-CD28 family [111]. This glycoprotein is known to interact with host defenses in certain cancers, being recognized by the monoclonal antibody 8H9 [112] that binds to a vast array of different tumours. Among primary brain tumors, for example, it bound to 15 of 17 glioblastomas, three of four mixed gliomas, and six of eight astrocytomas, among others; however, it did not bind to normal neurons or glial cells [113]. Moreover, extremely favourable results were observed in a study in which 21 children with recurrent stage IV neuroblastoma — like gliomas, a neuroectodermal tumor — were administered compartmental intra-thecal antibody-based radio-immunotherapy [114]. The therapy consisted of ^{131}I-monoclonal antibodies targeting B7-H3. Among the 21 children treated, 17 (81%) remained alive between seven and 74 months later (median 33 months), significantly longer than the expected, post-disease-recurrence median survival of six months. For all these reasons, the potential is there for B7-H3 to be a future therapeutic target for diffuse intrinsic brainstem gliomas. Considerable interest also has focussed on the epidermal growth factor receptor (EGFR), which has been the target of several chemotherapeutic drugs currently undergoing early phase trials, like gefitinib and erlotinib [115-117]. Another drug currently undergoing early phase testing is vandetanib, a tyrosine kinase inhibitor of both the EGFR and vascular endothelial growth factor receptor (VEGFR) [118]. To date, one-year survival rates have ranged from 38 to 56% [115-118], not significantly better than the median survival of 9 to 12 months reported elsewhere [79].

Promising results were observed when data were combined across four phase II trials [119] in which 18 mostly paediatric (age range 2 – 42 years, median=10) patients with brainstem gliomas were treated with anti-neoplaston A10 (A10I) and AS2-1 injections over a median of five months [120]. Fourteen of the 18 patients had diffuse intrinsic tumors; four were glioblastomas and 14 anaplastic gliomas. Prior to treatment, twelve patients had suffered a relapse and six had never received either radiation or chemotherapy. Contrary to the expected 2-year survival rate of roughly 10%, 39% remained alive at two years, and 22% at five years, including one patient with an anaplastic astrocytoma who remained alive for 17 years and another with a glioblastoma for more than five years. The only adverse event was a single case of reversible anaemia.

Another potential boon to the treatment of all CNS malignancies may be the development of nanotherapeutic approaches, which include an entire new generation of novel targeted-delivery devices — 'smart' nanoparticles — that facilitate the transfer of a variety of therapies, from drugs to thermotherapy, across the blood-brain barrier [121], a barrier that has traditionally hampered the delivery of most anti-neoplastic drugs. Stem cells that are themselves drawn to tumour cells are another potential vehicle that is being explored for the treatment of high-grade gliomas [122;123] and may have applications in the treatment of inoperable brainstem gliomas. Some investigators are also examining the potential to test the effectiveness of anti-neoplastic drugs *ex vivo* prior to patient administration via the use of *in vitro* assays [124]. In this way, drug regimens might be more appropriately taylorized to each patient, and *in vivo* drug effectiveness more accurately predicted prior to initiating therapy, thereby minimizing unnecessary toxicity and enhancing the likelihood of initial treatment response.

Finally, as mentioned earlier, advanced imaging techniques are now allowing for enhanced prospective monitoring of treatment response and the earlier detection of disease recurrence and progression [87;88]. Another previously-unexplored means by which to accomplish such monitoring might be via the analysis of various bodily fluids — like blood, urine and cerebrospinal fluid (CSF) — to identify and estimate levels of various CNS tumour markers, similar to how prostate-specific antigen (PSA) is being used to detect and monitor prostate cancer. For example, Saratsis et al. recently performed protein profiling by mass spectrometry of 76 specimens — including CSF, serum, urine, and normal and tumor brainstem tissue [125] — from 10 patients with diffuse intrinsic brainstem gliomas and four healthy controls. CSF proteomic analysis revealed selective up-regulation of both cyclophillin A (CypA) and dimethylarginase 1 (DDAH1) in patients relative to controls. Protein expression was validated further via Western blot analysis and immunohistochemical assays. Immunohistochemical staining exhibited selective up-regulation of secreted but not cytosolic CypA and DDAH1 in patients. The authors proposed that the detection of secreted CypA and DDAH1 in serum and urine could have clinical applications in the monitoring of treatment response and disease recurrence in patients with brainstem gliomas [125].

As such, although the prognosis for patients with inoperable brainstem gliomas remains bleak for the time being, beliefs regarding the potential for enhanced survival certainly are changing with the emergence of targeted therapies, better delivery systems, and enhanced imaging and other techniques to monitor disease regression and progression. But what will the neurosurgeon's role be in all this?

3.3. Emerging role of the neurosurgeon in the management of diffuse brainstem tumours

Nothing has changed in terms of neurosurgeons' reluctance to operate on diffuse intrinsic brainstem gliomas; nor does it seem likely to anytime soon, given the known aggressiveness of the vast majority of these tumours, their high degree of infiltration that would preclude anything more than partial resection, and the extreme risks of such surgery, given the anatomical compactness of vital structures and neural pathways. Consequently, the main change in current surgical practices relates to the stereotactic biopsy of these lesions, a practice that this year was formally recommended in a published, multi-disciplinary consensus statement concerning surgical approaches to low-and high-grade astrocytomas and diffuse intrinsic pontine gliomas in childhood [82].

There also has been a clear swing in the route selected for brainstem biopsy access, at least in studies involving paediatric patients. For example, over the decade of the nineteen nineties, 82% of reported brainstem biopsies were accessed via a trans-frontal route, versus just 18% trans-cerebellar. Since the year 2000, however, these percentages have completely reversed, with 82% of reported biopsies trans-cerebellar and 18% trans-frontal. In the five studies published since 2006 in which paediatric patients were identified among those biopsied [81;126-129], every one of the ninety biopsies were performed through the cerebellum. Across these ninety biopsies, 77 of them in children, there was one intra-operative complication (1.1%), nine post-operative complications (10%), two inconclusive biopsies (2.2%) and no deaths. The reason(s) for this shift in surgical approach is not entirely clear. In 2012, Dellaretti et al. published the results of their study comparing the two approaches over twenty-three years of practice (1984-2007), and no significant differences were noted [130]; however, whether any children were included within the sample of 142 patients is not stated in the manuscript. Moreover, there was a clear preference for trans-frontal biopsies, which were performed in 123 of the patients versus just 19 via the cerebellum, and no explanation for this preference was offered.

Cage et al. described their trans-cerebellar surgical approach in nine children with diffuse intrinsic brainstem tumours as follows [81]: "Preoperatively, patients all completed an MRI with and without gadolinium intravenous contrast of the brain according to Brainlab (Brainlab AG, Germany) protocols to allow for intraoperative neuronavigation. Patients were positioned either supine (n=3) or in the lateral decubitus position (n=6) opposite the side of their lesion with neck flexion in the same direction. The head was then fixed using both a horseshoe head-holding device and further immobilized with Mayfield pin fixation. For all stereotactic procedures, the Brainlab neuronavigation system was used to plan the trajectory from the skull to target locations in the brainstem. The biopsy entry point was transcerebellar, either right (n=4) or left (n=5) for all patients. A side-cutting biopsy needle was then passed along the trajectory path. Between one and four samples were obtained from within the lesion.... Target selection was designed to minimize the trajectory through the brainstem. If there was an obvious area of enhancement suggesting a pathologically-aggressive area of the tumour, then this was chosen as the biopsy target. Otherwise, the target was usually just deep to the cerebellar peduncle. Care was taken to avoid the lateral edge of the fourth ventricle and the ventral corticospinal tracts." [81]

Otherwise, surgeons continue to operate successfully on patients with focal, exophytic and cystic brainstem tumours, with survival and quality of life enhanced even by subtotal resections, as well as by cyst drainage procedures and the insertion of shunts when necessary [61]. But here too, stereotactic biopsies play a significant role, as some apparent tumours are found to be focal areas of inflammation, infectious lesions, vascular anomalies, or some other pathology necessitating different treatment [29;131]. As such, neurosurgeons now appear to have a role to play in all paediatric patients with brainstem tumours, a far cry from forty years ago, when they seemed to have no role at all.

4. Conclusions

Over the past forty years, much has changed in the way in which brainstem tumours are treated in children. Though these lesions continue to be the most common cause of CNS cancer-related death in the paediatric population, the discovery of a brainstem tumour is no longer a death sentence. Formerly thought to be pathologically homogeneous and/or of no pathological interest since they were not surgically accessible, paediatric brainstem tumours are now understood to be highly heterogeneous; and knowing the pathology is now considered critical to management decisions. For the minority of children who have focal, exophytic or cystic lesions, long-term survival is now the rule, with 5-and 10-year survival rates often 90% or higher. For those children in the future who will develop diffuse brainstem lesions, mostly high-grade gliomas, emerging therapies are now providing multiple reasons to hope. Besides providing competent, compassionate care to each child and their families, what is critical, from the current neurosurgeon's standpoint, is to assist in the collection of tissue, either by biopsy while a child is alive, or at autopsy via respectful conversations with parents and other caregivers, so that future targeted therapies can be developed, tested and ultimately approved for widespread use.

Author details

Adrianna Ranger*, Navjot Chaudhary and Jonathan Lau

London Health Sciences Center-Department of Clinical Neurological Sciences; Division of Neurosurgery, Western University, London, Ontario, Canada

References

[1] Ellison LF, De P, Mery LS, Grundy PE, Canadian Cancer Society's Steering Committee for Canadian Cancer Statistics.: Canadian cancer statistics at a glance: cancer in children. CMAJ 2009;180:422-424.

[2] Bunin GR, Feuer EJ, Witman PA, Meadows AT: Increasing incidence of childhood cancer: report of 20 years experience from the greater Delaware Valley Pediatric Tumor Registry. Paediatr Perinat Epidemiol 1996;10:319-338.

[3] Linet MS, Ries LA, Smith MA, Tarone RE, Devesa SS: Cancer surveillance series: recent trends in childhood cancer incidence and mortality in the United States. J Natl Cancer Inst 1999;91:1051-1058.

[4] Centers for Disease Control and Prevention (CDC): Trends in childhood cancer mortality--United States, 1990-2004. MMWR Morb Mortal Wkly Rep 2007;56:1257-1261.

[5] Rendon-Macias ME, Ramos-Becerril C, Bernadez-Zapata I, Iglesias-Leboreiro J: [Cancer epidemiology in children and adolescents at private health care (1995-2004)] [Article in Spanish]. Rev Med Inst Mex Seguro Soc 2008;46:353-360.

[6] Barr RD, Greenberg ML, Shaw AK, Mery L: The Canadian Childhood Cancer Surveillance and Control Program (CCCSCP): a status report. Pediatr Blood Cancer 2008;50:518-519.

[7] Stiller C: Population based survival rates for childhood cancer in Britain 1980-1991. BMJ 1994;309:1612-1616.

[8] La Vecchia C, Levi F, Lucchini F, Lagiou P, Trichopoulos D, Negri E: Trends in childhood cancer mortality as indicators of the quality of medical care in the developed world. Cancer 1998;83:2223-2227.

[9] Chatenoud L, Bertuccio P, Bosetti C, Levi F, Negri E, La Vecchia C: Childhood cancer mortality in America, Asia, and Oceania, 1970 through 2007. Cancer 2010;116:5063-5074.

[10] Dolecek TA, Propp JM, Stroup NE, Kruchko C: CBTRUS statistical report: primary brain and central nervous system tumors diagnosed in the United States in 2005-2009. Neuro Oncol 2012;14:1-49.

[11] Allen J: Brain stem glioma. Neurol Neurosurg Update Series 1983;2-7.

[12] Fisher PG, Carson BS: Management of brainstem gliomas in children. Contemp Neurosurg 1996;18:1-7.

[13] Walker DA, Punt JA, Sokal M: Clinical management of brain stem glioma. Arch Dis Child 1999;80:558-564.

[14] Russell DS, Rubenstein LJ: Pathology of Tumours of the Nervous System, ed Fourth Edition. Baltimore, Wilkins & Williams, 1977.

[15] Tumor Types. National Brain Tumor Society.

[16] Recinos PF, Sciubba DM, Jallo GI: Brainstem tumors: where are we today? Pediatr Neurosurg 2007;43:192-201.

[17] Shuper-A, Kornriech L, Loven D, Michowitz S, Schwartz S, Cohen IJ: Diffuse brain stem gliomas. Are we improving outcome? Childs Nerv Syst 1998;14:578-581.

[18] Freeman CR, Farmer JP: Pediatric brain stem gliomas: a review. Int J Radiat Oncol Biol Phys 1998;40:265-271.

[19] Laigle-Donadey F, Doz F, Delattre JY: Brainstem gliomas in children and adults. Curr Opin Oncol 2008;20:662-667.

[20] Mauffrey C: Paediatric brainstem gliomas: prognostic factors and management. J Clin Neurosci 2006;13:431-437.

[21] Matson D: Tumors of the posterior fossa.; in Thomas C (ed): Neurosurgery of Infancy and Childhood. Springfield, MA, Charles C. Thomas Publishing, 1969, pp 469-477.

[22] Gold JA, Smith KRJr: Childhood brain tumors: a 15-year survey. South Med J 1975;68:1337-1344.

[23] Klimo PJr, Pai Panandiker AS, Thompson CJ, Boop FA, Qaddoumi I, Gajjar A, et al.: Management and outcome of focal low-grade brainstem tumors in pediatric patients: the St. Jude experience. J Neurosurg Pediatr 2013;11:274-281.

[24] Lamm AF, Elaimy AL, Lamoreaux WT, MacKay AR, Fairbanks RK, Demakas JJ, Cooke BS, Lee CM: A review of the clinical outcomes for patients diagnosed with brainstem metastasis and treated with stereotactic radiosurgery. ISRN Surg 2013 Apr 11;2013:652895 doi: 10 1155/2013/652895 Print 2013.

[25] Duffner PK: Diagnosis of brain tumors in children. Expert Rev Neurother 2007;7:875-885.

[26] Albright AL, Pollack IF: Brainstem Gliomas; in Winn HD (ed): Youman's Neurological Surgery, Volume 3. Philadelphia, PA, Saunders, 2004, pp 3663-3669.

[27] Epstein F, Wisoff JH: Intrinsic brainstem tumors in childhood: surgical indications. J Neurooncol 1988;6:309-317.

[28] Pierre-Kahn A, Hirsch JF, Vinchon M, Payan C, Sainte-Rose C, Lelouch-Tubiana A, Fermanian J, et al.: Surgical management of brain-stem tumors in children: results and statistical analysis of 75 cases. J Neurosurg 1993;79:845-852.

[29] Pinero-Gonzalez de la Pena P, Rodriguez-Romero R: Nonglial tumors of the brainstem. Semin Ultrasound CT MR 2013;34:113-122.

[30] Bailey P, Buchanan DN, Buoy PC: Intracranial Tumors of Infancy and Childhood. Chicago, University of Chicago Press, 1939.

[31] Tomita T, McLone DG, Naidich TP: Brain stem gliomas in childhood. Rational approach and treatment. J Neurooncol 1984;2:117-122.

[32] Golden GS, Ghatak NR, Hirano A, French JH: Malignant glioma of the brain-stem. A clinicopathological analysis of 13 cases. J Neurol Neurosurg Psychiatry 1972;35:732-738.

[33] Greenberger JS, Cassady JR, Levene MB: Radiation therapy of thalamic, midbrain and brain stem gliomas. Radiology 1977;1:2-463.

[34] Lassiter KR, Alexander EJr, Davis CHJr, Kelly DLJr: Surgical treatment of brain stem gliomas. J Neurosurg 1971;34:719-725.

[35] Hara M, Takeuchi K: A temporal study of survival of patients with pontine gliomas. J Neurol 1977;216:189-196.

[36] Eisenhardt L: Long post-operative survivals in cases of intracranial tumor. Proc Ass Res Nerv Ment Dis 1937;16:390-416.

[37] Patton WB, Craig WM: Glioma of the pons: report of a case. Proc Staff Meet Mayo Clin 1940;15:506-508.

[38] Pool JL: Gliomas in the region of the brain stem. J Neurosurg 1968;29:164-167.

[39] Gilday DL, Ash J: Accuracy of brain scanning in pediatric craniocerebral neoplasms. Radiology 1975;117:93-97.

[40] Alvisi C, Cerisoli M, Maccheroni ME: Long-term results of surgically treated brain-stem gliomas. Acta Neurochir (Wien) 1985;76:12-17.

[41] Hoffman HJ, Becker L, Craven MA: A clinically and pathologically distinct group of benign brain stem gliomas. Neurosurgery 1980;7:243-248.

[42] Renier WO, Gabreels FJ: Evaluation of diagnosis and non-surgical therapy in 24 children with a pontine tumour. Neuropediatrics 1980;11:262-273.

[43] Epstein F: A staging system for brain stem gliomas. Cancer 1985;56:1806.

[44] Epstein F, McCleary EL: Intrinsic brain-stem tumors of childhood: surgical indications. J Neurosurg 1986;64:11-15.

[45] Stroink AR, Hoffman AJ, Hendrick EB, Humphreys RP, Davidson G: Transependymal benign dorsally exophytic brain stem gliomas in childhood: diagnosis and treatment recommendations. Neurosurgery 1987;20:439-444.

[46] Reigel DH, Scarff TB, Woodford JE: Biopsy of pediatric brain stem tumors. Childs Brain 1979;5:329-340.

[47] Strange P, Wohlert L: Primary brain stem tumours. Acta Neurochir (Wien) 2013;62:219-232.

[48] James AEJr: The efficacy of the brain scan in diagnosis of brainstem gliomas. Radiology 1975;116:117-120.

[49] Seeger JF, Gabrielsen TO: Angiography of eccentric brain stem tumors. Radiology 1972;105:343-351.

[50] Brnini FP, Calabro A, Corrado A, De Rosa G, Elefante R, Fucci G, et al.: [Radiological diagnosis of tumours of brain stem (author's transl)] [Article in Italian]. Radiol Med 1977;63:497-526.

[51] Baker HIJr, Howser OW: Computed tomography in the diagnosis of posterior fossa lesions. Radiol Clin North Am 1976;14:129-147.

[52] Gado M, Huete I, Mikhael M: Computerized tomography of infratentorial tumors. Semin Roentgenol 1977;12:109-120.

[53] Kazner E, Meese W, Kretzschmar K: The role of computed tomography in the diagnosis of brain tumors in infants and children. Neuroradiology 1978;16:10-12.

[54] Thomson JL: Computerised axial tomography in posterior fossa lesions. Clin Radiol 1978;29:233-250.

[55] Barkovich AJ, Krischer J, Kun LE, Packer R, Zimmerman RA, Freeman CR, et al.: Brain stem gliomas: a classification system based on magnetic resonance imaging. Pediatr Neurosurg 1990;16:73-83.

[56] Fischbein NJ, Prados MD, Wara W, Russo C, Edwards MS, Barkovich AJ: Radiologic classification of brain stem tumors: correlation of magnetic resonance imaging appearance with clinical outcome. Pediatr Neurosurg 1996;24:9-23.

[57] Choux M, Lena G, Do L: Brainstem tumors; in Choux M, Di Rocco C, Hockley A (eds): Pediatric Neurosurgery. New York, NY, Churchill Livingstone, 2000, pp 471-491.

[58] Albright AL: Brain stem gliomas; in J Y (ed): Neurological Surgery. Philadelphia, PA, Saunders, 1996, pp 2603-2611.

[59] Fisher PG, Breiter SN, Carson BS, Wharam MD, Williams JA, Weingart JD, et al.: A clinicopathologic reappraisal of brain stem tumor classification. Identification of pilocystic astrocytoma and fibrillary astrocytoma as distinct entities. Cancer 2000;89:1569-1576.

[60] Mehta VS, Chandra PS, Singh PK, Garg A, Rath GK: Surgical considerations for 'intrinsic' brainstem gliomas: proposal of a modification in classification. Neurol India 2009;57:274-281.

[61] Ramos A, Hilario A, Lagares A, Savador E, Perez-Nunez A, Sepulveda J: Brainstem gliomas. Semin Ultrasound CT MR 2013;34:104-112.

[62] Fasano VA, Urciuoli R, Ponzio RM, Lanotte MM: The effects of new technologies on the surgical management of brainstem tumors. Surg Neurol 1986;25:219-226.

[63] Teo C, Siu TL: Radical resection of focal brainstem gliomas: is it worth doing? Childs Nerv Syst 2008;24:1307-1314.

[64] Dellaretti M, Reyns N, Touzet G, Dubois F, Gusmao S, Pereira JL, Blond S: Diffuse brainstem glioma: prognostic factors. J Neurosurg 2012;117:810-814.

[65] Poussaint TY, Kowal JR, Barnes PD, Zurakowski D, Anthony DC, Goumnerova L, Tarbell NJ: Tectal tumors of childhood: clinical and imaging follow-up. AJNR Am J Neuroradiol 1998;19:977-983.

[66] Milstein JM, Geyer JR, Berger MS, Bleyer WA: Favorable prognosis for brainstem gliomas in neurofibromatosis. J Neurooncol 1989;7:367-371.

[67] Cohen ME, Duffner PK, Heffner RR, Lacey DJ, Brecher M: Prognostic factors in brainstem gliomas. Neurology 1986;36:602-605.

[68] Blatt J, Jaffe R, Deutsch M, Adkins JC: Neurofibromatosis and childhood tumors. Cancer 1986;57:1225-1229.

[69] Ilgren EB, Kinnier-Wilson LM, Stiller CA: Gliomas in neurofibromatosis: a series of 89 cases with evidence for enhanced malignancy in associated cerebellar astrocytomas. Pathol Annu 1985;20:331-358.

[70] Pascual-Castroviejo I, Pascual-Pascual SI, Viano J, Carceller F, Gutierrez-Molina M, Morales C, Frutos-Martinez R: Posterior fossa tumors in children with neurofibromatosis type 1 (NF1). Childs Nerv Syst 2010;26:1599-1603.

[71] Albers AC, Guttman DH: Gliomas in patients with neurofibromatosis type 1. Expert Rev Neurother 2009;9:535-539.

[72] Fried I, Hawkins C, Scheinemann K, Tsangaris E, Hesselson L, Bartels U, et al.: Favorable outcome with conservative treatment for children with low grade brainstem tumors. Pediatr Blood Cancer 2012;58:556-560.

[73] Hottinger AF, Khakoo Y: Neuro-oncology of Neurofibromatosis Type 1. Curr Treat Options Neurol 2009;11:306-314.

[74] Lopes Ferraz Filho JR, Munis MP, Soares Souza A, Sanches RA, Goloni-Bertollo EM, Pavarino-Bertelli EC: Unidentified bright objects on brain MRI in children as a diagnostic criterion for neurofibromatosis type 1. Pediatr Radiol 2008;38:305-310.

[75] Leonard JR, Perry A, Rubin JB, et al.: The role of surgical biopsy in the diagnosis of glioma in individuals with neurofibromatosis-1. Neurology 2006;67:1509-1512.

[76] Lesniak MS, Klem JM, Weingart J, Carson BSSr: Surgical outcome following resection of contrast-enhanced pediatric brainstem gliomas. Pediatr Neurosurg 2003;39:314-322.

[77] Sandri A, Sardi N, Genitori L, Giordano F, Peretta P, Basso ME, et al.: Diffuse and focal brain stem tumors in childhood: prognostic factors and surgical outcome. Experience in a single institution. Childs Nerv Syst 2006;22:1127-1135.

[78] Tokurika Y, Handa H, Yamashita J, Okumura T, Paine JT: Brainstem glioma: an analysis of 85 cases. Acta Neurochir (Wien) 1986;79:67-73.

[79] Jansen MH, van Vuurden DG, Vandertop WP, Kaspers GJ: Diffuse intrinsic pontine gliomas: a systematic update on clinical trials and biology. Cancer Treat Rev 2012;38:27-35.

[80] Hargrave D, Bartels U, Bouffet E: Diffuse brainstem glioma in children: critical review of clinical trials. Lancet Oncol 2006;7:241-248.

[81] Cage TA, Samagh SP, Mueller S, Nocolaides T, Haas-Kogan D, Prados M, et al.: Feasibility, safety, and indications for surgical biopsy of intrinsic brainstem tumors in children. Childs Nerv Syst 2013;29:1313-1319.

[82] Walker DA, Liu J, Kieran M, Jabado N, Picton S, Packer R, St.Rose C, CPN Paris 2011 Conference Consensus Group: A multi-disciplinary consensus statement concerning surgical approaches to low-grade, high-grade astrocytomas and diffuse intrinsic pontine gliomas in childhood (CPN Paris 2011) using the Delphi method. Neuro Oncol 2013;15:462-468.

[83] Wagner S, Warmuth-Metz M, Emser A, Gnekow AK, Strater R, Rutkowski S, et al.: Treatment options in childhood pontine gliomas. J Neurooncol 2006;79:281-287.

[84] Mann SD, Danesh BJ, Kamm MA: Intractable vomiting due to a brainstem lesion in the absence of neurological signs or raised intracranial pressure. Gut 1998;42:875-877.

[85] Guillamo JS, Doz F, Delattre JY: Brain stem gliomas. Curr Opin Neurol 2001;711.

[86] Jallo GI, Biser-Rohrbaugh A, Freed D: Brainstem gliomas. Childs Nerv Syst 2004;20:143-153.

[87] Laprie A, Pirzkall A, Haas-Kogan DA, Cha S, Banerjee A, Le TP, et al.: Longitudinal multivoxel MR spectroscopy study of pediatric diffuse brainstem gliomas treated with radiotherapy. Int J Radiat Oncol Biol Phys 2005;62:20-31.

[88] Barajas RF, Chang JS, Sneed PK, Segal MR, McDermott MW, Cha S: Distinguishing recurrent intra-axial metastatic tumor from radiation necrosis following gamma knife radiosurgery using dynamic susceptibility-weighted contrast-enhanced perfusion MR imaging. AJNR Am J Neuroradiol 2009;30:367-372.

[89] Thakur SB, Karimi S, Dunkel IJ, Koutcher JA, Huang W: Longitudinal MR spectroscopic imaging of pediatric diffuse pontine tumors to assess tumor aggression and progression. AJNR Am J Neuroradiol 2006;27:806-809.

[90] Porto L, Hattingen E, Pilatus U, Kieslich M, Yan B, Schwabe D, et al.: Proton magnetic resonance spectroscopy in childhood brainstem lesions. Childs Nerv Syst 2007;23:305-314.

[91] Kovacs A, Toth L, Glavak C, Liposits G, Hadjiev J, Antal G, Emri M, et al.: Integrating functional MRI information into conventional 3D radiotherapy planning of CNS tumors. Is it worth it? J Neurooncol 2011;105:629-637.

[92] Pirotte B, Acerbi F, Lubansu A, Goldman S, Brotchi J, Leviver M: PET imaging in the surgical management of pediatric brain tumors. Childs Nerv Syst 2007;23:739-751.

[93] Leitch JK, Figley CR, Stroman PW: Applying functional MRI to the spinal cord and brainstem. Magn Reson Imaging 2010;28.

[94] Nadvi SS, Ebrahim FS, Corr P: The value of 201thallium-SPECT imaging in childhood brainstem gliomas. Pediatr Radiol 1998;28:575-579.

[95] Oriuchi N, Tamura M, Shibazaki T, Ohye C, Watanabe N, Tateno M, Tomiyoshi K, et al.: Clinical evaluation of thallium-201 SPECT in supratentorial gliomas: relationship to histologic grade, prognosis and proliferative activities. J Nucl Med 1993;34:2085-2089.

[96] Adams WS: Investigations in Stellar Spectroscopy: III. Application of a Spectroscopic Method of Determining Stellar Distances to Stars of Measured Parallax. Proc Natl Acad Sci U S A 1916;2:152-157.

[97] Carr JJ, Hemler PF, Halford PW, Freimanis RI, Choplin RH, Chen MY: Stereotactic localization of breast lesions: how it works and methods to improve accuracy. Radiographics 2001;21:463-473.

[98] Becker W: Stereotactic localization of breast lesions. Radiology 1979;133:238-240.

[99] Lewander R, Bergstrom M, Boethius J, Collins VP, Edner G, Greitz T, Willems J: Stereotactic computer tomography for biopsy of gliomas. Acta Radiol Diagn (Stockh) 1978;19:867-888.

[100] Boethius J, Collins VP, Edner G, Lewander R, Zajicek J: Stereotactic biopsies and computer tomography in gliomas. Acta Neurochir (Wien) 1978;40:223-232.

[101] Coffey RJ, Lunsford LD: Stereotactic surgery for mass lesions of the midbrain and pons. Neurosurgery 1985;17:12-18.

[102] Rajshekhar V, Chandy MJ: Computerized tomography-guided stereotactic surgery for brainstem masses: a risk-benefit analysis in 71 patients. J Neurosurg 1995;82:976-981.

[103] Kondziolka D, Lunsford LD: Results and expectations with image-integrated brainstem stereotactic biopsy. Surg Neurol 1995;43:558-562.

[104] Rachinger W, Grau S, Holtmannspotter M, Herms J, Tonn JC, Kreth FW: Serial stereotactic biopsy of brainstem lesions in adults improves diagnostic accuracy compared with MRI only. J Neurol Neurosurg Psychiatry 2009;80:1134-1139.

[105] Paugh BS, Qu C, Jones C, Liu Z, Adamowicz-Brice M, Zhang J, et al.: Integrated molecular genetic profiling of pediatric high-grade gliomas reveals key differences with the adult disease. J Clin Oncol 2010;28:3061-3068.

[106] Paugh BS, Broniscer A, Qu C, Miller CP, Zhang J, Tatevossian RG, et al.: Genome-wide analyses identify recurrent amplifications of receptor tyrosine kinases and cell-cycle regulatory genes in diffuse intrinsic pontine glioma. J Clin Oncol 2011;29:3999-4006.

[107] Monje M, Mitra SS, Freret ME, Raveh TB, Kim J, Masek M, et al.: Hedgehog-responsive candidate cell of origin for diffuse intrinsic pontine glioma. Proc Natl Acad Sci U S A 2011;108:4453-4458.

[108] Zhou Z, Luther N, Ibrahim GM, Hawkins C, Vibhakar R, Handler MH, Souweidane MM: B7-H3, a potential therapeutic target, is expressed in diffuse intrinsic pontine glioma. J Neurooncol 2013;111:257-264.

[109] Puget S, Philippe C, Bax DA, Job B, Varlet P, Junier MP, et al.: Mesenchymal transition and PDGFRA amplification/mutation are key distinct oncogenic events in pediatric diffuse intrinsic pontine gliomas. PLoS One 2012;7:e30313.

[110] Hashizume R, Smirnov I, Liu S, Phillips JJ, Hyer J, McKnight TR, et al.: Characterization of a diffuse intrinsic pontine glioma cell line: implications for future investigations and treatment. J Neurooncol 2012;110:305-313.

[111] Chapoval AI, Ni J, Lau JS, Wilcox RA, Flies DB, Liu D, et al.: B7-H3: a costimulatory molecule for T cell activation and IFN-gamma production. Nat Immunol 2001;2:269-274.

[112] Xu H, Cheung IY, Guo HF, Cheung NK: MicroRNA miR-29 modulates expression of immunoinhibitory molecule B7-H3: potential implications for immune based therapy of human solid tumors. Cancer Res 2009;69:6275-6281.

[113] Modak S, Kramer K, Gultekin SH, Guo HF, Cheung NK: Monoclonal antibody 8H9 targets a novel cell surface antigen expressed by a wide spectrum of human solid tumors. Cancer Res 2001;61:4048-4054.

[114] Kramer K, Kushner BH, Modak S, Pandit-Taskar N, Smith-Jones P, Zanzonico P, et al.: Compartmental intrathecal radioimmunotherapy: results for treatment for metastatic CNS neuroblastoma. J Neurooncol 2010;97:409-418.

[115] Geoerger B, Hargrave D, Thomas F, Ndiaye A, Frappaz D, Andreiuolo F, et al.: Innovative Therapies for Children with Cancer pediatric phase I study of erlotinib in brainstem glioma and relapsing/refractory brain tumors. Neuro Oncol 2011;13:109-118.

[116] Geyer JR, Stewart CF, Kocak M, Broniscer A, Phillips P, Douglas JG, et al.: A phase I and biology study of gefitinib and radiation in children with newly diagnosed brain stem gliomas or supratentorial malignant gliomas. Eur J Cancer 2010;46:3287-3293.

[117] Pollack IF, Stewart CF, Kocak M, Poussaint TY, Broniscer A, Banerjee A, et al.: A phase II study of gefitinib and irradiation in children with newly diagnosed brainstem gliomas: a report from the Pediatric Brain Tumor Consortium. Neuro Oncol 2011;13:290-297.

[118] Broniscer A, Baker JN, Tagen M, Onar-Thomas A, Gilbertson RJ, Davidoff AM, et al.: Phase I study of vandetanib during and after radiotherapy in children with diffuse intrinsic pontine glioma. J Clin Oncol 2010;28:4762-4768.

[119] Burzynski SR: The present state of antineoplaston research (1). Integr Cancer Ther 2004;3:47-58.

[120] Burzynski SR, Janicki TJ, Weaver RA, Burzynski B: Targeted therapy with antineoplastons A10 and AS2-1 of high-grade, recurrent, and progressive brainstem glioma. Integr Cancer Ther 2006;5:40-47.

[121] Del Burgo LS, Hernandez RM, Orive G, Pedraz JL: Nanotherapeutic approaches for brain cancer management. Nanomedicine 2013 Oct 14 pii: S1549-9634(13)00555-8 doi: 10 1016/j nano 2013 10 001 [Epub ahead of print] 2013.

[122] Binello E, Germano IM: Stem cells as therapeutic vehicles for the treatment of high-grade gliomas. Neuro Oncol 2012;14:256-265.

[123] Kosztowski T, Zaida HA, Quinones-Hinojosa A: Applications of neural and mesenchymal stem cells in the treatment of gliomas. Expert Rev Anticancer Ther 2009;9:597-612.

[124] Costello PC, MacDonald D, McDonald R, Hammond R, Sloby V, Faubert B, Megyesi J: Determination of human brain tumour therapy response using an ex vivo invasion assay provides a potential step toward individualized treatment. J Clin Oncol 2006;24:18S.

[125] Saratsis AM, Yadavilli S, Magge S, Rood BR, Perez J, Hill DA, et al.: Insights into pediatric diffuse intrinsic pontine glioma through proteomic analysis of cerebrospinal fluid. Neuro Oncol 2012;14:547-560.

[126] Perez-Gomez JL, Rodriguez-Alvarez CA, Marhx-Bracho A, Rueda-Franco F: Stereotactic biopsy for brainstem tumors in pediatric patients. Childs Nerv Syst 2010;26:29-34.

[127] Patel P, Balamurugan M: Transcerebellar stereotactic biopsy for brainstem lesions in children. J Pediatr Neurosci 2009;4:17-19.

[128] Sanai N, Wachorst SP, Gupta NM, McDermott MW: Transcerebellar stereotactic biopsy for lesions of the brainstem and peduncles under local anesthesia. Neurosurgery 2008;63:460-466.

[129] Roujeau T, Machado G, Garnett MR, Miquel C, Puget S, Geoerger B, et al.: Stereotactic biopsy of diffuse pontine lesions in children. J Neurosurg 2007;107:1-4.

[130] Dellaretti M, Reyns N, Touzet G, Dubois F, Gusmao S, Pereira JL, Blond S: Stereotactic biopsy for brainstem tumors: comparison of transcerebellar with transfrontal approach. Stereotact Funct Neurosurg 2012;90:79-83.

[131] Valdez-Gorcia J, Espinoza-Diaz DM, Paredes-Diaz E: Stereotactic biopsy of brain stem and posterior fossa lesions in children. Acta Neurochir (Wien) 1998;140:899-903.

Section 2

New Diagnostic Approaches – CNS Tumors

Spatial Relationships of MR Imaging and Positron Emission Tomography with Phenotype, Genotype and Tumor Stem Cell Generation in Glioblastoma Multiforme

Davide Schiffer, Consuelo Valentini, Antonio Melcarne, Marta Mellai, Elena Prodi, Giovanna Carrara, Tetyana Denysenko, Carola Junemann, Cristina Casalone, Cristiano Corona, Valentina Caldera, Laura Annovazzi, Angela Piazzi, Paola Cassoni, Rebecca Senetta, Piercarlo Fania and Angelina Cistaro

Additional information is available at the end of the chapter

http://dx.doi.org/10.5772/58391

1. Introduction

Glioblastoma multiforme (GBM), the most malignant and frequent glioma, is a heterogeneous tumor in which areas of different histological aspect, aggressiveness, genetic expression and regressive events coexist so that one region of the tumor is not representative of the entire neoplasia. The consequences of the heterogeneity reflect on the diagnostics, prognostics and therapies. As a matter of fact, unguided surgical biopsies can lead to sampling error and to undergrade the tumor up to 30% of cases [1]. From the surgical, but also prognostic and therapeutic point of view, it is of great importance to know in advance the composition of the tumor and the biological significance of the different imaging aspects. Neuro-imaging is the only and fundamental source of information for the neurosurgeon and it has progressed today from the simple anatomic recognition of the tumor to that of functional and metabolic significance of its different regions, contributing greatly to a better approach to tumor surgery, prognosis and therapy. The detection of highly malignant regions and the definition of the tumor extent are crucial before the operation, when they are the main concern of neurosurgeons.

GBM is composed, as it is universally known, of three zones: central necrosis, proliferation and infiltration zones (Figures 1,2). Proliferation region is characterized by high indices of cell

INTECH
open science | open minds

© 2014 The Author(s). Licensee InTech. This chapter is distributed under the terms of the Creative Commons Attribution License (http://creativecommons.org/licenses/by/3.0), which permits unrestricted use, distribution, and reproduction in any medium, provided the original work is properly cited.

density, proliferation, mitoses, vessel density or angiogenesis and circumscribed necroses. In the spectrum of the many aspects of the tumor, with the term disruption one indicates the passage from the uniform and quiescent appearance of an astrocytoma to the rupture of the structure, forms and dimensions of GBM (Figure 3A). Circumscribed necroses and angiogenesis are the absolute features of GBM and their occurrence is needed for its recognition, because they are direct signs of malignancy (Figures 3B,4A-C). Angiogenesis in gliomas represents the intervened transformation, whereas it depends on the imbalance between the high proliferation potential of tumor cells and the low reproduction capacity of endothelial cells [2]. When the diagnosis has to be carried out on small tumor samples, as for example in stereotactic biopsies, the diagnosis cannot be of certainty. When close to central necrosis, circumscribed necroses merge with it. Infiltration zone represents the invasion into the brain of tumor cells that acquire a particular phenotypic and molecular signature. It is not uniform along the tumor borders and often it is so mild that it is hardly detectable, also histologically. Frequently, it is discovered in histological sections only after counting the cells and this happens either when it affects the white matter or the cortex, where tumor cells must be distinguished from normal cells. In the latter, perineuronal satellitosis may be of help. Isolated tumor cells (ITCs) in the normal nervous tissue make the problem of the tumor delimitation very hard. They cannot be detected, of course, in the samples removed during intervention, but only in the study of the brain at autopsy and they can be found very far from the tumor borders; the classic example is the passage of normally looking corpus callosum by ITCs [3,4]. Regressive events are frequent and include haemorrhages, large necroses, vascular thrombosis, *etc* and they contribute to the so-called disruption of the tissue.

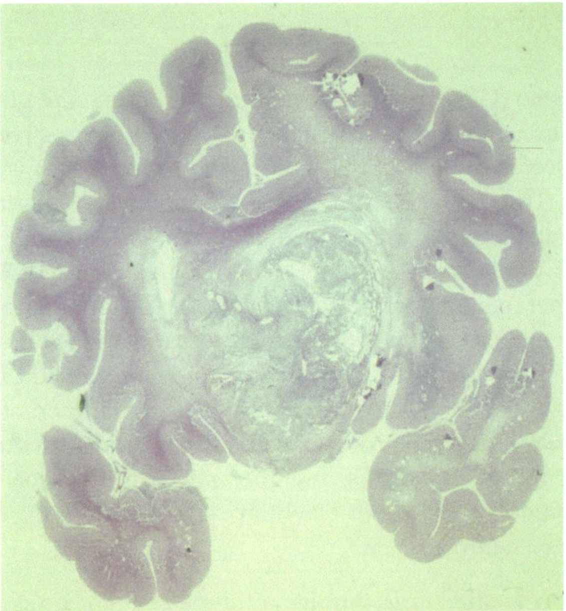

Figure 1. Coronal section of a brain with GBM. The borders of the tumor show different nervous structures. H&E.

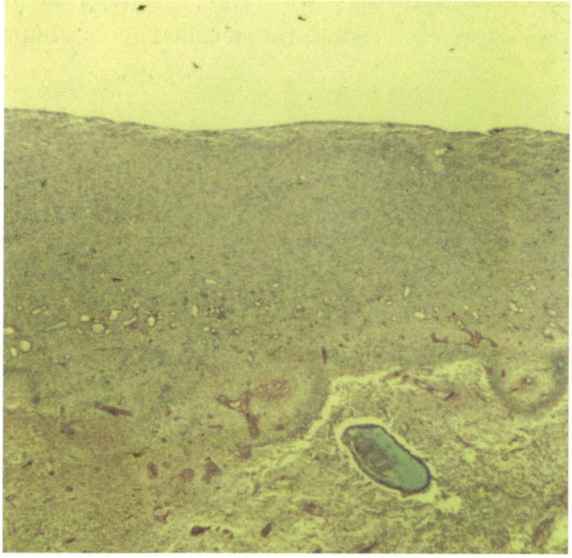

Figure 2. Three zones can be recognized: central necrosis, proliferation, and infiltration zone. H&E, 25x.

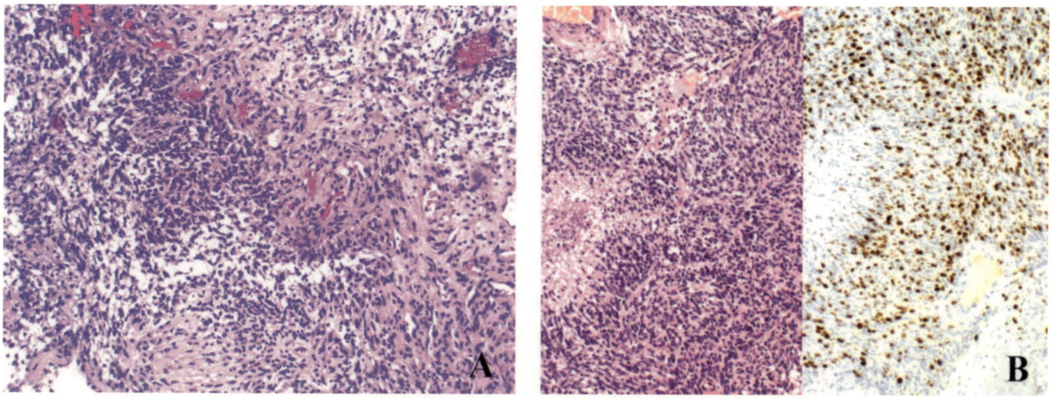

Figure 3. A – Area of disrupture with high cell density, vessels of different size and edema dissociation of the tissue; B – Circumscribed necrosis with pseudo-palisading in an area with high cell density (H&E, 100x) and area with a high Ki-67/MIB.1 proliferation index (DAB, 100x).

Beside the classic T1 and T2 imaging of GBM, supplied by the anatomy based magnetic resonance (MR), physiology-based MR imaging methods, namely diffusion-weighted imaging (DWI), perfusion-weighted imaging (PWI) and proton MR spectroscopy imaging (MRSI), together with the positron emission tomography (PET), which is highly correlated with the degree of malignancy [5,6], improved the tumor characterization. Today, the advancement of the knowledge in molecular biology and cell biology, associated with new surgical procedures, radiation techniques and therapeutic possibilities ask the neuro-imaging to answer three main questions: the identification *in vivo* of the tumor sites with the highest malignancy grade, the extension of tumor invasion and the sites where the capacity of the tumor to reproduce, to recur and to resist therapies resides, *i.e.* where the so-called glioblastoma stem cells (GSCs) are located.

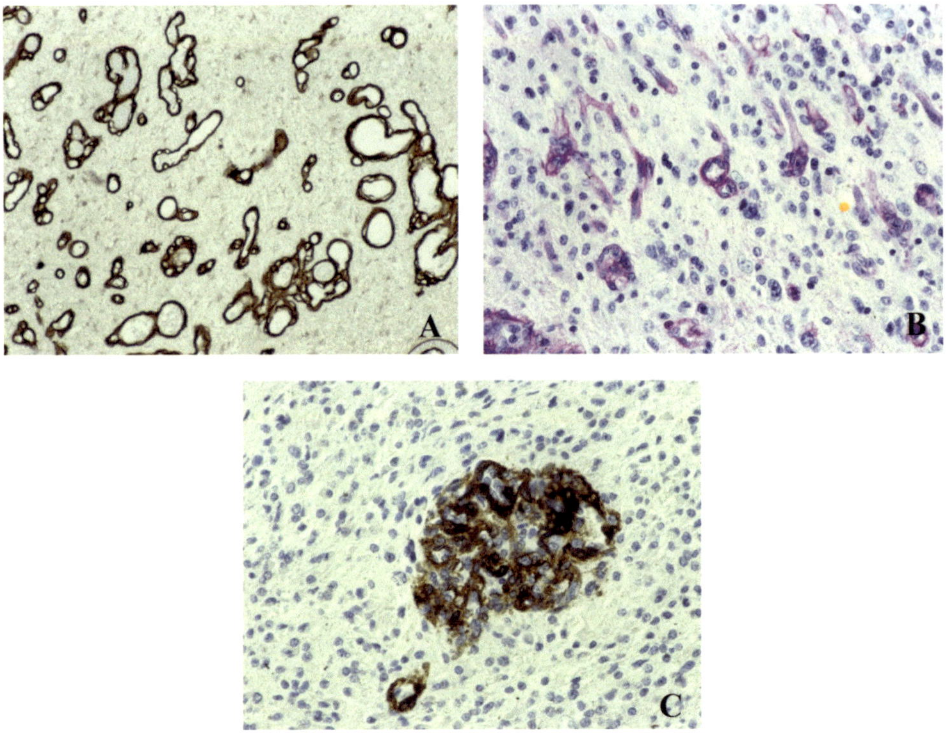

Figure 4. A – High vessel density. Laminin, DAB, 100x; B – Neoformed vessels and endothelial buds. PAS, 200x; C – Glomeruloid structure. α-sm-actin, DAB, 200x.

2. Physiology based MRI and PET

DWI rationale is to quantify the brownian movement of water protons within tissues that depends on the complex interaction between the intracellular and extracellular compartments, but also on cell density, cell membrane permeability and tissue structure. Water diffusivity within the extracellular compartment is inversely related to cell size and cell number. The greater the volume of the intracellular space and also the higher the cell density, the lower is the water diffusivity in the extracellular space, resulting in a low apparent diffusion coefficient (ADC), a measure of water diffusion. Diffusivity within tumors is heterogeneous due to different tumor components, being reduced in areas with high cellular density and increased in necrotic regions. Restricted ADC values in a tumor can also be related to ischemic changes, haemorragic or calcific components.

Although several reports have shown that glioma grade inversely correlates with intra-tumor minimum ADC [7], reflecting the presence of areas with high cell density in high grade tumors [8,9], the clinical significance of ADC measurement is limited as a consequence of the tissue heterogeneity within a tumor and because of substantial overlap in ADC values among different grades of glioma [10,11]. The range of ADC values within a given glioma, therefore, can vary markedly [11] and there is no final confirmation that minimum ADC always correlates with cell density.

PWI is used to measure vascularization and perfusion of brain lesions. Different PWI techniques are available, namely dynamic susceptibility contrast (DSC) and dynamic contrast-enhanced (DCE), widely used in the clinical setting. DSC perfusion measures T2-weighted signal-intensity loss occurring dynamically over a bolus injection of contrast medium, from which relative cerebral blood volume (rCBV), a marker of tumor angiogenesis, can be computed. DCE is a T1-weighted sequence that measures vascular permeability in tumors during a bolus injection of contrast medium; rCBV values are then calculated from DCE data. rCBV values have shown good correlation with the World Health Organization (WHO) tumor grading [12,13]; exceptions are represented by low-grade glial neoplasms with oligodendroglial features and grade I pilocytic astrocytoma, that may have markedly elevated rCBV (Figure 5).

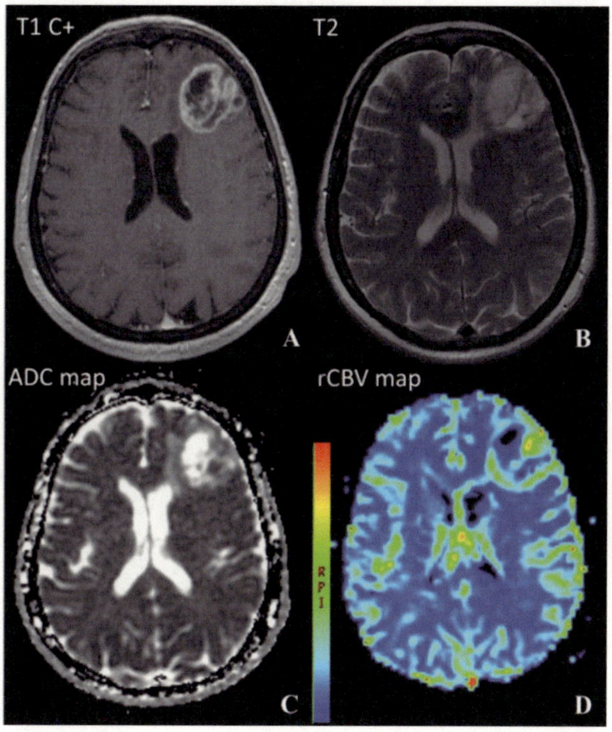

Figure 5. A –T1C MRI; B – T2 MRI; C – Diffusion MRI; D – Perfusion MRI.

Arterial spin-labeling (ASL) is a more recent perfusion technique that uses water of the blood entering the brain as an endogenous tracer to evaluate perfusion. ASL is emerging as an alternative to gadolinium based techniques in the evaluation of tumor perfusion.

MRSI is another advanced technique that provides metabolic information of the brain tissue. The predominant metabolites are choline (Cho), N-acetylaspartate (NAA), creatine (Cr), glutamate and glutamine (Glx), myo-inositol (MI) and lactate/lipids (LL). The Cho peak contains contributions from several different choline-containing compounds, which are involved in membrane synthesis and degradation; NAA is marker of neuronal integrity; Cr is a marker of cellular energetics; MI is considered a glial cell marker; LL are markers of tissue breakdown and anaerobic glycolysis. Glx is a complex peak from glutamate (Glu), glutamine (Gln) and gamma-aminobutyric acid (GABA). Glu is an important excitatory neurotransmitter and it also plays a role in the redox cycle. In brain tumors, as malignancy increases, NAA signal decreases, as a consequence of loss, dysfunction or displacement of normal neurons, while Cho levels increase as a consequence of rapid cell membrane turnover. Malignant tumors also have reduced Cr due to high metabolic activity that depletes the energy stores; this is associated to anaerobic glycolysis leading to the appearance of lactate. Necrotic portions of tumor show the presence of lipid peaks. Elevated concentration of Gln can be found in high grade tumors.

Metabolite concentrations are usually expressed as ratios (*i.e.* Cho/Cr, Cho/NAA, NAA/Cr) rather than as absolute concentrations.

Such spectra can be obtained using single voxel or multi-voxel 2D or 3D technique. Multi-voxel spectroscopy is the best to detect infiltration of malignant cells beyond the enhancing margins of tumors [14,15] (Figures 6,7).

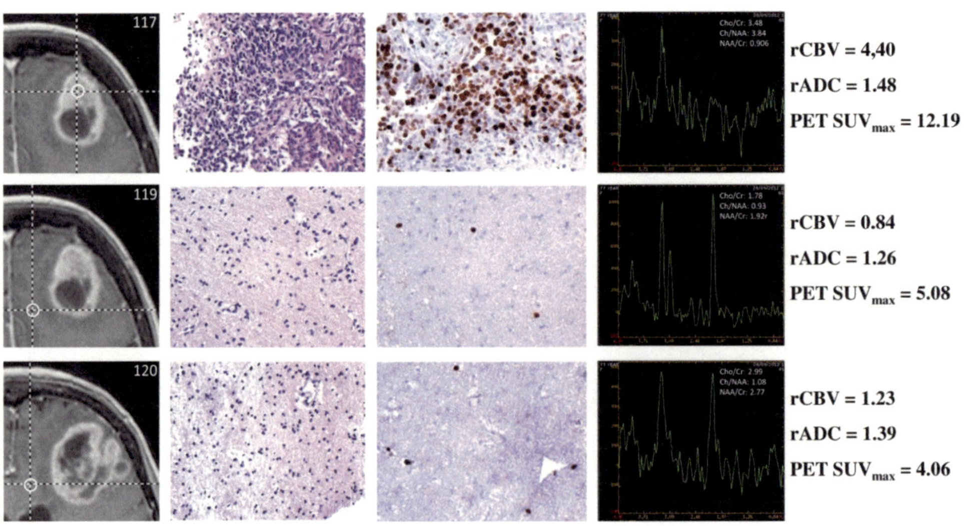

Figure 6. Case CTO3. Correlation among histopathology, Ki-67/MIB.1 proliferation marker, MRSI, physiologic MRI and PET values. Column 1 – ROIs on T1C MRI; Column 2 – Histopathology of a hyper-proliferating area and two areas differently infiltrated. H&E, 200x; Column 3 – Ki-67/MIB.1 proliferation index, DAB, 200x; Column 4 – MRSI values; Column 5 – PET values.

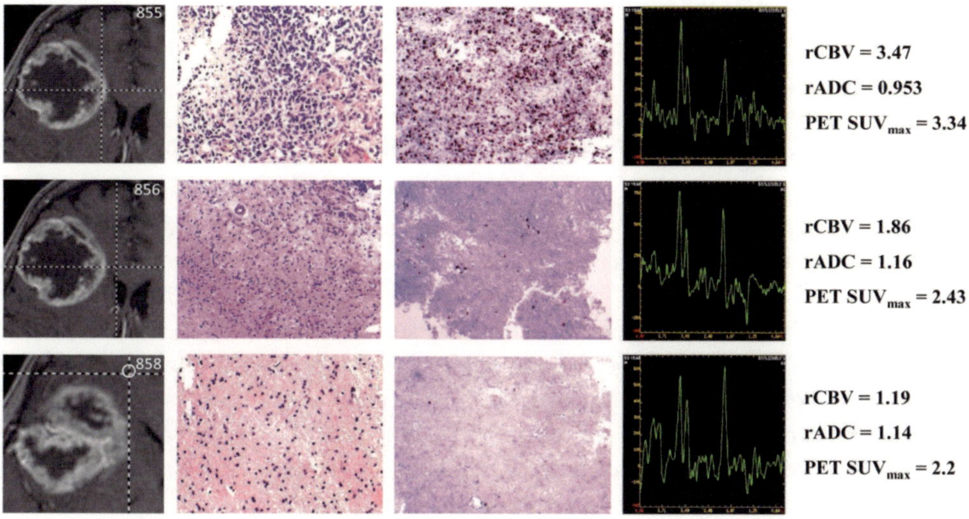

Figure 7. Case CTO5. Correlation among histopathology, Ki-67/MIB.1 proliferation marker, MRSI, physiologic MRI and PET values. Column 1 – ROIs on T1C MRI; Column 2 – Histopathology of a hyper-proliferating area and two areas differently infiltrated. H&E, 200x; Column 3 – Ki-67/MIB.1 proliferation index, DAB, 200x; Column 4 – MRSI values; Column 5 – PET values.

Diffusion tensor imaging (DTI) is an advanced MRI technique that describes the movement of water molecules using two metrics, mean diffusivity (MD) and fractional anisotropy (FA), that represent the magnitude and directionality of water diffusion, respectively. FA technique measures the preferential direction of proton movement and varies among values between 0 (isotropic diffusion, *i.e.* random diffusion such as in brain gray matter) and 1 (anisotropic diffusion, such as in brain white matter where proton diffusion is constrained along myelin fibres). MD technique gives information on the whole diffusivity in the brain; the reduction of nervous fibres results in an increased MD because of a higher degree of freedom of movement of water molecules. The degree of anisotropy depends on many factors, such as fibre density and diameter, myelin sheath integrity and the intercellular space characteristics. In the presence of a structural alteration of the nervous fibre tract, the anisotropic value reduces.

Anisotropy is reduced in cerebral lesions due to the loss of structural organisation. The measurement of FA allows prediction of histological characteristics such as cellularity, vascularity, or fibre structure. This technique is useful to differentiate normal white matter from edematous brain tissue and occult white matter invasion around the enhancing portion of the tumor.

DTI may help to determine the white matter fibre displacement by tumor. This technique, in combination with functional neuro-imaging methods, permits to map the individual anatomo-functional connectivity and represents a useful tool for surgical planning [16-18].

PET is currently the most powerful method of molecular imaging, as it has been emphasized in a recent review [19] (Figure 8). Depending on the radiotracer, various molecular processes can be visualized by PET, most of them relating to an increased cell proliferation within gliomas. Radiolabeled 2-[18F]fluoro-2-deoxy-D-glucose ([18F]FDG), methyl-[11C]-L-methionine ([11C]MET) and 3-deoxy-3-[18F]fluoro-L-thymidine ([18F]FLT) are taken up by proliferating gliomas depending on their tumor grade as the consequence of an increased activity of membrane transporters for glucose ([18F]FDG), amino acids ([11C]MET), and nucleosides ([18F]FLT) as well as increased expression of cellular hexokinase ([18F]FDG) and thymidine kinase ([18F]FLT) genes, which specifically phosphorylate [18F]FDG and [18F]FLT, respectively [20]. Imaging of brain tumors with [18F]FDG was the first oncologic application of PET. [18F]FDG is actively transported across the blood-brain barrier (BBB) into the brain where it is phosphorylated and trapped into cells. Since 1982 [5,21], PET with [18F]FDG has been accepted and widely used in the grading of brain tumors; its uptake is generally high in high-grade tumors and it has a good prognostic value, because increased intra-tumoral glucose consumption correlates with tumor grade [22], biological aggressiveness and survival of patients in both primary and recurrent gliomas. Pathology and survival can be predicted by [18F]FDG-PET in gliomas [6]. In addition, a tumor-to-white matter ratio and tumor-to-gray matter ratio were found to increase the sensitivity of the grading evaluation [22]. Since intra-tumor heterogeneity of brain tumors is not adequately revealed in conventional MRI, because evaluation of the contrast enhancing lesion can either under-or overestimate the presence of active tumor, MRSI and PET are requested to gain additional information on metabolic and molecular tumor markers. In a tumor, the grading can be heterogenous with low-and high-grade areas, as it happens frequently in GBM. This may affect the choice of the site for stereotactic biopsy, which must direct towards tumor sites with the highest tumor grade. Therefore, suitable targets for biopsy will have positive contrast enhancement on T1-weighted MRI, a high choline-peak on MRSI and hypermetabolism on [18F]FDG-PET, the uptake of which is much higher in high-grade component of tumors. As a matter of fact, the [18F]FDG-PET improved the diagnostic yield of stereotactic biopsies by detecting metabolically active areas of tumor [23].

However, [18F]FDG-PET can have some diagnostic limitations, because of the high rate of physiologic glucose metabolism in normal brain tissue. In the brain cortex it is particularly high [24,25], so when a hypermetabolic lesion is close to the cortex or the subcortical white matter, the distinction of the tumor from the normal tissue may be difficult [22]. Moreover, it must be taken into account that [18F]FDG accumulation can be non-specific, because it is also observed in inflammatory or granulation tissues [26]. A later PET image acquisition [27] and a co-registration of PET images with MR images greatly improves the performance of [18F]FDG-PET [28]. Technologic advances have allowed to merge PET and MR images, combining the high resolution of MR imaging with the low-resolution functional capability of PET [23], defined as a reduction of intracellular oxygen pressure (pO2), because of decreased supply and of increased demand for oxygen. It predicts poor treatment response of malignant tumors. Two different forms of tumor hypoxia are recognized. Diffusion-limited chronic hypoxia may develop as a result of increased intercapillary distances, and acute hypoxia can result from occlusion of large tumor vessels [29]. Both forms of hypoxia have several implications for the further evolution of tumors (induction of signaling cascades that promote angiogenesis, growth, and cell migration) [30]. Tumor hypoxia may also lead to necrosis, which is mandatory to establish the diagnosis of GBM. The **([18F]Fluoromisonidazole) ([18F]FMI-**

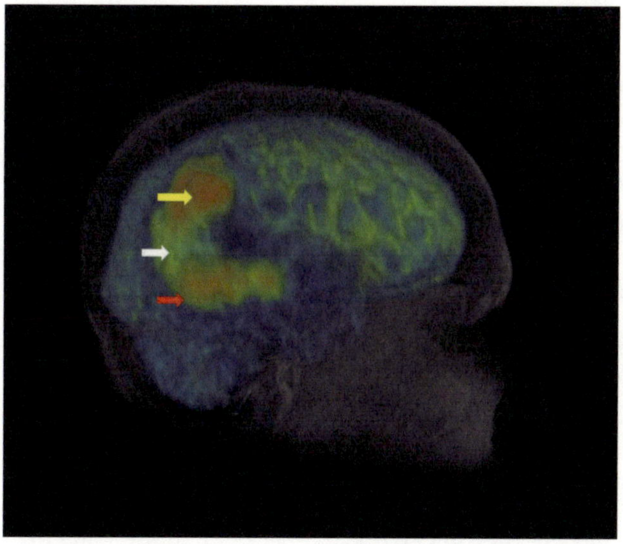

Figure 8. Female 22-year-old affected by GBM. Maximum intensity projection (MIP) fusion PET/3D spgr MRI image showing extensive lesion involving the right parietal-temporal lobe with heterogeneous increased [18F]FDG uptake, due to the lesion heterogeneity: high-grade component presenting elevated [18F]FDG activity with standardized uptake value $(SUV)_{max=}17$ (yellow arrow), intermediate-grade component presenting $SUV_{max}=12$ (white arrow), low-grade component $SUV_{max}=4$ (red arrow).

SO) is a nitroimidazole derivative, a PET agent used for hypoxia detection. [18F]FMISO-PET can image tumor hypoxia by increased [18F]FMISO tumor uptake, because [18F]FMISO metabolites are trapped exclusively in hypoxic cells. It accumulates in both hypo-and hyper-perfused tumor regions, suggesting that hypoxia in GBM may develop irrespective of the magnitude of perfusion [31].

3. Biological significance of MRI variables in GBM

Basically, three conditions can be detected with anatomy-based MRI: iso-hypo-intensity in TC1 (tumor, edema), hyper-intensity in TC2 (edema) and contrast enhancement (malignancy). The contrast enhancing regions (CERs) of untreated GBM correspond to the most histologically malignant areas of the tumor with architectural disruption, high cell density, proliferation, vessel density and angiogenesis with circumscribed necroses. Many other properties are revealed by physiology-based MRI. In CERs, in comparison with non-enhancing regions (NERs), physiologic MRI variables show higher values of rT1C, relative fast spin echo (rFSE), rCBV, relative peak height (rPH) and relative recovery factor (rRF), whereas rADC, relative fractional anisotropy (rFA) and fluid attenuated inversion recovery (rFLAIR) do not differ from NERs. All these observations have been shown and confirmed in recent studies of many cases of GBM planning pre-operatively tissue sampling sites and marking them on the anatomic images used by the surgical navigation work station. A comparison between MRI variables and histology of the samples corresponding to the MRI regions of interest (ROIs) in

CERs and NERs has been made [32,33]. A correlation of histopathologic features and DWI and DSC variables prevailed in enhancing areas and rCBV and Cho/NAA index (CNI) above and rADC below a certain value could indicate the occurrence of tumor cells. Neoangiogenesis could be recognized and distinguished from simple endothelial hyperplasia, even though the permeability of the region is limited. Interestingly, also T2 rFSE and rFLAIR hyperintensity areas could show histopathologic features of malignancy. On the whole, it was demonstrated by gene microarray that the genetic expression patterns between CERs and NERs were different, with genes associated with mitosis, angiogenesis and apoptosis clustered in CER surgical samples [32].

The values of MRSI variables such as Cho/Cr and Cho/NAA showed a parallel variation as those of DWI and PWI. In spite of the possibility of a misregistration between biopsy sites and MRI uploaded to the neuronavigation device if a brain shift occurs, GBM histologic features could be usefully identified by physiology-based MRI [33].

Using the same technique, *i.e.* combining physiology-based MRI, MRSI and [18F]FDG-PET imaging with neuronavigation work station in a series of gliomas, mainly GBMs, we observed that the values of rCBV, ADC, Cho/Cr, CNI were useful for recognizing tumor areas and their phenotypic variations, as for both the number of cells and vascular pathologic structures (Figures 6,7). A possible source of error was the mismatch between the MRI registration and the sampling by the navigator, so that a dissociation between the variable values of the ROIs and histopathology occurred. For example, a ROI on central necrosis could erroneously correspond to a high rCBV value and histologically to the occurrence of tumor tissue in the sample. However, this was a rare event and it did not prevent from recognizing the biological significance of the imaging values contained in the ROIs, also by extrapolation among all the samples.

Malignant gliomas are hypermetabolic in comparison with normal brain. The glycolytic metabolism is increased as well as protein and membrane synthesis to maintain the rapidly dividing tumor cells. MRSI in spite of an intra-or inter-subject variability can identify the tumor. There are two patterns clearly distinct: one is that corresponding to the ROIs on necrotic regions and the other that on the enhancing ring. In the first one, two patterns have been in turn described: "necrosis" and "cystic necrosis" with variable Ch and high LL peak and with no peaks and variable LL, respectively. The ROIs on the ring show a high Cho and Cho/NAA ratio, whereas very variable are those on regions around the ring [34]. In our series Cho, Cho/Cr and Cho/NAA values were constantly high in CERs in comparison with NERs.

Fusing MRI and [11C]MET-PET it was shown that the volume of the radio-compound uptake is greater than that of gadolinium enhancement on T1, even though smaller than T2 volume; it extends beyond in most cases [35,36] correlating with the proliferation markers [37,38], increased Cho/NAA and DTI abnormalities in the white matter [28,39]. However, there could be an underestimation of the tumor extension, because infiltrating cells do not proliferate [3,40].

The number of genetic alterations decreased from the most malignant areas of the tumor to the peripheral areas, correlating fairly well with the MRI variable values and indicating the occurrence or not of tumor cells. In particular, Epidermal Growth Factor Receptor (EGFR) amplification, the occurrence of EGFRvIII and Tumor Protein p53 (TP53) mutations were more frequent in CERs than in NERs, corresponding to a malignant histology. The genetic variability in the different samples was interpreted as due to polyclonality and not only to a genetic heterogeneity supported by the occurrence in the same tumor of different non-tumor cells of various species. Polyclonality means cell complexity, formed by tumor cells that differ among themselves for a series of phenotypic and molecular characteristics of cell proliferation, invasion, *etc.* [41,42]. This observation can be a warning against the use of small tumor samples to characterize the genotype of the entire tumor. Heterogeneity has been explained either by the hierarchic model mechanism [43] or by the stochastic mechanism [44] of tumor development. The two models, however, cannot be mutually exclusive, because their cells should derive from a common ancestor [45]. As for EGFR amplification, the possibility that its variation could depend on an asymmetrical distribution during mitoses must be mentioned [46,47], even if it is already included in the clone formation. The neurosphere assay produces neurospheres (NS), characterized by stemness antigens (Figure 9A,C,E), and adherent cells (AC), characterized by differentiation antigens (Figure 9B,D,F).

However, their phenotype is not the same in the different tumor sites, differing for the quota of the two types of antigens. There must be a different capacity of the tumor areas to host or to generate GSCs and this is in line with the concept that a GSCs hierarchy exists for their potential [48-52]. GSCs have been interpreted as the top of a hierarchy of tumor cells for stemness and, therefore, for self-renewing, clonogenicity, *etc.* They occur in tumor niches and are under the control of microenviroments with their intrinsic and extrinsic signaling [53,54]. The niches can be perivascular or perinecrotic [53] and for a series of observations and considerations they must develop in the most malignant sites of the tumor [51,55]. Stemness and differentiation are the opposite poles of a spectrum in which a hierarchy exists of GSCs as for their potential [48-52]. Going from areas of the highest malignancy, such those of CERs, to differentiated ones, the stem-cell potential decreases [55]. In this way the distribution of GCS in GBM could be explained. The NS and AC degree of differentiation or stemness, demonstrated by the relevant antigens, represents an interesting subject of study that has been pursued by us by confocal microscopy (unpublished data).

Confocal microscopy is an advanced technique of optical imaging used to obtain high resolution images [56,57]. In tissue and cells derived from GBM, it is possible to distinguish the emission signal of different markers and to perform study of both co-localization and quantification of the luminous signal related to the protein marker expression. The cellular heterogeneity is a hallmark of GBM. Using differentiation and stemness markers it is possible to identify hypothetical immature or dedifferentiated elements in the whole tumor cell population, as well as in NS or AC by the neurosphere assay. Confocal images of glioma cells by double immunofluorescence allow to distinguish the expression pattern of the markers above mentioned. Their expression levels, related to the intensity of the emitted signal, show variable Nestin and glial fibrillary acidic protein (GFAP) positivity, depending on the tumor site. The method has a paramount importance in the study of the spectrum from stemness to differentiation.

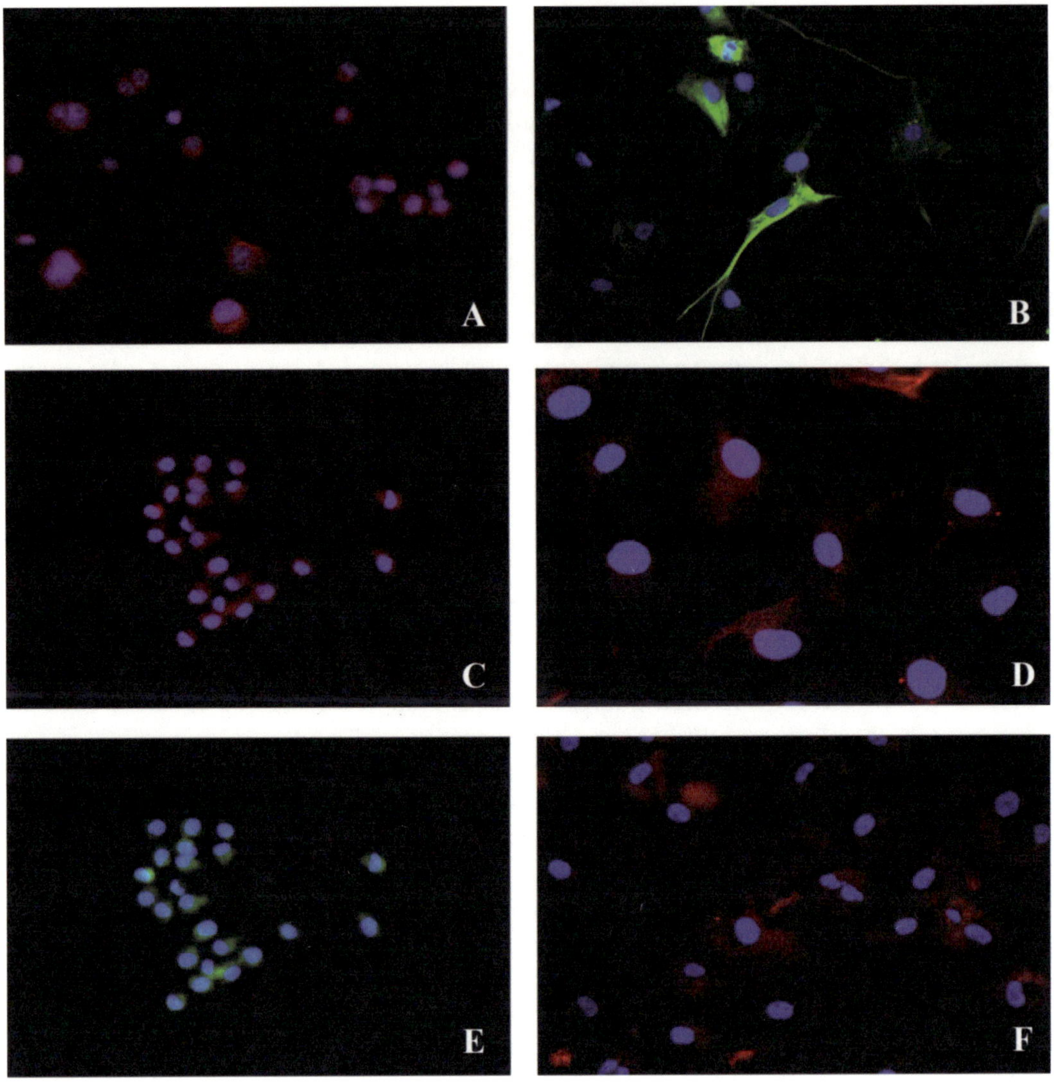

Figure 9. Immunofluorescence (IF) for stemness antigens in NS. A – Nestin, 200x; C – CD133, 200x; E – Musashi1, 200x. IF for differentiation antigens in AC. B – GFAP, 400x; D – GalC, 400x; F – β-III Tubulin, 400x. Nuclei are counterstained with DAPI.

4. The tissue around the tumor — Cell invasion and edema

Beside resistance to chemo-and radiotherapy, the failure of a local control of GBM by therapies is due to the modalities of tumor cell invasion into the brain. Surgical resection cannot prevent recurrence because of the occurrence of infiltrating cells; recurrence usually starts from the resection margin. The target volume for radiotherapy, therefore, conventionally includes the tissue within 2 cm from the MRI border of the tumor. This is for sparing normal nervous tissue from irradiation damage, but also for including in it infiltrating cells. Nevertheless, 80% of tumors relapses within 2-cm margin around the enhanced region [58]; another adverse characteristic of infiltrating cells is that they do not proliferate [3,40], escaping thus detection and being less sensitive to treatments.

Tumor invasion is not uniform along its borders. It can be non-existent where the tumor sharply abuts against the normal nervous tissue (Figure 10A), as it may happen with the white matter, or it gradually progresses from the tumor outwards (Figure 10B). Typical is the invasion of the cortex from a tumor located in the white matter, even with the typical picture of perineuronal satellitosis (Figure 10C). The different invasion modalities have been codified [59] and a distinction between diffuse and local tumors has even been proposed [60], but it was not confirmed by the observation of substantially different outcomes.

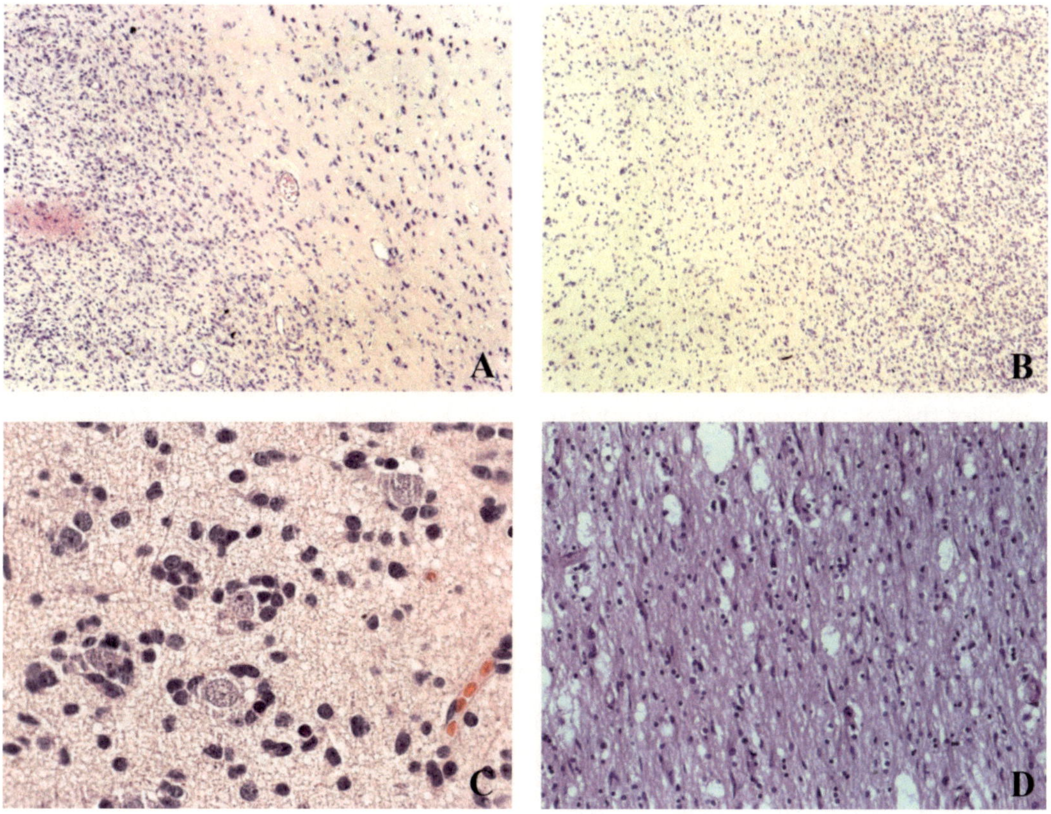

Figure 10. A – Sharp tumor border. Ki-67/MIB.1, DAB, 100x; B – Invasion gradient toward the cortex. H&E, 100x; C – Perineuronal satellitosis. H&E, 400x; D – Infiltration along corpus callosum. H&E, 200x.

Letting aside the mechanisms of tumor cell migration and invasion of which there is today a good knowledge [61-63], some information about neuropathologic findings on peritumor tissue are relevant. First of all, it has been demonstrated that patients with absence of tumor cells in the adjacent normal nervous tissue had better survival than those with tumor cells [64]. This is not in contrast with the observation that the removal of edematous peritumor tissue does not improve the outcome of operated patients [65]. In this regard, residual cells after surgery have been interpretated as distinct from the cells found in routinely resected GBM tissue, as if they would represent a distinct, malignant GBM subentity [66]. A second important point is how to recognize invading cells. Beside nuclear abnormalities, there are only the counts of cells, as will be said. Nestin expression [67] and mainly Isocitrate Dehydrogenase isoforms 1 and 2 (IDH1/2) mutations [68] have been proposed, but it must be taken into account that primary GBM cells are IDH1/2 wild-type.

Cell infiltration, as it is usually seen in histological sections of tumor surgically removed, can be very mild and not easily recognizable without cell counts or decidedly evident (Figure 11A,B). Its aspects largely depend on the various modalities of GBM spreading and three main possibilities are recognized [69]: the distant spreading through corpus callosum (Figure 10D), septum pellucidum, *etc.*, the sub-pial invasion (Figure 11C) and the invasion of the cortex from the white matter where the tumor is located (Figures 11C). Also sub-arachnoidal seeding is frequent [70,71], sometimes as small clusters of tumor cells, visible at naked eyes from which tumor cells go down along penetrating vessels to invade the cortex (Figure 11D). It is very important to remark that invading cells do not proliferate, as it has been demonstrated *in vitro* [72,73] and *in vivo* [3,41,74]. Two other cell types can be found in peritumor tissue: macrophages/microglia and reactive astrocytes, both in edematous and non-edematous tissue. The former, independently of their influence on immunoregulation and tumor growth [61], are abundant in both tumor and peritumor tissue [75]; it has been calculated that up to one third of cells in glioma biopsies are represented by macrophages [75,76] (Figure 12B,C). Incidentally, a positive or negative relationship between microglia/macrophages and TICs is today discussed [77]. The same can be said for the possibility that microglia can be exploited in tumor therapy. It remains today "in its infancy" [78] as it happens for the possibility to inhibit microglia/macrophages in order to prevent their promotion of tumor progression [79].

Reactive astrocytes can be sometimes confused with tumor cells, mainly because their phenotype changes over time until complete maturation (Figure 12A). There are analogies between glial reaction and physiological maturation of astrocytes during embryogenesis. In initial phases, the fine processes originate directly from the cell soma and then from the thick and long processes [80]. Nestin and Vimentin would be the main intermediate filaments of immature astrocytes, whereas GFAP of the mature ones [81,82].

It is long debated whether infiltrated tissue can be recognized by MRI, not only when adjacent to tumor, but also at a distance. It has been observed, for example, that low-grade gliomas, which preferentially locate in the insula and the supplementary motor area, spread along distinct sub-cortical fasciculi [83]. Analyzing different peritumor areas with different MRI methods, it has been shown that FA and not apparent diffusion coefficient can be used to evaluate glioma cell invasion. An attempt to classify different peritumoral tissues by a voxel-wise analytical solution using serial diffusion MRI has been made [84].

Peritumoral reactive gliosis has a particular importance because of three main characteristics: reactive astrocytes divide by mitosis as tumor cells; they progressively lose Nestin and they increase GFAP expression as during development, and they may exert regionally a series of metabolic and molecular influences [61]. The most important point is that reactive astrocytes

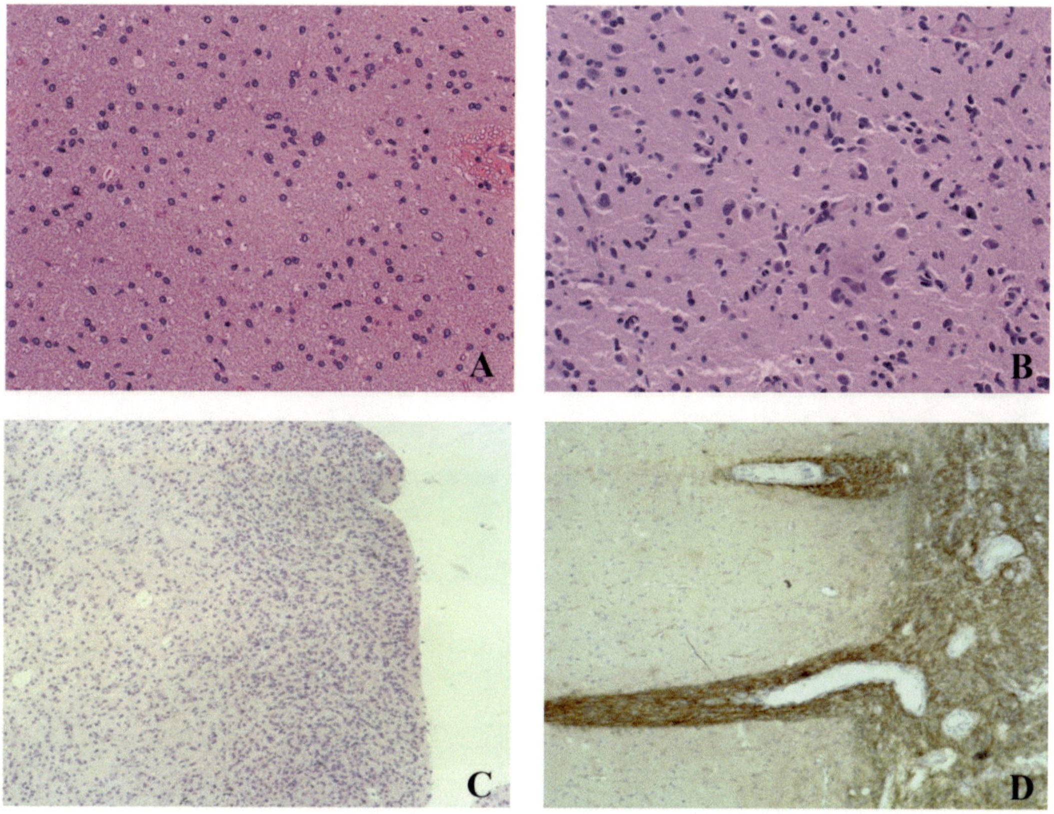

Figure 11. A – Mild infiltration. H&E, 200x; B – Strong infiltration. H&E, 200x; C – Sub-pial infiltration and growth. H&E, 100x; D – Infiltration along penetrating vessels from a tumor seeding in sub-arachnoidal space. PCNA, DAB, 100x.

may be included in the advancing tumor in which they progressively become no more recognizable from tumor cells. The question is whether they disappear suffocated by the high density of tumor cells or if they remain, unrecognizable from tumor cells, contributing to the pleomorphic aspect of gliomas, or if they are transformed into tumor cells [85].

Practically, two important points are that the tumor extends beyond the area of enhancement and that tumor cells can be found in peritumor edema [86]. In 20% of stereotactic biopsies tumor cells have been found in normal areas [87]. With the MRI era, detection of tumor infiltrating cells did not improve and it was shown that they can occur either in the T2-hyperintense areas or beyond them [88] or even in areas apparently normal in T1 or edematous in T2.

GBM spreads frequently along white matter tracts and their disruption can be detected by DTI. Observations have been made, but without any histological control. For example, infiltrated white matter shows a decrease of FA and an increase of ADC as when it is edematous. Displacement of white matter tracts with decreased FA can be recognized [89]. Many studies have been dedicated to FA reduction, but it did not appear to be sensitive enough to detect infiltration [90]. The problem has not yet been resolved and it is still under discussion, because new techniques have been proposed [91,92], even though ADC values, lower in the tumor than in peritumor tissue, were not interpreted by others as significant [93]. Nevertheless, DTI is going to be accepted in the evaluation of tumor margins and invasiveness [94].

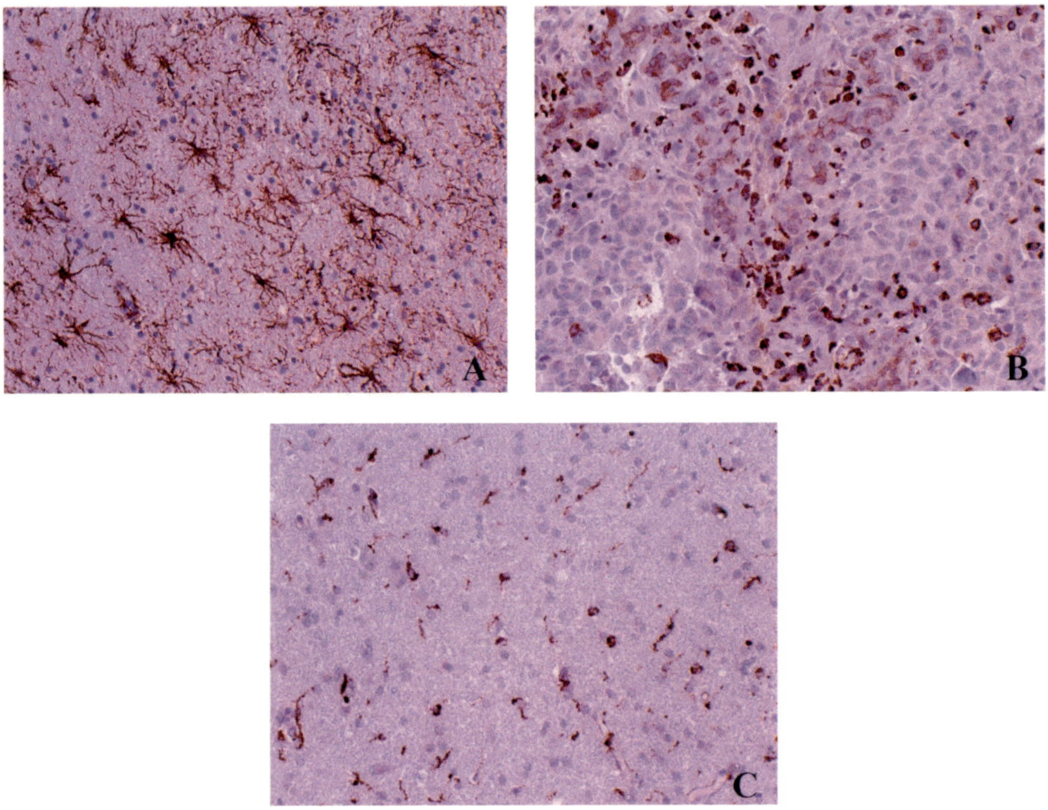

Figure 12. A – Reactive astrocytes at regular inter-distance. GFAP; B – Macrophages/microglia in the tumor. CD68; C – *id.* in peritumor area. CD68. All DAB, 200x.

Edema on T2-weighted imaging may have a high Cho/NAA ratio as in tumors [95] and this would indicate the occurrence of tumor cell infiltration [96] (Figure 13). It can be demonstrated by Aquaporin-4 antibody method (Figure 14A), but in the tissue this is not suitable for quantitative assessments. However, the real problem is how to detect mild infiltration, either alone or with edema. Some observations were supported by histological examination of peritumor edematous areas with or without cell infiltration. Three spectral patterns in peri-enhancing apparently edematous ROIs have been described: high Cho and abnormal Cho/NAA ratio in presumed tumor areas, normal Cho/NAA ratio in presumed edematous areas and Cho levels similar to normal, but with abnormal Cho/NAA ratio in tumor edema. In ROIs on peri-enhancing normal tissue, the patterns therefore could be: presumed infiltration with high Cho and abnormal Cho/NAA ratio and presumed normality with normal values.

These findings are in agreement with those indicating that tumor cells could be detected beyond the margin of the tumor by MRSI [97] and this has been substantiated by histopathology studies [88,96].

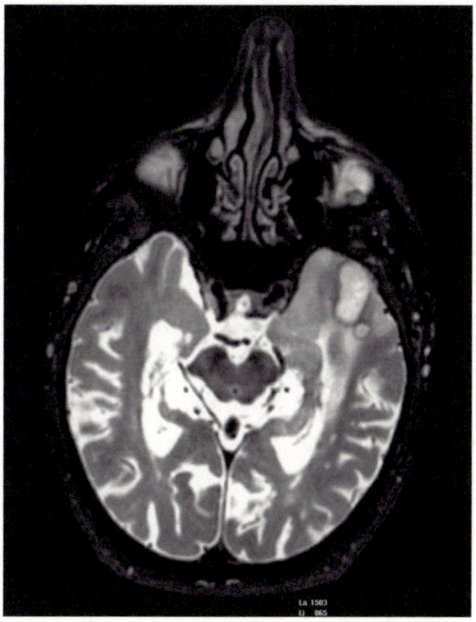

Figure 13. Axial contrast enhanced T1-weighted image, T2-weighted image, ADC and rCBV maps showing a lesion in the left frontal lobe with heterogeneous signal and diffusion properties, peripheral and irregular contrast enhancement. Perfusion is increased in the peripheral portion of the lesion.

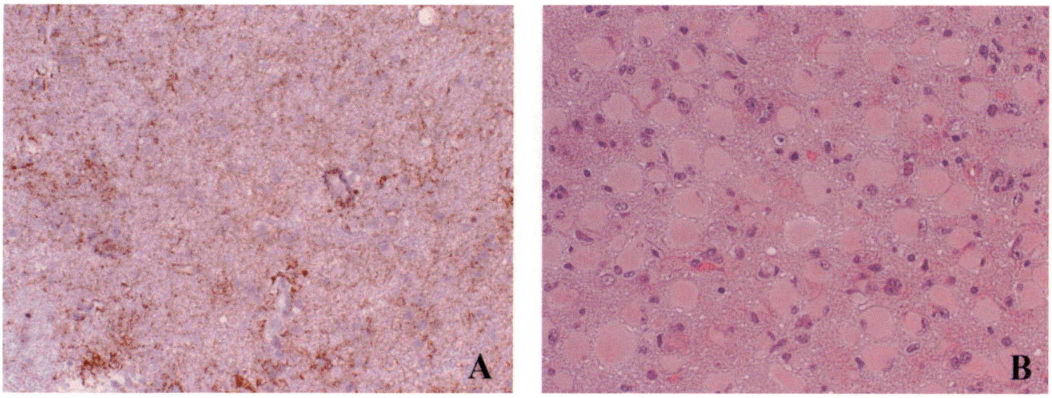

Figure 14. A – Aquaporin-4 in a peritumor area with astrocyte and vessel positive staining. DAB, 200x; B – Aspect of a gemistocytic astrocytoma found in a T2 hyper-intense area. H&E, 200x.

The overlapping of tumor cell infiltration and edema remains a major problem in the brain adjacent to tumor (BAT), because of the difficulty of their distinction [98,99], even though somebody supports that white matter fibre tract infiltration can be recognized [97]. In experimental tumors transplanted into mice, it has been observed by superimposing immunohistochemistry to MRI that in edema districts around the tumor, reactive astrocytes and activated microglia increased Aquaporin-4 expression and invasive tumor cells coexist [100]. Aquaporin-4 has been observed to correlate in peritumor tissue with edema and in the tumor with Hypoxia-Inducible Factor-1 (HIF-1), Vascular Endothelial Growth Factor (VEGF) and the grade of malignancy [101], whereas NAA seemed to be more suitable to detect low tumor infiltration in peritumor edema [102]. Of course, in the latter a damage to myelin sheaths takes place and it is detectable by MRSI [103].

In the recognition of tumor cell infiltration in edematous areas by MRI, histological examination of the surgical samples corresponding to the ROIs on rFSE or rFLAIR areas, is of great importance, in spite of the demonstration that removing T2 hyperintense non-enhancing areas and areas possibly containing ITCs, survival did not change [65]. It must be known that a T2 hyper-intense area may well correspond to a tumor (Figure 14B). A distinction would be possible, provided that there is no mismatch between the ROIs and sample removal. Usually, the cells composing edematous areas can be: tumor, normal or endothelial cells, macrophages or inflammatory cells and mainly reactive astrocytes. In our experience, the cell count is of paramount importance, especially when the number of non-tumor cells largely exceeds that of tumor cells, including in the former reactive astrocytes, microglia and endothelial cells. By comparing the number of cells in H&E stained sections and of GFAP+and CD68+cells with MRI variables, it has been found that normal cells, reactive astrocytes and microglia cells represent a rather stable quota of cells, so that variations of the total number of cells of a given area could be attributed to tumor cells. Reactive astrocytes, once no more proliferating, become fibrillogenetic and mature; usually, they do not exceed a certain number *per* field (Figure 12A). Therefore, they may influence the total number of cells only when tumor cell infiltration is mild. When the number of infiltrating cells is high, the astrocytic quota becomes insignificant. The same can be said for microglia/macrophages. Inside the tumor these cells are often found in perivascular or perinecrotic masses, but in peritumor tissue they are more regularly distributed and they too do not exceed a certain number *per* field (Figure 12B,C). CBV or Cho/NAA values will be influenced by macrophages/microglia only when the total number of cells is very low, *i.e.* when tumor cell infiltration will be really mild, below a certain percentage of the total number of cells, taking into account that the number of reactive astrocytes plus that of microglia/macrophages usually corresponds to the half of that of normal cells (unpublished data).

ITCs can be detected only after a systemic study of the brain at autopsy, as in the whole mounting preparation technique (Figure 15); they cannot be detected in surgical material because this usually cannot include them [4]. ITCs remain as a sword of Damocles in regard to tumor recurrence.

http://dx.doi.org/10.5772/58391

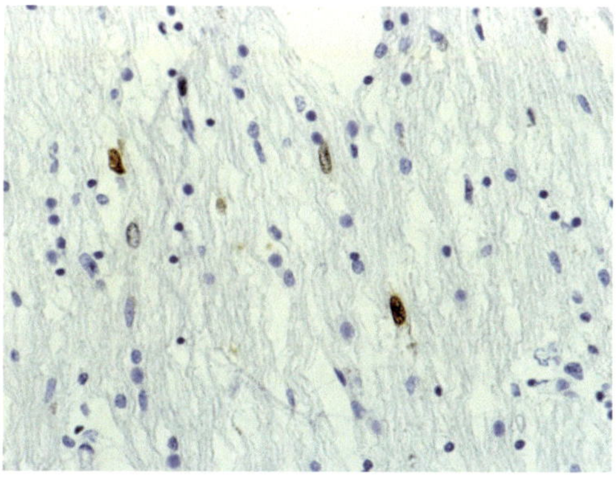

Figure 15. Isolate tumor cells in a white matter bundle. PCNA, DAB, 400x.

5. GSCs in the tumor: Target of therapies?

In the last decades, the aphorism is that the eradication of the tumor cannot be obtained by directing chemo-and radiotherapies to the entire tumor mass, composed of non-proliferating, differentiated and insensitive cells; on the contrary, such therapies would be successful if addressed to the cells responsible for growth, recurrence and resistance, *i.e.* GSCs. Therefore, the question is whether these cells can be *in vivo* detected by neuro-imaging and where are they located or generated in the tumor. To answer this question, a short discussion on the origin and nature of GSCs is necessary.

The hypothesis of GSCs is based on the concept that a rare subset of cells within GBM may have significant expansion capacity and the ability to generate new tumors. The remainder of tumor cells, which predominantly make up GBM, may represent partially differentiated cells with limited progenitor capacity or terminally differentiated cells that cannot form new tumors. Following the model of glioma origin from sub-ventricular zone (SVZ) after nitrosourea derivatives [104], the most important hypothesis on gliomagenesis is today that GSCs derive by the transformation of Normal Stem Cells (NSCs) or progenitors, *i.e.* from B or C cells of the SVZ niche [105]. There is a great similarity between SVZ NSCs or progenitors and TICs and malignant gliomas most probably originate from the SVZ [106,107]. The concept is supported by the observation that GBM is almost always in contact with lateral ventricles [108]. This hypothesis cannot be applied to benign gliomas that should derive from mature glia. According to other hypotheses, also GBMs could derive from mature glial cells by acquiring stemness properties through a dedifferentiation process [109] or from stem cells of the white matter, NG2 cells. This origin would fit better with tumors far from the ventricles or with secondary GBM [110]. Also reactive astrocytes can be candidate for glioma origin [111,112], considering that they can acquire a stem-like phenotype [113].

GSCs develop in niches that can be perivascular or perinecrotic [114]. In perivascular niches there is a close contact between endothelial cells and Nestin+and CD133+cells [115]; the former would favor the self-renewal of the latter, mainly by Notch, and the opposite would happen for angiogenesis through VEGF and hypoxia/HIF-1 [115-120]. In perinecrotic niches, GSCs are generated by hypoxia through HIF-1. Really, in the niches there can be a complicated relationship among different cell types, such as macrophages, pericytes, astrocytes, *etc.* with a multiple signalling [54,121,122]. In our experience, perinecrotic GSCs could be the remnants of GSCs that populated hyper-proliferating areas before the development of circumscribed necroses within them; this would take place because of the imbalance between the high proliferation capacity of tumor cells and the low one of endothelial cells [2,123]. GSCs, either as NS or AC, are heterogeneous as for stemness properties, clonogenicity and tumorigenicity and they have been regarded as at the top of a cell hierarchy for some molecular signs [49,50]. Stemness among tumor cells could be distributed in a spectrum with a *crescendo* from quiescent highly differentiated cells, where it is nil, to those in which it reaches the highest degree of expression. Stemness would be regulated by the microenvironment [53] and it could be the feature of a functional status rather than of a subset of cells [124,125]. As it is lost during differentiation of normal cytogenesis beyond the stage of progenitors, in the opposite way it is gained by dedifferentiating tumor cells when they reach the stage of progenitors.

The heterogeneity of GBM, before discussed, conditions different genetic assets of the cells in the different clones; going from the samples of the most malignant areas of the tumor to those of tumor periphery, the potential of generating NS or AC decreases. The conclusion is that stem cells are kept as such by microenvironments and these are realized in the most malignant sites of the tumor [51,55].

6. Location of GSCs in the tumor and their detection by neuro-imaging

If GSCs were considered as a subset of special cells, they should be located somewhere in the tumor and therefore their search *in vivo* could be justified. According to the hypothesis that they represent a functional status, they should appear in the tumor when and where, as the consequence of the transformation process, tumor cells reach the threshold of stemness. In some experience, NS would be generated from whatever part of GBM [126], whereas in some other experiences [48], different subsets of GSCs arise from regions of GBM with different malignancy potential, showing different tumorigenic potential and genetic abnormalities, even though originating from the same ancestor cell. Since GSCs reside in niches, their distribution in the tumor should follow that of niches which in turn with their microenvironments develop where malignancy occurs [52]. On the other hand, it has been observed that GSCs occur in the hypoxic area between the central necrosis and the proliferating zone of GBM [127].

Until today, the only mean to detect GSCs is to apply the neurosphere assay to the surgical samples removed from different parts of the tumor. Their recognition can be therefore achieved only after surgery. It would be highly useful to know in advance where in tumor GSCs are located or generated in order to try to annihilate them without surgery and to cure the patient. Can they be detected by MRI or other procedures *in vivo*?

Animal *in vivo* imaging techniques have been applied to some stem cell populations – hematopoietic and leukemic stem cells – but the application to solid tissues has been limited [41].

Using intravital microscopy, labelled GSCs could be followed in their propagation and responsibility in producing glioma heterogeneity [41], but data are not available by MRI techniques. Bone marrow-derived endothelial precursors, labelled by super-paramagnetic iron oxide nanoparticles, could be demonstrated in glioma-bearing immunodeficient SCID mice by MRI [128], but no similar procedure has been adopted for GSCs. The only possibility is to use the spatial relationship between MRI variables and tumor phenotypes [33] including into the phenotype the expression of GSC stemness status.

Acknowledgements

This work was supported by Grant n. 4011 SD/cv 2011-0438 from Compagnia di San Paolo, Turin, Italy.

Author details

Davide Schiffer[1], Consuelo Valentini[2], Antonio Melcarne[3], Marta Mellai[1], Elena Prodi[2], Giovanna Carrara[2], Tetyana Denysenko[1,3], Carola Junemann[3], Cristina Casalone[4], Cristiano Corona[4], Valentina Caldera[1], Laura Annovazzi[1], Angela Piazzi[1], Paola Cassoni[5], Rebecca Senetta[5], Piercarlo Fania[6] and Angelina Cistaro[6,7]

1 Neuro-bio-oncology Center of Policlinico di Monza Foundation, Vercelli, Italy

2 Neuroradiology Unit, CTO Hospital, Turin, Italy

3 Neurosurgery Unit, CTO Hospital, Turin, Italy

4 Istituto Zooprofilattico, Turin, Italy

5 Department Medical Sciences, University of Turin, Turin, Italy

6 Positron Emission Tomography Center IRMET S.p.A, Euromedic inc., Turin, Italy

7 Institute of Cognitive Sciences and Technologies, National Research Council, Rome, Italy

References

[1] Coons SW, Johnson PC, Scheithauer BW, Ytes AJ, Pearl DK. Improving diagnostic accuracy and interobserver concordance in the classification and grading of primary gliomas. Cancer 1997; 79(7): 1381-1393.

[2] Schiffer D, Chiò A, Giordana MT, Mauro A, Migheli A, et al. The vascular response to tumor infiltration in malignant gliomas. Morphometric and reconstruction study. Acta Neuropathologica 1989; 77(4): 369-378.

[3] Schiffer D. Brain tumors: biology, pathology and clinical references. Berlin, Heidelberg, New York: Springer; 1997.

[4] Schiffer D. Brain tumor pathology. Current diagnostic hotspots and pitfalls. Dordrecht: Springer; 2006.

[5] Alavi JB, Alavi A, Chawluk J, Kushner M, Powe J, et al. Positron emission tomography in patients with glioma. A predictor of prognosis. Cancer 1988; 62(6): 1074-1078.

[6] Padma MV, Said S, Jacobs M, Hwang DR, Dunigan K, et al. Prediction of pathology and survival by FDG PET in gliomas. Journal of Neuro-Oncology 2003: 64(3): 227-237.

[7] Kitis O, Altay H, Calli C, Yunten N, Akalin T, et al. Minimum apparent diffusion coefficients in the evaluation of brain tumors. European Journal of Radiology 2005; 55(3): 393-400.

[8] Murakami R, Hirai T, Sugahara T, Fukuoka H, Toya R, at al. Grading astrocytic tumors by using apparent diffusion coefficient parameters: superiority of a one-versus two-parameter pilot method. Radiology 2009; 251(3): 838-845.

[9] Kang Y, Choi SH, Kim YJ, Kim KG, Sohn CH, et al. Gliomas: histogram analysis of apparent diffusion coefficient maps with standard-or high-b-value diffusion-weighted MR imaging-correlation with tumor grade. Radiology 2011; 261(3): 882-890.

[10] Castillo M, Smith JK, Kwock L, Wilber K. Apparent diffusion coefficients in the evaluation of high-grade cerebral gliomas. AJNR American Journal of Neuroradiology 2001; 22(1): 60-64.

[11] Cha S. Update on brain tumor imaging: from anatomy to physiology. American Journal of Neuroradiology 2006; 27(3): 475-487.

[12] Law M, Cha S, Knopp EA, Johnson G, Arnett J, et al. High-grade gliomas and solitary metastases: differentiation by using perfusion and proton spectroscopic MR imaging. Radiology 2002; 222(3): 715-721.

[13] Yang S, Zhang C, Zhu T, Cai L, Gao S, et al. Resection of gliomas using positron emission tomography/computer tomography neuronavigation. Neurologia Medico-Chirurgica (Tokyo) 2007; 47(9): 397-401.

[14] Howe FA, Barton SJ, Cudlip SA, Stubbs M, Saunders DE, et al. Metabolic profiles of human brain tumors using quantitative in vivo 1H magnetic resonance spectroscopy. Magnetic Resonance in Medicine 2003; 49(2): 223-232.

[15] Al-Okaili RN, Krejza J, Wang S, Woo JH, Melhem ER. Advanced MR imaging techniques in the diagnosis of intraaxial brain tumors in adults. Radiographics 2006; 26(Suppl 1): S173-189.

[16] Jellison BJ, Field AS, Medow J, Lazar M, Salamat MS, et al. Diffusion tensor imaging of cerebral white matter: a pictorial review of physics, fiber tract anatomy, and tumor imaging patterns. American Journal of Neuroradiology 2004; 25(3): 356-369.

[17] Lu S, Ahn D, Johnson G, Law M, Zagzag D, et al. Diffusion-tensor MR imaging of intracranial neoplasia and associated peritumoral edema: introduction of the tumor infiltration index. Radiology 2004; 232(1): 221-228.

[18] White ML, Zhang Y, Yub F, Jaffar Kazmi SA. Diffusion tensor MR imaging of cerebral gliomas: evaluating fractional anisotropy characteristics. American Journal of Neuroradiology 2011; 32(2): 374-381.

[19] Shuyuan Y, Chuan Z, Shuyuan Y, Li C, Shuo G, et al. Preoperative estimation and resection of gliomas using positron emission tomography/computed tomography neuronavigation. In: Garami M. (ed.) Management of CNS tumors. Rijeka: InTech; 2012. p179-196.

[20] Jacobs AH, Kracht LW, Gossmann A, Rüger MA, Thomas AV, et al. Imaging in neurooncology. The Journal of the American Society of Experimental NeuroTherapeutics 2005; 2(2): 333-347.

[21] Di Chiro G, DeLaPaz RL, Brooks RA, Sokoloff L, Kornblith PL, et al. Glucose utilization of cerebral gliomas measured by [18F] fluorodeoxyglucose and positron emission tomography. Neurology 1982; 32(12): 1323-1329.

[22] Delbeke D, Meyerowitz C, Lapidus RL, Maciunas RJ, Jennings MT, et al. Optimal cutoff levels of F-18 fluorodeoxyglucose uptake in the differentiation of low-grade from high-grade brain tumors with PET. Radiology 1995; 195(1): 47-52.

[23] Stanescu L, Ishak GE, Khanna PC, Biyyam DR, Shaw DW, et al. FDG PET of the brain in pediatric patients: imaging spectrum with MR imaging correlation. Radiographics 2013; 33(5): 1279-1303.

[24] Bénard F, Romsa J, Hustinx R. Imaging gliomas with positron emission tomography and single-photon emission computed tomography. Seminars in Nuclear Medicine 2003; 33(2): 148-162.

[25] Chen W. Clinical applications of PET in brain tumors. Journal of Nuclear Medicine 2007; 48(9): 1468-1481.

[26] Kato T, Shinoda J, Oka N, Miwa K, Nakayama N, et al. Analysis of 11C-methionine uptake on low-grade gliomas and correlation with proliferative activity. American Journal of Neuroradiology 2008; 29(10): 1867-1871.

[27] Cistaro A. Atlas of PET/CT in pediatric patients. Dordrecht: Springer; 2013.

[28] Stadlbauer A, Prante O, Nimsky C, Salomonowitz E, Buchfelder M, et al. Metabolic imaging of cerebral gliomas: spatial correlation of changes in O-(2-18F-fluoroethyl)-L-tyrosine PET and proton magnetic resonance spectroscopic imaging. Journal of Nuclear Medicine 2008; 49(5): 721-729.

[29] Airley RE, Monaghan JE, Jane N. Hypoxia and disease: opportunities for novel diagnostic and therapeutic prodrug strategies. Pharmaceutical Journal 2000; 264(7094): 666-673.

[30] Bernsen HJ, Rijken PF, Peters H, Raleigh JA, Jeuken JW, et al. Hypoxia in a human intracerebral glioma model. Journal of Neurosurgery 2000; 93(3): 449-454.

[31] Bruehlmeier M, Roelcke U, Schubiger PA, Ametamey SM. Assessment of hypoxia and perfusion in human brain tumors using PET with 18F-fluoromisonidazole and 15O-H2O. Journal of Nuclear Medicine 2004; 45(11): 1851-1859.

[32] Barajas RF Jr, Hodgson JG, Chang JS, Vandenberg SR, Yeh RF, et al. Glioblastoma multiforme regional genetic and cellular expression patterns: influence on anatomic and physiologic MR imaging. Radiology 2010; 254(2): 564-576.

[33] Barajas RF Jr, Phillips JJ, Parvataneni R, Molinaro A, Essock-Burns E, et al. Regional variation in histopathologic features of tumor specimens from treatment-naive glioblastoma correlates with anatomic and physiologic MR Imaging. Journal of Neuro-Oncology 2012; 14(7): 942-954.

[34] Di Costanzo A, Scarabino T, Troisi F, Popolizio T, Catapano D, et al. Proton MR spectroscopy of cerebral gliomas at 3 T: spatial heterogeneity, and tumour grade and extent. European Radiology 2008; 18(8): 1727-1735.

[35] Miwa K, Shinoda J, Yano H, Okumura A, Iwama T, et al. Discrepancy between lesion distribution on methionine PET and MR images in patients with glioblastoma multiforme: insight from a PET and MR fusion image study. Journal of Neurology, Neurosurgery and Psychiatry 2004; 75(10): 1457-1462.

[36] Jacobs AH, Thomas A, Kracht LW, Li H, Dittmar C, et al. 18F-fluoro-L-thymidine and 11C-methylmethionine as markers of increased transport and proliferation in brain tumors. Journal of Nuclear Medicine 2005; 46(12): 1948-1958.

[37] Chen W, Cloughesy T, Kamdar N, Satyamurthy N, Bergsneider M, et al. Imaging proliferation in brain tumors with 18F-FELT PET: comparison with 18F-FDG. Journal of Nuclear Medicine 2005; 46(6): 945-952.

[38] Price SJ, Fryer TD, Cleij MC, Dean AF, Joseph J, et al. Imaging regional variation of cellular proliferation in gliomas using 3'-deoxy-3'-[18F]fluorothymidine positron emission tomography: an image-guided biopsy study. Clinical Radiology 2008; 64(1): 52-63.

[39] Stadlbauer A, Pölking E, Prante O, Nimsky C, Buchfelder M, et al. Detection of tumour invasion into the pyramidal tract in glioma patients with sensorimotor deficits

by correlation of (18)F-fluoroethyl-L-tyrosine PET and magnetic resonance diffusion tensor imaging. Acta Neurochirurgica (Wien) 2009; 151(9): 1061-1069.

[40] Giese A, Loo MA, Tran N, Haskett D, Coons SW, et al. Dichotomy of astrocytoma migration and proliferation. International Journal of Cancer 1996; 67(2): 275-282.

[41] Lathia JD, Gallagher J, Myers JT, Li M, Vasanji A, et al. Direct in vivo evidence for tumor propagation by glioblastoma cancer stem cells. Public Library of Science One 2011; 6(9): e24807.

[42] Mazzoleni S, Galli R. Gliomagenesis: a game played by few players or a team effects? Frontiers in Neuroscience 2012; 4(1): 205-213.

[43] Reya T, Morrison SJ, Clarke MF, Weissman IL. Stem cells, cancer, and cancer stem cells. Nature 2001; 414(6859): 105-108.

[44] Adams JM, Strasser A. Is tumor growth sustained by rare cancer stem cells or dominant clones? Cancer Res 2008; 68(11): 4018-4021.

[45] de Almeida Sassi F, Lunardi Brunetto A, Schwartsmann G, Roesler R, Abujamra AL. Glioma revisited: from neurogenesis and cancer stem cells to the epigenetic regulation of the niche. Journal of Oncology 2012; 2012: 537861.

[46] Sun Y, Goderie SK, Temple S. Asymmetric distribution of EGFR receptor during mitosis generates diverse CNS progenitor cells. Neuron 2005; 45(6): 873-886.

[47] De Bacco F, Casanova E, Medico E, Pellegatta S, Orzan F, et al. The MET oncogene is a functional marker of a glioblastoma stem cell subtype. Cancer Research 2012; 72(17): 4537-4550.

[48] Piccirillo SG, Combi R, Cajola L, Patrizi A, Redaelli S, et al. Distinct pools of cancer stem-like cells coexist within human glioblastomas and display different tumorigenicity and independent genomic evolution. Oncogene 2009; 28(15): 1807-1811.

[49] Chen R, Nishimura MC, Bumbaca SM, Kharbanda S, Forrest WF, et al. A hierarchy of self-renewing tumor-initiating cell types in glioblastoma. Cancer Cell 2010; 17(4): 362-375.

[50] Mazzoleni S, Politi LS, Pala, M. Cominelli M, Franzin A, et al. Epidermal growth factor receptor expression identifies functionally and molecularly distinct tumor-initiating cells in human glioblastoma multiforme and is required for gliomagenesis. Cancer Research 2010; 70(19): 7500-7513.

[51] Caldera V, Mellai M, Annovazzi L, Piazzi A, Lanotte M, et al. Antigenic and genotypic similarity between primary glioblastomas and their derived neurospheres. Journal of Oncology 2011; 2011: 314962.

[52] Schiffer D, Mellai M, Annovazzi L, Piazzi A, Monzeglio O, et al. Glioblastoma cancer stem cells: basis for a functional hypothesis. Stem Cell Discovery 2012; 2(3): 122-131.

[53] Charles NA, Holland EC, Gilbertson R, Glass R, Kettenmann H. The brain tumor microenvironment. Glia 2012; 60(3): 502-514.

[54] Filatova A, Acker T, Garvalov BK. The cancer stem cell niche(s): the crosstalk between glioma stem cells and their microenvironment. Biochimica et Biophysica Acta 2013; 1830(2): 2496-2508.

[55] Schiffer D, Mellai M, Annovazzi L, Caldera V, Piazzi A, et al. Stem cell niches in glioblastoma. A neuropathological view. Submitted.

[56] Dunn KW, Kamocka MM, McDonald JH. A practical guide to evaluating colocalization in biological microscopy. American Journal of Physiology. Cell Physiology 2011; 300(4): C723-742.

[57] Adler J, Parmryd I. Quantifying colocalization by correlation: the Pearson correlation coefficient is superior to the Mander's overlap coefficient. Cytometry 2010; 77(8): 733-742.

[58] Górska-Chrzastek M, Grzelak P, Bieńkiewicz M, Tybor K, Zakrzewska E, et al. Assessment of clinical usefulness of 131I alpha-methyl-tyrosine and fused SPECT/MRI imaging for diagnostics of recurrent cerebral gliomas. Nuclear Medicine Review. Central & Eastern Europe 2004; 7(2): 135-141.

[59] Burger PC, Heinz ER, Shibata T, Kleihues P. Topographic anatomy and CT correlations in untreated glioblastoma multiforme. Journal of Neurosurgery 1988; 68(5): 698-704.

[60] Shapiro WE. Current therapy for brain tumors: back to the future. Archives of Neurology 1999; 56(4): 429-432.

[61] Schiffer D, Annovazzi L, Caldera V, Mellai M. The brain adjacent to tumor (BAT). In: Garami M. (ed.) Management of CNS tumors. Rijeka, InTech; 2011. p197-224.

[62] Caffo M, Barresi V, Caruso G, La Fata G, Pino MA, et al. Gliomas biology: angiogenesis and invasion. In: Lichtor T. (ed.) Evolution of the molecular biology of brain tumors and the therapeutic implications. Rijeka, InTech; 2013. p37-103.

[63] Province P, Griguer CE, Han X, Louis NB, Shaykh HF. Hypoxia, angiogenesis and mechanisms for invasion of malignant gliomas. In: Lichtor T. (ed.) Evolution of the molecular biology of brain tumors and the therapeutic implications. Rijeka, InTech; 2013. p105-123.

[64] Mangiola A, de Bonis P, Maira G, Balducci M, Sica G, et al. Invasive tumor cells and prognosis in a selected population of patients with glioblastoma multiforme. Cancer 2008; 113(4): 841-846.

[65] Ramakrishna R, Barber J, Kennedy G, Rizvi A, Goodkin R, et al. Imaging features of invasion and preoperative and postoperative tumor burden in previously untreated

glioblastoma: correlation with survival. Surgical Neurology International 2010; 1(1): 40-51.

[66] Glas M, Rath BH, Simon M, Reinartz R, Schramme A, et al. Residual tumor cells are unique cellular targets in glioblastoma. Annals of Neurology 2010; 68(2): 264-269.

[67] Kitai R, Horita R, Sato K, Yoshida K, Arishima H, et al. Nestin expression in astrocytic tumors delineates tumor infiltration. Brain Tumor Pathology 2010; 27(1): 17-21.

[68] Capper D, Weissert S, Balss J, Habel A, Meyer J, et al. Characterization of R132H mutation-specific IDH1 antibody binding in brain tumors. Brain Pathology 2010; 20(1): 245-254.

[69] Schiffer D. Neuropathology and imaging: the ways in which gliomas spreads and varies in its histological aspects, In: Walker and DGT Thomas (ed.) Biology of brain tumors. Boston, Nijhoff: 1986. p286-290.

[70] Nishio S, Korosue K, Tateishi J, Fukui M, Kitamura K. Ventricular and subarachnoid seeding of intracranial tumors of neuroectodermal origin-a study of 26 consecutive autopsy cases with reference to focal ependymal defect. Clinical Neuropathology 1982; 1(2): 83-91.

[71] Rosenblum ML. Factors influencing tumor cell traffic in the central nervous system. Surgical Neurology 1995; 43(6): 595.

[72] Pilkington GJ. Glioma heterogeneity in vitro: the significance of growth factor and gangliosides. Neuropathology and Applied Neurobiology 1992; 18(5): 434-432.

[73] Merzak A, Koochekpour S, Dkhissi F, Raynal S, Lawrence D, et al. Synergism between growth-factors in the control of glioma cell-proliferation, migration and invasion in-vitro. International Journal of Oncology 1995; 6(5): 1079-1085.

[74] Dalrymple SJ, Parisi JE, Roche PC, Ziesmer SC, Scheithauer BW, et al. Changes in proliferating cell nuclear antigen expression in glioblastoma multiforme cells along a stereotactic biopsy trajectory. Neurosurgery 1994; 35(6): 1036-1044.

[75] Roggendorf W, Strupp S, Paulus W. Distribution and characterization of microglia/ macrophages in human brain tumors. Acta Neuropathologica 1996; 92(3): 288-293.

[76] Morimura T, Neuchrist C, Kitz K, Budka H, Scheiner O, et al. Monocyte subpopulations in human gliomas: expression of Fc and complement receptors and correlation with tumor proliferation. Acta Neuropathologica 1990; 80(3): 287-294.

[77] Yi L, Xiao H, Xu M, Ye X, Hu J, et al. Glioma-initiating cells: A predominant role in microglia/macrophages tropism to glioma. Journal of Neuroimmunology 2011; 232(1-2): 75-82.

[78] Graeber MB, Scheithauer BW, Kreutzberg GW. Microglia in brain tumors. Glia 2002; 40(2): 252-259.

[79] Zhai H, Heppner FL, Tsirka SE. Microglia/macrophages promote glioma progression. Glia 2011; 59(3): 472-485.

[80] Bushong EA, Martone ME, Ellisman MH. Maturation of astrocyte morphology and the establishment of astrocyte domains during postnatal hippocampal development. International Journal of Developmental Neuroscience 2004; 22(2): 73-86.

[81] Clarke SR, Shetty AK, Bradley JL, Turner DA. Reactive astrocytes express the embryonic intermediate neurofilament nestin. Neuroreport 1994; 5(15): 1885-1888.

[82] Eliasson C, Sahlgren C, Berthold CH, Stakeberg J, Celis JE, et al. Intermediate filament protein partnership in astrocytes. The Journal Biological Chemistry 1999; 274(34): 23996-24006.

[83] Mandonnet E, Capelle L, Duffau H. Extension of paralimbic low grade gliomas: toward an anatomical classification based on white matter invasion patterns. Journal of Neuro-Oncology 2006; 78(2): 179-185.

[84] Ellingson BM, LaViolette PS, Rand SD, Malkin MG, Connelly JM, Mueller, et al. Spatially quantifying microscopic tumor invasion and proliferation using a voxel-wise solution to a glioma growth model and serial diffusion MRI. Magnetic Resonance in Medicine 2011; 65(4): 1131-1143.

[85] Tamagno I, Schiffer D. Nestin expression in reactive astrocytes of human pathology. J Neuro-Oncology 2006; 80(3): 227-233.

[86] Selker RG, Mendelow H, Walker M, Sheptak PE, Phillips JG. Pathological correlation of CT ring in recurrent previously treated gliomas. Surgical Neurology 1982; 17(4): 251-254.

[87] Kelly PJ, Daumas-Duport C, Kispert DB, Kall BA, Scheithauer BW, et al. Imaging-based stereotaxic serial biopsies in untreated intracranial glial neoplasms. Journal of Neurosurgery 1987; 66(6): 865-874.

[88] Watanabe M, Tanaka R, Takeda N. Magnetic resonance imaging and histopathology of cerebral gliomas. Neuroradiology 1992; 34(6): 463-469.

[89] Witwer BP, Moftakhar R, Hasan KM, Deshmukh P, Haughton V, et al. Diffusion-tensor imaging of white matter tracts in patients with cerebral neoplasm. Journal of Neurosurgery 2002; 97(3): 568-575.

[90] Price SJ, Gillard JH. Imaging biomarkers of brain tumour margin and tumour invasion. The British Journal of Radiology 2011; 84(Spec No 2): S159-167.

[91] Zhou XJ, Leeds NE, Poonawalla AH, Weinberg J. Assessment of tumor cell infiltration along white matter fiber using diffusion tensor imaging. Proceedings of the International Society for Magnetic Resonance in Medicine 2003; 11: 2238.

[92] Price SJ, Peña A, Burnet NG, Pickard JD, Gillard JH. Detecting glioma invasion of the corpus callosum using diffusion tensor imaging. The British Journal of Neurosurgery 2004; 18(4): 391-395.

[93] Pauleit D, Langen KJ, Floeth F, Hautzel H, Riemenschneider MJ, et al. Can the apparent diffusion coefficient be used as a non invasive parameter to distinguish tumor tissue from peritumoral tissue in cerebral gliomas? Journal of Magnetic Resonance Imaging 2004; 20(5): 758-764.

[94] Price SJ, Jena R, Burnet NG, Carpenter TA, Pickard JD, et al. Predicting patterns of glioma recurrence using diffusion tensor imaging. European Radiology 2007; 17(7): 1675-1684.

[95] McKnight TR, von dem Bussche MH, Vigneron DB, Lu Y, Berger MS, et al. Histopathological validation of three-dimensional magnetic resonance spectroscopy index as a prediction of tumor presence. Journal of Neurosurgery 2002; 97(4): 794-802.

[96] Croteau D, Scarpace L, Hearshen D, Gutierrez J, Fisher JL, et al. Correlation between magnetic resonance spectroscopy imaging and image-guided biopsies: semiquantitative and qualitative histopathological analyses of patients with untreated glioma. Neurosurgery 2001; 49(4): 823-829.

[97] Pirzkall A, Li X, Oh J, Chang S, Berger MS, et al. 3D MRSI fro resected high-grade gliomas before RT: tumor extent according to metabolic activity in relation to MRI. International Journal of Radiation Oncology, Biology, Physics 2004; 59(1): 126-137.

[98] Law M, Cha S, Knopp EA, Johnson G, Arnett J, et al. High-grade gliomas and solitary metastases: differentiation by using perfusion and proton spectroscopy MR imaging. Radiology 2002; 222(3): 715-722.

[99] Nelson SJ. Multivoxel magnetic resonance spectroscopy of brain tumors. Molecular Cancer Therapeutics 2003; 2(5): 497-507.

[100] Engelhorn T, Savaskan NE, Schwarz MA, Kreutzer J, Meyer EP, et al. Cellular characterization of the peritumoral edema zone in malignant brain tumors. Cancer Science 2009; 100(10): 1856-1862.

[101] Mou K, Chen M, Mao Q, Wang p, Ni R, et al. APQ-4 in peritumoral edematous tissue is correlated with the degree of glioma and with expression of VEGF and HIF-alpha. Journal of Neuro-Oncology 2010; 100(3): 375-383.

[102] Stadlbauer A, Nimsky C, Buslei R, Pinker K, Gruber S, et al. Proton magnetic resonance spectroscopic imaging in the borderzone of gliomas. Correlation of metabolic and histological changes at low tumor infiltration-initial results. Investigative Radiology 2007; 42(4): 218-223.

[103] Ricci R, Bacci A, Tugnoli V, Battaglia S, Maffei M, et al. Metabolic findings on 3T 1H-MR spectroscopy in peritumoral brain edema. AJNR American Journal of Neuroradiology 2007; 28(7): 1287-1291.

[104] Schiffer D, Annovazzi L, Caldera V, Mellai M. On the origin and growth of gliomas. Anticancer Research 2010; 30(6): 1977-1998.

[105] Holland EC. Progenitor cells and glioma formation. Current Opinion in Neurology 2001; 14(6): 683-688.

[106] Alcantara Llaguno S, Chen J, Kwon CH, Jackson EL, Li Y, et al. Malignant astrocytomas originate from neural stem/progenitor cells in a somatic tumor suppressor mouse model. Cancer Cell 2009; 15(1): 45-56.

[107] Jaques TS, Swales A, Brzozowski MJ, Henriquez MV, Linehan JN, et al. Combinations of genetic mutations in the adult neural stem cell compartment determine brain tumour phenotypes. The EMBO Journal 2010; 29(1): 222-235.

[108] Barami K, Sloan AE, Rojiani A, Schell MJ, Staller A, et al. Relationship of gliomas to the ventricular walls. Journal of Clinical Neuroscience 2009; 16(2): 195-201.

[109] Sanai N, Alvarez-Buylla, Berger MS. Neural stem cells and the origin of gliomas. The New England Journal of Medicine 2005; 353(8): 811-822.

[110] Siebzehnrubl FA, Reynolds BA, Vescovi A, Steindler DA, Deleyrolle LP. The origins of glioma: e pluribus unum? Glia 2011; 59(8): 1135-1147.

[111] Dufour C, Cadusseau J, Varlet P, Surena AL, de Faira GP, et al. Astrocytes reverted to a neural progenitor-like state with transforming growth factor alpha are sensitized to cancerous transformation. Stem Cells 2009; 27(10): 2373-2382.

[112] Silver DJ, Steindler DA. Common astrocytic programs during brain development, injury and cancer. Trends in Neurosciences 2009; 32(6): 303-311.

[113] Buffo A, Rite I, Tripathi P, Lepier A, Colak D, et al. Origin and progeny of reactive gliosis: a source of multipotent cells in the injured brain. Proceedings of the Natural Academy of Sciences USA 2008; 105(9): 3581-3586.

[114] Li L, Neaves WB. Normal stem cells and cancer stem cells: the niche matters. Cancer Research 2006; 66(9): 4553-4557.

[115] Calabrese C, Poppleton H, Kokac M, Hogg TL, Fuller C, et al. A perivascular niche for brain tumor stem cells. Cancer Cell 2007; 11(1): 69-82.

[116] Bao S, Wu S, Sathornsumetee S, Hao Y, Li Z, et al. Stem cell-like glioma cells promote tumor angiogenesis through vascular endothelial growth factor. Cancer Research 2006; 66(16): 7843-7848.

[117] Jensen RL, Ragel BT, Whang K, Gillespie D. Inhibition of hypoxia inducible factor-1 alpha (HIF-1 alpha) decreases vascular endothelial growth factor (VEGF) secretion and tumor growth in malignant gliomas. Journal of Neuro-Oncology 2006; 78(3): 233-247.

[118] Folkins C, Shaked Y, Man S, Tang T, Lee CR, et al. Glioma tumor stem-like cells promote tumor angiogenesis and vasculogenesis via vascular endothelial growth factor and stromal-derived factor 1. Cancer Research 2009; 69(18): 7243-7251.

[119] Bar EE, Lin A, Mahairaki V, Matsui W, Eberhart CG. Hypoxia increases the expression of stem-cell markers and promotes clonogenicity in glioblastoma neurospheres. The American Journal of Pathology 2010; 177(3): 1491-1502.

[120] Charles N, Holland EC. The perivascular niche microenvironment in brain tumor progression. Cell Cycle 2010; 9(15): 3012-3021.

[121] Christensen K, Schrøder HD, Kristensen BW. CD133 identifies perivascular niches in grade II-IV astrocytomas. Journal of Neuro-Oncology 2008; 90(2): 157-170.

[122] Seidel S, Garvalov BK, Wirta V, von Stechow L, Schänzer A, et al. A hypoxic niche regulates glioblastoma stem cells through hypoxia inducible factor 2 alpha. Brain 2010; 133(Pt4): 983-995.

[123] Kargiotis O, Rao JS, Kyritsis AP. Mechanisms of angiogenesis in gliomas. Journal of Neuro-Oncology 2006; 78(3): 281-293.

[124] Zipori D. The nature of stem cells: state rather than entity. Nature Review Genetics 2004; 5(11): 873-878.

[125] Reynolds BA, Vescovi AL. Brain cancer stem cells: think twice before going flat. Cell Stem Cell 2009; 5(5): 466-467.

[126] Pallini R, Ricci-Vitiani L, Banna GL, Signore M, Lombardi D, et al. Cancer stem cell analysis and clinical outcome in patients with glioblastoma multiforme. Clinical Cancer Research 2008; 14(24): 8205-8212.

[127] Persano L, Rampazzo E, Della Puppa A, Pistollato F, Basso G. The three-layer concentric model of glioblastoma: cancer stem cells, microenvironmental regulation, and therapeutic implications. TheScientificWorldJournal 2011; 11: 1829-1841.

[128] Anderson S, Glod J, Arbab AS, Noel M, Ashari P, et al. Noninvasive MR imaging of magnetically labelled stem cells in directly identify neovasculature in a glioma model. Blood 2005; 105(1): 420-425.

Chapter 4

New Application of ^{123}I-Iodoamphetamine SPECT for the Diagnosis of Primary Central Nervous System Lymphoma

Yasushi Shibata

Additional information is available at the end of the chapter

http://dx.doi.org/10.5772/58321

1. Introduction

^{123}I-iodoamphetamine (IMP) single photon emission computed tomography (SPECT) is used to evaluate the cerebral blood flow (CBF) in patients with either cerebrovascular or neurodegenerative diseases [3, 6]. However, its application for patients with brain tumors has so far only been rarely reported [2, 8, 11]. Primary central nervous system lymphoma (PCNSL) is a rare tumor that shows a delayed IMP uptake [1, 5, 7, 9, 10]. The relatively low spatial resolution of SPECT is a clinical problem when it is used to diagnose brain tumors.

Anatomical standardized statistical mapping is a useful method for improving the diagnostic ability of SPECT. We examined the statistical mapping of IMP SPECT in patients with brain lesions. In this report, we analyzed the diagnostic performance of the usual reconstructed images and statistical mapping of IMP SPECT of patients with brain tumors.

2. Patients and methods

This study included IMP SPECT images for 49 patients with brain lesions: 20 with PCNSL, one with Burkitt's lymphoma, 15 with glioma, two with meningioma, one with a metastatic tumor, two with multiple sclerosis (MS), five with cerebritis and three without any pathological diagnosis, but a clinical diagnosis of PCNSL. No patients had received prior radiation or chemotherapy for brain tumors. Three patients had previously received steroid medication at the time of IMP SPECT examination.

INTECH
open science | open minds

© 2014 The Author(s). Licensee InTech. This chapter is distributed under the terms of the Creative Commons Attribution License (http://creativecommons.org/licenses/by/3.0), which permits unrestricted use, distribution, and reproduction in any medium, provided the original work is properly cited.

We examined the normal reconstructed images and statistical mapping of IMP SPECT. After the intravenous injection of 222 Megabecquerel (MBq) of ^{123}I-IMP, the early (15 minutes) and delayed (3 hours) images were acquired using a multi-detector SPECT machine (E.CAM, Siemens Medical, Erlangen, Germany) and a high resolution collimator (LEHR, Siemens Medical, Erlangen, Germany). The Butterworth pre-correction filter and the Chang method were used for pre- and post-attenuation corrections. The Ramp filter was used for reconstruction. The image matrices, the pixel sizes and the slice thickness of the IMP SPECT were 128 x 128, 3.31 mm and 6.62 mm, respectively. All SPECT data were saved in the Digital Imaging and Communication in Medicine (DICOM) format. The DICOM data were transferred to a newly developed software program, the iNeurostat+ (Nihon Medi-physics, Hyogo, Japan), which runs on a Windows personal computer. The SPECT data were anatomically standardized on normal brain images. The increased uptakes of IMP were statistically mapped on the tomographic images of the normal brain. The image quality, diagnostic ability and imaging artifacts were evaluated by a visual inspection (Figure 1).

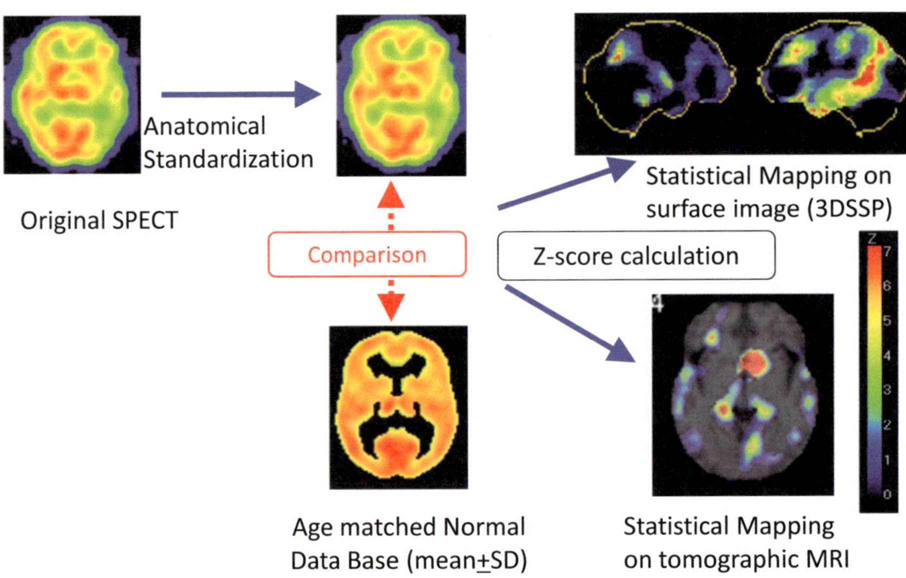

Figure 1. Automatic Process Flow of iNeurostat+

Magnetic resonance imaging (MRI) data were acquired with 1.5 Tesla instrument (Gyroscan NT Intera, Philips, Amsterdam, The Netherlands). The tumor diameters and size were measured using gadolinium-diethyltriaminepentaacetic acid (Gd-DTPA)-enhanced T1-weighted MRI.

http://dx.doi.org/10.5772/58321

The statistical analysis was performed with the Chi-square test. Values of $p < 0.05$ were considered to be significant.

3. Representative cases

3.1. Case 1 (Figure 2)

A 58-year-old female had a Gd-enhanced MRI scan, which showed a homogenously enhanced tumor at the left putamen. Delayed IMP SPECT showed tumor uptake, however, other normal brain uptake was also detected. Statistical mapping of IMP SPECT data demonstrated hot tumor uptake and no uptake into the normal brain. A tumor biopsy revealed a pathological diagnosis of PCNSL.

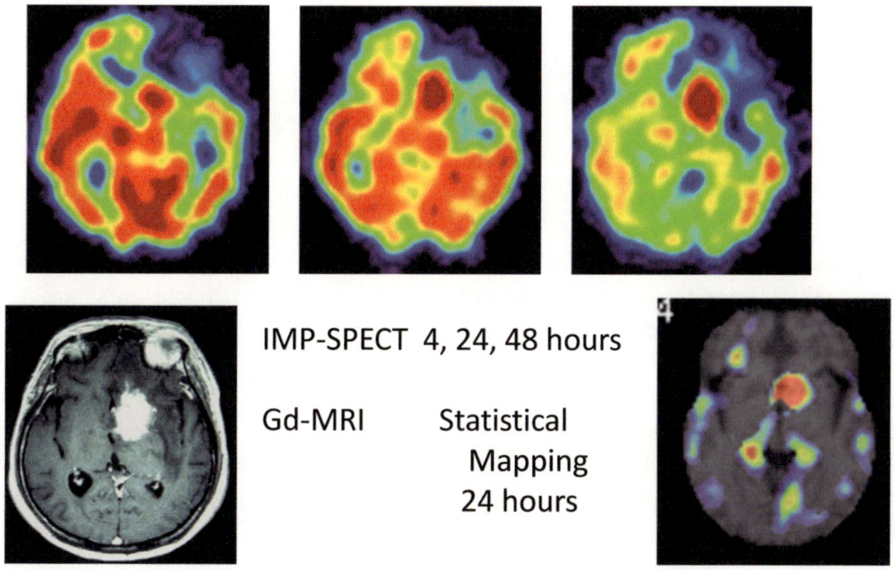

Figure 2. 58 Woman: PCNSL

3.2. Case 2 (Figure 3)

A 71-year-old female underwent a Gd-enhanced MRI scan, which showed a homogeneously enhanced tumor at the left cerebellum. Delayed IMP SPECT did not show clear uptake into the cerebellar lesion. Statistical mapping of IMP SPECT demonstrated clear uptake of IMP into the tumor. The tumor was pathologically diagnosed as PCNSL by biopsy.

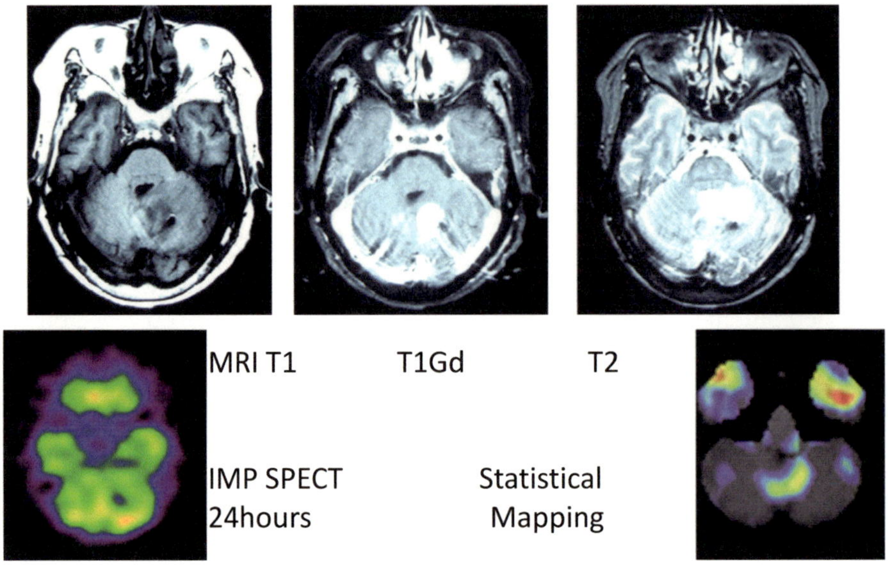

Figure 3. 71 Woman: PCNSL

4. Results

Eighteen patients showed a high uptake in the delayed IMP SPECT images (16 PCNSL, two unknown). All unknown patients were successfully treated with steroids and radiation therapy, so their clinical diagnosis was PCNSL. Other tumors or lesions did not show a high uptake on delayed IMP SPECT, so there were no false positives (Table 1). Four patients with pathologically proven PCNSL showed no uptake in the original IMP SPECT. These tumors were either too small to detect by IMP SPECT or the IMP SPECT images were taken after the administration of steroids. However, statistical mapping revealed the IMP uptake in two of these four patients. A heterogeneous IMP uptake was seen in homogenous tumors in MRI. For patients with a hot IMP uptake, statistical mapping showed clearer uptake. The sensitivity and specificity of original IMP SPECT were 80 and 100% (Chi-test $p<0.01$), respectively. Those of statistical mapping were 90 and 100% (Chi-test $p<0.01$), respectively.

The patients who had received steroid treatment showed negative of IMP SPECT findings. However, patients with glioma, MS and Burkitt's lymphoma did not show a high uptake of delayed IMP SPECT. IMP SPECT is therefore useful for the diagnosis of PCNSL, especially for the differentiation from glioma, MS and Burkitt's lymphoma. A heterogeneous IMP uptake was seen in homogenous tumors in MRI. For patients with a hot IMP uptake, statistical mapping showed an even clearer uptake. There were some artifacts on the statistical mapping, however, these artifacts did not result in diagnostic problems due to comparisons of the statistical mapping and original SPECT or MRI findings.

http://dx.doi.org/10.5772/58321

Original IMP	PCNSL	other	unknown
uptake +	16	0	2
uptake −	4	26	1

Sensitivity 80%, specificity 100%, Chi-test p<0.01

Statistical Mapping	PCNSL	other	unknown
uptake +	18	0	2
uptake −	2	26	1

Sensitivity 90%, specificity 100%, Chi-test p<0.01

5. Discussion

5.1. Sensitivity and specificity of IMP SPECT

Our results revealed a high sensitivity (80%) and high specificity (100%) of IMP SPECT in the diagnosis of PCNSL. Our IMP SPECT of 3.31 mm in pixel size could not detect one small supratentorial tumor less than 5 mm. Because our patient series included only one patient with a tumor less than 20 mm in diameter, the detection threshold could not be demonstrated. However, two cerebellar tumors more than 30 mm in diameter could be detected with the usual IMP SPECT, while two cerebellar tumors smaller than 25 mm in diameter could not be detected. Based on our results, the detection threshold of cerebellar tumors seems to be around 25 to 30 mm in diameter.

Akiyama reported that the PCNSL larger than 3 ml could be detected in delayed IMP SPECT [1]. Their patient series included some patients with brain stem tumors and no patients with cerebellar tumor. Shinoda reported the IMP SPECT findings in 10 patients with PCNSL [9]. There were two patients with cerebellar tumors in their study, but the tumor size or volume was not described.

SPECT has some physical and radiological limitations. The absorption of gamma rays in each tissue decreases the detected signal. Scattering radiation from the gamma ray source leads to low spatial resolution of the reconstructed SPECT images. The posterior fossa is covered by a thick area of the skull, so the signal from the brain stem and cerebellum is attenuated more than that from the cerebrum. Homogeneous attenuation correction could not correct for the low signal from the posterior fossa. These reasons might underlie the low sensitivity at the cerebellum. Some methods of correcting the absorption and scattering have been employed, however, all of these correction methods are associated with some limitations [4]. In our facility, the scatter was corrected with a Butterworth filter, and the absorption and attenuation were corrected with the chang method. The chang method assumes homogenous attenuation, however, the head is not homogenously attenuated. Therefore, using the Chang method leads to an overestimation of the regional CBF values in IMP SPECT in low CBF regions and an underestimation in high CBF regions [4]. The cerebellum is a high CBF region. Therefore, the tumors at the cerebellum might be less detectable by IMP SPECT than the tumors at the brain stem.

5.2. Mechanism of IMP uptake

The mechanisms underlying the uptake and retention of IMP in PCNSL are not fully understood. The amine receptor is one of the IMP binding sites [6]. A specific amine receptor in PCNSL was hypothesized to be responsible for the IMP retention in PCNSL [10] [11]. Most IMP binding is considered to be mainly associated with high capacity, relatively nonspecific binding sites in brain synaptosomes [6]. The IMP SPECT findings suggested that there is strong IMP binding to PCNSL. In the future, the mechanisms of IMP uptake and the retention in PCNSL may be revealed by clinical and basic studies of PCNSL.

5.3. Standardization of SPECT images

The CBF is dependent on the patient age. Each patient's CBF should therefore be evaluated in comparison with a normal standardized database for specific age groups. Each patient also has different cerebral morphology. In order to compare the SPECT data of each patient with the normal standardized database, each patient's SPECT data should be transformed to fit standard SPECT data. Using the iNeurostat+ software program, a statistical evaluation of an anatomically standardized tomographic image is possible. Anatomical standardization and statistical mapping are useful methods to reduce the differences based on the individual brain morphology and to objectively evaluate the image findings.

Based on our results, the IMP uptake into PCNSL was highly specific. At present, the final definite diagnosis of PCNSL should be determined by biopsy and pathological examination. However, a biopsy is an invasive surgical procedure. Therefore, there is currently no definitive non-invasive method for diagnosing PCNSL. Some patients, such as those with tumors in the brain stem, or who are in poor general condition, are not candidates for surgical procedures. In such cases, IMP SPECT may be helpful to diagnose PCNSL without the surgical risk associated with a biopsy. Our results warrant further clinical prospective research to evaluate the clinical significance of IMP SPECT for the diagnosis of PCNSL.

The statistical mapping method was especially useful to detect small tumors that were not detected using usual IMP SPECT. Statistical mapping has the same spatial resolution as the original SPECT images. The detectability of tumors at the posterior fossa and skull base is affected by absorption and scattering corrections. Statistical mapping method reduces these affects, and as a result, improves the detectability of tumors at the posterior fossa or skull base.

Reconstructed SPECT images include some error and artifacts by nature. A statistical analysis can reduce some errors and artifacts, however, it can also lead to new errors and artifacts. In our study, some artifacts were observed in the statistical mapping results that were not seen in original SPECT images. These artifacts were recognizable as artifacts by comparing the statistical mapped images with original reconstructed SPECT images. However, it should be

http://dx.doi.org/10.5772/58321

kept in mind that the statistical mapping images are not original images, and should not be overrated. The final clinical evaluation should be based on careful image interpretation.

5.4. Study limitations

Our study has some limitations. The patient population was small and selected based on the criteria of suspected PCNSL. All patients with brain lesions were not included in this study. However, the patient population in this study represents the actual target population who need a differential diagnosis. Therefore, this study demonstrated the actual clinical usefulness of IMP SPECT for the differential diagnosis of PCNSL.

IMP SPECT is useful for the diagnosis of PCNSL because the uptake is specific, as shown in our results. The gold standard for the diagnosis of PCNSL is the pathological examination of surgical specimens. There is currently no definitive non-invasive diagnostic method. Because some patients with PCNSL are contraindicated for surgery, IMP SPECT may represent an alternative to biopsy for obtaining a diagnosis. Further collection of experiences and improvements of the diagnostic methods will increase the reliability and decrease the limitations of diagnostic imaging using IMP SPECT for PCNSL. In the actual clinical diagnosis of PCNSL, we generally acquire additional information from other examinations, including tumor marker levels and gallium and/or thallium scintigraphy. In our patient population, we also examined the findings by these modalities. A detailed discussion of the results of these examinations is not within the scope of this paper, but such combined evaluations may help overcome some of the limitations of IMP SPECT.

6. Conclusion

IMP-SPECT and statistical mapping are considered to be useful for the diagnosis of PCNSL. Multi-modal images should be taken before steroid therapy, because steroids affect the diagnostic performance of both of MRI and SPECT. Statistical mapping is useful for detecting small tumors which cannot be detected by usual IMP SPECT. However, some artifacts also exist in statistical mapping images. The careful interpretation of such image findings is essential. Anatomical standardized statistical mapping is thus considered a useful method for improving the diagnostic sensitivity, specificity and accuracy of IMP SPECT for brain lesions.

Author details

Yasushi Shibata*

Address all correspondence to: yshibata@md.tsukuba.ac.jp

Department of Neurosurgery, Mito Medical Center, University of Tsukuba, Mito, Ibaraki, Japan

References

[1] Akiyama Y, Moritake K, Yamasaki T, Kimura Y, Kaneko A, Yamamoto Y, Miyazaki T, Daisu M: The diagnostic value of 123I-IMP SPECT in non-Hodgkin's lymphoma of the central nervous system. *J Nucl Med.* 41:1777-1783., 2000.

[2] Fukahori T, Tahara T, Mihara F, Kato A, Masumoto H, Kudo S, Tsuji T, Tabuchi K: [Diagnostic value of high N-isopropyl-p-[123I] iodoamphetamine (IMP) uptake in brain tumors]. *Nippon Igaku Hoshasen Gakkai Zasshi.* 56:53-59., 1996.

[3] Greenberg JH, Kushner M, Rango M, Alavi A, Reivich M: Validation studies of iodine-123-iodoamphetamine as a cerebral blood flow tracer using emission tomography. *J Nucl Med* 31:1364-1369, 1990.

[4] Hayashi M, Deguchi J, Utsunomiya K, Yamada M, Komori T, Takeuchi M, Kanna K, Narabayashi I: Comparison of methods of attenuation and scatter correction in brain perfusion SPECT. *J Nucl Med Technol* 33:224-229, 2005.

[5] Kitanaka C, Eguchi T, Kokubo T: Secondary malignant lymphoma of the central nervous system with delayed high uptake on 123I-IMP single-photon emission computerized tomography. Case report. *J Neurosurg.* 76:871-873., 1992.

[6] Nishizawa S, Tanada S, Yonekura Y, Fujita T, Mukai T, Saji H, Fukuyama H, Miyoshi T, Harada K, Ishikawa M, Kikuchi H, Konishi J: Regional Dynamics of N-Isopropyl-(123I)p-iodo-Amphetamine in Human Brain. *J Nucl Med* 30:150-156, 1989.

[7] Ohkawa S, Yamadori A, Mori E, Tabuchi M, Ohsumi Y, Yoshida T, Yoneda Y, Furumoto M: A case of primary malignant lymphoma of the brain with high uptake of 123I-IMP. *Neuroradiology.* 31:270-272., 1989.

[8] Sagiuchi T, Oka H, Utsuki S, Sato K, Kobayashi I, Asano Y, Ishii K, Fujii K: Increased accumulations of N-isopropyl-p-[123I]-iodoamphetamine related to tumefactive multiple sclerosis. *Ann Nucl Med* 19:603-606, 2005.

[9] Shinoda J, Yano H, Murase S, Yoshimura S, Sakai N, Asano T: High 123I-IMP retention on SPECT image in primary central nervous system lymphoma. *J Neurooncol.* 61:261-265., 2003.

[10] Yamamoto Y, Nishiyama Y, Kawakita K, Toyama Y, Ohkawa M, Tanabe M: Malignant lymphoma of the central nervous system with delayed increased accumulation on I-123 IMP SPECT. *Clin Nucl Med.* 26:105-108., 2001.

[11] Yoshikai T, Fukahori T, Ishimaru J, Kato A, Uchino A, Tabuchi K, Kudo S: 123I-IMP SPET in the diagnosis of primary central nervous system lymphoma. *Eur J Nucl Med* 28:25-32, 2001.

Section 3

Neurobiochemical – Considerations for the Future

Chapter 5

Biochemical and Surgical Aspects of Epilepsy Related to Brain Tumors — Appraising Redox Biology and Treatments

Pinar Atukeren, Taner Tanriverdi and
M. Ramazan Yigitoglu

Additional information is available at the end of the chapter

http://dx.doi.org/10.5772/58343

1. Introduction

Oxidative stress appears when prooxidant-antioxidant balance is altered in the direction of the former, causing neuronal cell death and dysfunction, so resulting in oxidative damage lending to disease pathogenesis. Brain tissue have a very high metabolic rate as it consumes approximately 20% of the inhaled oxygen due to the fact that neurons need high amounts of ATP for sustaining ionic gradients across cell membranes and so as for neurotransmission and as most of the ATP is produced via oxidative metabolism, neurons are dependant on mitochondrial function supremely. Oxidative stress is known to act a part in mitochondrial dysfunction and brain damage associated with epileptic seizures. In recent studies it is implied that epileptic status alters the redox potential and diminishes ATP levels creating a break down in brain energy production and a damage to cellular targets such as protein, lipids and DNA is seen following persistent seizures. Thus a consecutive cell damage emerges after persistent seizures with an increase in mitochondrial oxidative stress status in epilepsy patients.

Brain tumours typically cause epileptic seizures. The life quality of patients with brain tumors having epileptic seizures are seriously effected owing to the factors not being clear and the problems confronted in the treatment. Antiepileptic treatment culminates with limited success due to drug interactions, adverse effects and pharmacoresistance frequently.The mechanism of epileptogenesis in patients having a brain tumour is not clarified obviously yet. Seizures are conferred as the initial symptom in around 30-50% of patients particularly with slow growing primary brain tumors [1]. Seizures are mostly seen in patients having low grade tumors while in patients with high grade brain tumors the insidance is lower. Also, the location of the tumor

INTECH
open science | open minds

© 2014 The Author(s). Licensee InTech. This chapter is distributed under the terms of the Creative Commons Attribution License (http://creativecommons.org/licenses/by/3.0), which permits unrestricted use, distribution, and reproduction in any medium, provided the original work is properly cited.

is an important deterministic of epileptic seizures. Due to the decreased intratumoral perfusion and increased metabolism, hypoxia occurs causing acidosis through metabolic requirements of the proliferating tissue and the disrupted oxidative energy metabolism, both inducing glial cell swelling and damage effecting the surrounding tissue [2]. It was implied that derangement between the excitatory and inhibitory balance leads to glioma associated seizures as there is an intimate relationship between seizure activity and increased extracellular glutamate levels in tumor related epilepsy. The involvement of tumor growth is not clear yet. Glutamate levels are shown to increase reaching neurotoxic levels during seizures. Epileptic activity is implied to be originating within the peritumoral border distant from the tumor tissue and it was shown that the glutamate levels were higher in peritumoral cortex when compared with health brain tissue parts in glioma patients. GABA receptor activity is thought to be an inhibitor as receptor down regulation seems causing hyperactivity in the surrounding microenvironment. There is also a close relationship between immunological and inflammatory changes with a diminished risks of glioma and epileptic seizures related to tumor presence as proinflammatory cytokines seem to be involved in epilepsy pathogenesis [3,4]. On the other hand, patients having epileptic seizures with brain tumors were reported having increased levels of ROS and the antioxidant status was found to be decreased. This seems to be recovered after treatment with antiepileptic drugs favoring the so called damaging effect of oxidative stress in epilepsy flashing the estimated possibility of preventing the seizures via antioxidant treatment. Alleviation of the oxidative damage utilizing antioxidant substances in epilepsy was shown experimentally.

These knowledge may highlight the possible future strategies in the medical treatment of tumor associated epilepsy. In terms of surgical aspects, removing the tumor to stop epileptic seizures might not assure a prosperous result alone considering that the neurons surrounder the tumor form an epileptogenic area [2]. On the other hand, when the lesion is removed, surrounding neurons may stop exciting aberrantly, returning to normal status. Thus the neurosurgeons are suggested to minimize the residual tumor volume where applicable. The conservation of the mitochondria and eventually decreasing oxidative stress related events seems to be reasonable therapeutic approach. Not only resecting the tumor but also combining an appropriate postoperative treatment should be the main aim in seizure control. As mentioned, therapy with antioxidants having a potential neuroprotective effect, should be intended to lower the conferred oxidative damage in epilepsy treatment where ketogenic diets were also shown to have beneficial effects in treating epileptic seizures as they seem to increase glutathione levels in mitochondria. It is clear that developing a mitochondria targeted antioxidant therapy would be promising approach in epilepsy, hopefully resulting in seizure control withdrawing treatment with antiepileptic drugs in long term.

2. The biochemical mechanisms transpiring in case of epileptic seizures

Epilepsy should be considered not only as a single disease, but also common symptomatic symptoms of brain abnormalities involving central nervous system infections, traumatic brain injuries, genetic syndromes or brain lesions such brain tumors are present. The relationship of inflammation in the pathophysiology of epilepsy is implied in various clinical studies [5,6].

The dysregulated homeostasis in the peritumoral tissue may cause to seizure somethesia as the tumor cells create an intrinsic epileptogenicity. The most vital mechanism inducing tumor related seizures is the alteration of amino acid neurotransmission where also an alteration in the extracellular ions is involved. These mechanisms should be enlightened to provide guidance for improving new strategies in the surgical and medical treatment for tumor associated epilepsy.

The tumor tissue might be epileptogenic due to excreting some molecules itself or the peritumoral tissue might be transformed into an epileptogenic zone as the microenvironment of brain tumors is considerably different from that of healthy brain tissue which is demonstrated via contemporary imaging techniques. On the other hand, the peritumoral tissue might turn into an epileptogenic zone because of the mechanic restrainment of the tumor as a result of hypoxia and ischemia. These lead to epileptic seizures following the alterations in neurotransmitters and their receptors, metabolic changes and inflammatory responses. Structural epileptogenic abnormalities in the cortex might also be attended as low levels of N-acetylaspartate which is a marker for the survival and functionality of the neurons, was shown in the epileptogenic cortex via magnetic resonance spectroscopy [7]. It was shown that damage in the subcortical network affecting the electrical transmission is effectuated mostly by high grade brain tumors [8] while a partial deafferentation in cortical regions is induced by low grade tumors causing an epileptogenic stage [9,10]. Inflammatory changes and gliosis in the peritumoral tissue also contribute. Derangements in the neurovascular entirety also cause hypersynchronization leading to epileptogenity. The emerge of decreased expression of junctional transmembrane proteins [11] and increased vascular endothelial growth factor (VEGF) release which aggrevates the edema in the surrounding of the lesion [12] is due to the impaired blood brain barrier through molecular alterations in brain tumors and hypoxia and acidosis, appearing sequentially, occur because of the enhanced metabolism and the diminished perfusion in the intratumoral tissue. Definitely, an adequate blood supply is obligatory for brain tumor growth [13] and in case of inadequate blood supply, acidosis followed by interstitial hypoxia appears extending to the surrounding tissue, as a consequence of both elevated metabolic requirements of the proliferating tissue and impaired oxidative energy metabolism. Also, peritumoral hypoxia comes out because of direct restrainment through large sized tumors. In either case, damage sequential to glial cell swelling occurs [14] where the membranes of the cells are vulnerable for inward sodium currents augmenting the risk of epilepsy [15]. In consequence of hypoxia, glucose catabolism picks up culminating excess lactate production which leads to acidosis and in tumor tissues increased lactate levels were also shown [16]. In the peritumoral area the increase in sodium and calcium levels contribute to neuronal hyperexcitability [17] and the change in the gating of calcium channels have been reported in epileptic tissue where calcium influx is blocked via NMDA receptor channels through stabilizing the neuronal excibility by magnesium. Also, mutations in the potassium channels were implied and the extracellular potassium concentrations are known to play a role in membrane potential [18,19].

Glutamate is an excitatory neurotransmitter which acts on postsynaptic membranes through interacting with ionotropic and metabotropic glutamate receptors [20]. There is a relationship between seizure activity and high levels of extracellular glutamate in tumor associated epilepsy. Increased levels of glutamate was shown in glioma patients with epilepsy [15,21]. The number of glutamate receptors are variable depending on the tumor degree. Ionotropic glutamate receptors, which induce intracellular calcium release when activated, are NMDA, AMPA and kainate receptors and with marred activity, in the peritumoral tissue differences in the expression are seen. GABA is also a neurotransmitter which inhibits neuronal discharge and when there is a down regulation in GABA receptors, which are GABAA, GABAB and GABAC, hyperactivity in the peritumoral zone is encountered. Alterations in the functions of GABA receptors in the peritumoral tissue, induce GABAergic neurotransmission alleviation and GABA levels are reported to be increased in tumor tissues [18,19]. GABAergic activity doesn't have a relationship with seizure somethesia directly yet the alterations in the levels seem causal for tumor related epilepsy. Also, in gliomas decreased kynurenic acid levels causing NMDA receptor disinhibition [22] and decreased noradrenaline and serotonin levels causing antiepileptogenic effects were reported [23].

Inflammation, either immune mediated or without infection, also play a crucial role in epileptic seizures and in tumor related epilepsy where proinflammatory cytokines being inflammatory mediators and their receptors are involved in the pathogenesis. High levels of cytokines such as interleukin (IL)-6, IL-1β and the IL-1, tumor necrosis factor (TNF)-α were implied [24]. Cytokine activation depends on both seizure severity and duration in epilepsy patients. [25, 26]. Activation of IL-1β system in glial cells expressing IL-1β and its receptor was reported in studies with chronic epileptic rats [27,28]. IL-4 and IL-6 were shown to be having modulating effects on neurotoxic neurotransmitters which are released during excitation and inflammation [29]. In the peritumoral tissue neurochemical alterations, coupled with the imbalance between stimulatory and inhibitory cytokines, which are immune mediated were shown in glioma [30-32] and reported to be related with tumor associated epilepsy. The activation of toll like receptor (TLR) signaling pathways, which are activated via pathogens or endogenous ligands released by damaged or stressor activated cells called as danger signals, is also a current subject in epilepsy [33,34] and in neurons and astrocytes TLR4 overexpression was demonstrated in chronic epileptic mice [33,35]. The inflammation in the brain tissue is thought to be contributing to the deterioration of the blood brain barrier leading to serum albumin and IgG accumulation. Albumin was reported to be inducing the long lasting hyperexcitability via impairing astrocyte buffering capacity of extracellular potassium and glutamate through activating transforming growth factor (TGF)-β pathway which leads to glutamate transporter downregulation [36-38]. These induced mechanisms through brain inflammation might explain the detention time occuring between the inflammatory complications and the inception of epilepsy.

3. The redox status in brain tumors

Brain is considered to be intensely vulnerable to oxidative damage having a high content of peroxidizable unsaturated fatty acids, high oxygen consumption per unit weight, high content of iron which is a key in lipid peroxidation and a shortage of antioxidant defense systems [39], so a crucial and unique target for both oxidative stress effects compared to other tissues and for metastatic growth being surrounded by the blood brain barrier. Reactive oxygen species (ROS), or free radicals, may exceed the scavenging ability of endogenous antioxidants, resulting in a shift of the redox state of the brain to the oxidative state. Redox balance in neural tissue has an important role in the pathophysiology of neurotoxicity through the free radical generation. ROS are particularly active in the brain and neuronal tissue and very aggressive to glial cells and neurons. Endogenous antioxidant system plays a constitutive role in prevention of any damage due to free radicals. However, imbalanced defense mechanism of antioxidants, overproduction or incorporation of free radicals from environment to living system bring about a serious infliction and therefore to a neuronal death [40].

Tumor cells frequently demonstrate a change in redox status. The alterations in the redox environment enhancing oxidation can induce some of the factors that cause cell proliferation and malignant transformation. Cancer cells display increased glycolysis rate combined with a reduced respiration rate [41]. The enhanced requirements for ATP; generates oxygen free radicals and this causes oxidative stress conditions to come out which eventually promotes cell death. Neurons and cancer cells consume glucose as energy source to respond this issue and glycolytic metabolism rules over in tumor cells. The release of cytochrome c couples with the pentose phosphate pathway and this initiates cytochrome c mediated apoptosis [42]. Caspase activation is initiated by cytochrome c when released from mitochondria during apoptosis. So, the cancer cells and neurons control apoptosis through regulation of cytochrome c release, while utilizing glucose as a source of energy [43]. This marked changes in metabolism have been shown to be related with increased oxidative stress which is emphasized to be due to increased mitochondrial superoxide radical production [44].

Studies have been done to evaluate antioxidant enzyme activities in different types of brain tumors. However, most studies have emphasized decreased levels of antioxidant enzymes and vitamins in diverse malignancies but still the results are inconsistent. Elevated manganase superoxide dismutase (MnSOD) activities were shown in the serum samples of neuroblastoma patients in a study. In recent studies, MnSOD was found to be associated with loss of differentiation and increased clinical malignancy in neuroepithelial origined brain tumors. MnSOD was found significantly positive in Grade IV astrocytomas and medulloblastomas and negative in normal brain samples. It can be said that MnSOD is overexpressed in most brain tumor types and enhanced MnSOD expression is related with a poor prognosis. MnSOD seems to be a tumor suppressor in the proliferative stage. When tumor progresses more aggressive, MnSOD is upregulated. MnSOD level positively correlates with increased metastasis so MnSOD has an oncogene role. Increase in MnSOD level was seen during the progression of different types of tumors, including brain, to the metastatic stage. Tumorigenesis and metastasis are dependent on the levels of ROS. A cell having low levels of MnSOD is vulnerable to oxidative stress then it may turn its progression to a tumor cell. Oxidative gene polymorphism and brain tumor risk seems to be associated, the increased risk of glioma and meningioma type brain tumors were found to be related with variants in some antioxidant enzyme genes and in a study, MnSOD tissue expression is said to be a prognostic marker for glioblastoma. Superoxide dismutase (SOD) and glutathione peroxidase (GPx) activities showed a clear decrease proportionally with tumor malignancy, decrease of SOD activity with the increasing grades of malignancy in brain tumors were implied [45,46].

The GSH redox cycle is one of the most important antioxidative systems. GSH is a primary endogenous neuroprotectant for the brain. GSH protects neuron cells from lipid peroxidation and brain cells from peroxynitrite mediated oxidative damage. GSH is prevalantly seen in brain tissue, thus highly expressed in various primary brain tumors. GSH content was shown to be related to tumor response to nitrogen mustard therapy in human brain neoplasms. When glutathione-S-transferase (GST) isoenzymes in neoplastic and non-neoplastic astroglia were compared, GST3 isoenzyme was seen to be significantly higher in tumors. It is said that GST expression levels in brain tumors seems in association with the tumor histology as some tumor types express enhanced levels but some show only slight rise or decrease when compared to normal cells. GST was found to be active in high levels in benign tumors such as meningioma but only two-three folds higher compared to normal tissue but it was slightly increased in astrocytoma. In glioblastomas, GSH levels were found significantly lowered compared to normal tissue and merely elevated in meningioma. It has been reported that GPx and glutathione reductase (GR) enzyme activities decrease and protein oxidation levels increase in patients with glioblastoma multiforme and transitional meningioma; the two kinds of tumors which represent specially one of the most malignant and most benign tumors respectively and it was shown that there is a complex relationship between pro-and anti-apoptotic molecules in glioblastoma multiforme pathogenesis, thus targeting multiple pathways with advanced chemotherapeutic agents or radiotheraupetic regimens following total resections might be helpful in patients with glioblastoma multiforme and consistent differences in the levels of antioxidants in different types of brain tumors were emphasized in different studies. The decreased antioxidant levels in brain tumor patients reflect the enhanced oxidative damage and increased cancer developing possibility, stating the role of antioxidants in cancer prevention and role of oxidative injury as the of cancer. It was seen that β-carotene and α-tocopherol levels decreases when malignancy grade increases and the decrease was found significant for oligodendroglioma grade I-II, glioblastoma multiforme and medulloblastoma [45,46].

4. The pivotal role of oxidative stress during epileptic seizures

Epilepsy, being an excitotoxic brain disorder, causes neuronal destruction incrementally. The generation of ROS is distinctly implicated in a number of neurologic diseases including seizure disorders. Oxidative stress and mitochondrial dysfunction are indicated to be having a crucial role in the pathogenesis of epilepsy [47,48], contributing to the neuronal destruction through the activation of proapoptotic transcription factors [49,50]. Neuronal cell damage develops due to recurrent or obstinate seizures and abnormal increases in by products during seizures through the increased metabolic activity producing ROS with damage and leading to disruption of electrophysiologic integrity and instability of neuronal membranes. Fe^{3+}induces oxidative damage to neuronal plasma membranes and experimentally it was shown that this is related with the development of epileptic activity. Due to small bleedings, Fe^{3+}levels may increase in tumoral and peritumoral areas which also prospectively contribute to the development of tumor related seizures and this is mostly encountered in high grade gliomas [2]. In an experimental study, intracortical injection of Fe^{3+}induced the formation of epileptic areas in cerebral cortex. Also, increase in the peroxidation of membrane lipids is found to be related with the development of epileptic activity [51].

Mitochondrial dysfunction is associated with epilepsy and this was demonstrated both in humans [52,53] and in several experimental epilepsy models [54,55]. When complex I was inhibited, markers of oxidative damage; 3-nitrotyrosine, 4-hydroxynonenal and protein carbonyl levels were significantly increased and this was alleviated treating with a radical scavenger and an antioxidant enzyme [56,57]. It is suggested that the reduced activity of complex I is due to oxidative modification with an extreme sensitivity to ROS, on the other hand complex I is also an important source of ROS, especially when the enzyme complex is partially inhibited [58,59]. Thereby, when complex I is inhibited, enhanced production of ROS might lead to epileptogenesis [60]. The pivotal role of mitochondrial dysfunction in the pathogenesis of epileptic seizure generation seems to be the main topic appraising oxidative stress.

5. Contributing mitochondrial alterations

Seizure activity is considered to be inducing energy failure and leading to neuronal injury. Neuronal mitochondria, moving along axons and dendrites, are substantially dynamic [61]. Ca^{2+}regulation, redox signaling, developmental and synaptic plasticity are among the functions of mitochondria [62].The triggering influence of several mutations in the genes affecting oxidative phosphorylation in epilepsy implies the importance of mitochondria for neurons. The related mutations were demonstrated in the mitochondrial DNA polymerase γ (POLG1) [63,64], mitochondrial tRNALys (MT-TK) [65,66] and tRNAPhe (MT-TF) [67] genes in different phenotypes of epilepsy. Epilepsy is also appelled as a nonsyndromic mitochondrial disorder (MID) due to a novel classification and has a genetic or metabolic ground through a cerebral lesion or dysfunction [68]. Depending on the selection of MID patients, the prevalence seems to be lower in adulthood and the generalized seizures are remarkably more often compared to focal seizures.

Decreased ATP levels, changes in neuronal calcium homeostasis and modifications of ion channels and neurotransmitter transporters due to ROS damage are the main causes of impaired mitochondrial function and the increased neuronal excitability leading to epileptogenesis. In many studies, ATP depletion during seizures was indicated [69-71] entailing a decrease in neuronal plasma membrane potential leading to an increase in neuronal excitability as the major source of ATP for sodium potassium ATPase is the mitochondrial oxidative phosphorylation in neurons [72,73]. The interneurons, being mithochondria rich, expose a decreased synaptic transmission in inhibitory synapses, thereby the increased excitability in epilepsy due to mitochondrial dysfunction could be explained accordingly.

Mitochondria have a substantial role in intracellular Ca^{2+}sequestration in neurons so can be named as major calcium buffers [74,75]. Attributing to remarkable calcium flow in neuronal excitability, through ligand gated and voltage gated ion channels, cyclic calcium elevations are seen during epileptic activity. Referring to this, mitochondria can attenuate the altered neuronal excitability and synaptic transmission in epilepsy [76]. Yet another reason for the increased excitability encountered in epilepsy is, astroglial and neuronal glutamate transporters' being quite sensitive to oxidative damage which are known to be crucial for the maintenance of low synaptic glutamate levels [77]. and it was indicated that complex I activity induces the excess release of glutamate [78]. So it can be concluded by stating that oxidative stress has direct effects on neuronal excitability in the same time.

6. Surgical approach

The majority of surgical series showed that almost 60 to 90% of supratentorial benign gliomas present with epilepsy and surgical resection may be the only treatment option for both histopathological diagnosis and treatment [79]. There is still discussion whether epilepsy is a specific property of the tumor or the brain's reaction to the tumor. However, proximity to the functional areas such as primary motor strip or language or Broca's area increases the chance of having seizures. Advanced developments in the imaging technology, brain tumors, especially low-grade gliomas which were missed in the past, led the physicians to diagnose such lesions and early surgery is now performed without doubt. Since these gliomas are slow growing, seizures may occur late and any seizure in the adult life must raise the suspicion of a tumor until proven otherwise. Magnetic resonance imaging (MRI) is the gold standard diagnostic modality to diagnose brain tumors and sensitivity is higher than computerized tomography (CT). Especially T_2-weigted and FLAIR images (Figure 1) are important for visualize low grade tumors which are generally not enhanced with contrast agent. Additional imaging modalities such as MR spectroscopy may provide further evidence of the lesions true nature. In some patients electroencephalography (EEG) is needed because of discordant finding between the MRI and seizure semiology but there is no characteristic EEG pattern. However; EEG can lateralize the tumor in 70% of patients. Rarely, intracranial depth electrodes and/or electrocorticography (EcOG) is needed before and during surgery to expose the epileptogenic area. The most common location for these gliomas is the frontal lobe, followed by parietal, temporal lobes and insula. Occipital lobe alone is less involved and the reason is not clear.

Clinical experience has demonstrated that surgical removal of the lesion alone significantly reduces seizure frequency. It is interesting to note that lesionectomy alone or lesionectomy with corticectomy show similar good results so that there has been no standard resection among the centers. But we know very well that completeness of tumor removal is the most important prognostic factor for seizure control, recurrence, and improved quality of life. Surgical approach depends mainly on the proximity to the functional cortices which necessitated local anesthesia (awake craniotomy). On the other hand, when a tumor is located in silent area, general anesthesia is preferred.

Scalp incision and craniotomy is planned according to the location of the tumor and "question mark" incision has been extensively used for temporal, frontal tumors (Figure 2). For central

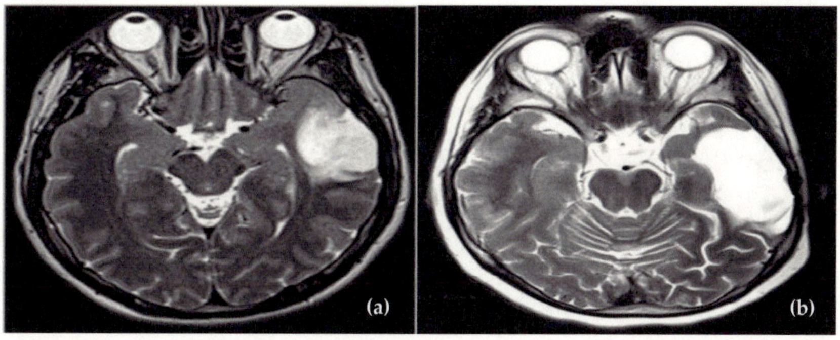

Figure 1. This 27-year-old male was presented with complex-partial seizure and MRI showed a mass in the left temporal lobe without involvement of the mesial temporal structures (hippocampus, parahippocampus and amygdala). The tumor margin is clearly seen in the preopretive T_2-weighted image (**a**) and histopathological diagnosis was astrocytoma grade-II and 3 years after the surgery the T_2-weighted image (**b**) shows no tumor recurrence and the patients is seizure free without antiepileptic medication.

and parietal located tumors an inverted"U-shaped" incision is usually sufficient. Particular attention should be paid to dural sinuses and large cortical veins when removing the bone flap and opening the dura. If awake craniotomy is performed, cortical mapping with intraoperative electrical cortical stimulation in order to figure out the functional area should be performed. The aim of the cortical mapping is to have maximum tumor removal with minimum neurological deficit by not causing any damage to the functional cortex (Figure 3).

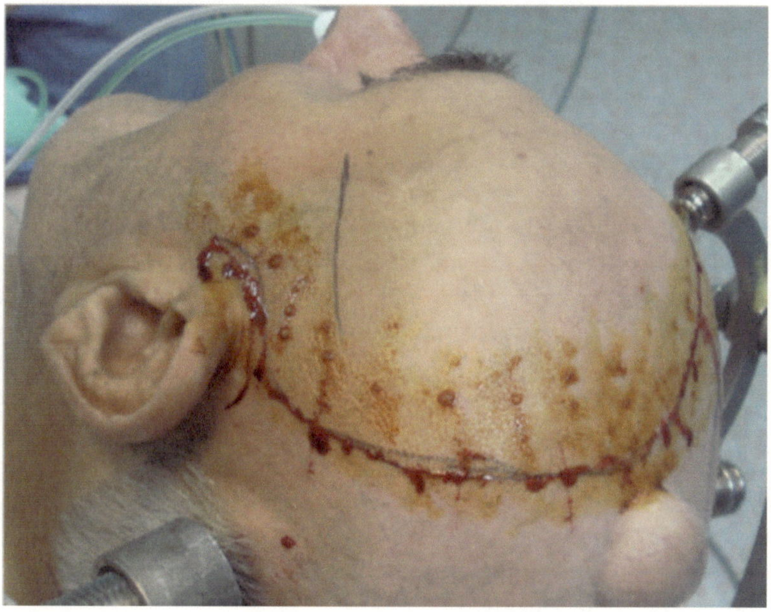

Figure 2. The picture showing a "question mark" scalp incision which is the commonest incision type used in the neurosurgical operations.

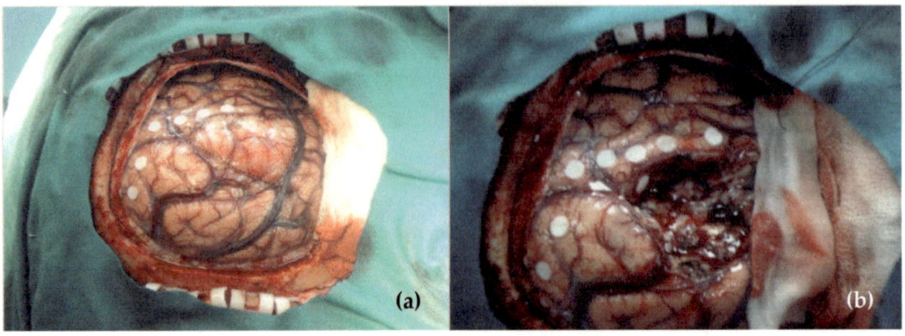

Figure 3. This picture shows an awake craniotomy and intraoperative electrical cortical stimulation (cortical mapping) for the identification of the motor cortex (white paper marks) which is close to the tumor (black dots depict the tumor) (**a**). The tumor was removed without any motor deficits (**b**) and the patient is seizure free at 1 year follow up.

The main surgical technique for the removal of these gliomas is "endopial" resection. By doing this technique, vessels running deep in the sulci and neighboring cortices are saved. Since these tumors are surrounded by the pial layers, respecting the pia avoids severe neurovascular damage during surgery and minimizes postoperative neurological deficits.

7. Potential neuroprotective and therapeutic strategies in tumor related epilepsy

Epileptic seizures related to brain tumors generally expose kind of focal seizures and around one third of the patients are resistive to medical antiepileptic treatment. Generally, neuronal voltage gated sodium and calcium channels, glutamate receptors and the GABA system are the main targets for antiepileptic drugs (AED) [80] which usually trend to treat through several mechanisms suppressing abnormal neuronal set off, solely none of the medications seems to be exhibiting an alteration neither in the progress of the disease not in the prevention [81] due to a number of reasons involving the biochemical context of the peritumoral zone and the drug drug interactions between the chemotherapeutics and AEDs inspiring an antiepileptic effectiveness revealing some side effects [82]. Also, the overexpression of the multidrug resistance proteins (MRPs) in tumors may restrict medicine diffusion into the brain as increased levels of MRPs were reported in brain tumor cells [82]. AEDs are known to be leading to cognitive impairment [83]. Moreoever, some patients under AED therapy exhibit poor seizure control as well as with undesireable side effects [84] embracing a high risk of teratogenicity in women [85], alterations in mood, hepatotoxicity, decrease in the mineral density of the bone, difficulties in weight management, dermal maladies etc. [86], thereby an increased tolerability towards new desiged AEDs should be the main intention in future studies. Currently, development of novel glial specific AEDs is considered to be a potential target promising to improve a good outcome.

Obviously, epileptogenesis is intimately associated with oxidative stress inducing ROS generation thus leading to membrane lipid peroxidation and impairment in the antioxidant defense system which also increase the risk of seizure recurrence [87]. In case, treatment with antioxidants is considered to be very profitable in inhibiting epileptic seizures without any adverse effect [88]. Selenium, an antioxidant protecting against ROS, is known to be causing an alteration in the rate of some neurotransmitters when deficient and depletion in selenium levels was reported to be leading to a failure in response to AEDs which act through GABAergic receptors due to an increased glutamate receptor activation [89] and utilization of selenium supplements reduce epileptic seizures [90]. Application of resveratrol, a meritorious antioxidant, was also demonstrated to be useful in seizure management and in reducing seizure incidence [91]. Similar findings were indicated experimentally where the prevention of seizures was concerned [92,93] Thymoquinone, another potent free radical and superoxide radical scavenger, exhibited an antiepileptic effect in children suggesting a lack of adverse effects even at high doses [94]. With respect to this point of view, the antiepileptic effect of curcumin, which is an active polyphenolic component, extracted from *Curcuma longa* called as turmeric, was also investigated being almost ten times more active than vitamin E as an antioxidant [95]. Implementation of curcumin which inhibits the transcription of inflammatory cytokines via nuclear factor kappa B (NF-κB),inducible nitric oxide synthase (iNOS), and cyclooxygenase 2 (Cox-2) [96], was demonstrated to be preventing the cognitive decline related to traumatic brain injury [97] and its antiepileptic potential was ascertained with short term treatment. Recently, inhibitors of mammalian target of rapamycin (mTOR), including rapamycin and its analogs, are pointed out and regular treatment with rapamycin is emphasized in preventing epileptogenesis experimentally [98,99], thereby, research relevant to inhibiting mTOR activity seems appreciable. Curcumin is also suggested as mTOR inhibitor suppressing epileptogenesis in experimental studies [100,101].

The ketogenic diet (KD), a subdued carbohydrate diet, is known to be effective in epilepsy treatment [102-104] being neuroprotective and antiepileptogenic. In children, seizures owing to GLUT-1 and pyruvate dehydrogenase deficiency are treated with KD [105], also a prosperous outcome is seen with other pediatric epilepsy syndromes [106] as it upregulates the neuronal gene expression of the enzymes in Krebs cyclus, oxidative phosphorylation and glycolysis and increases mitochondria density leading to enhanced brain metabolism [107,108], therefore, stimulating the Krebs cyclus seems to be an attractive strategy in seizure management via direct replenishment of energy substrates [109,110]. β-hydroxybutyrate, being a ketone body, protects against metabolic and excitotoxic insults in organotypic hippocampal cultures [111]. Considering the nutrient and energy sensing ability of mTOR, it has a role in pathophysiologic changes related to epileptogenesis and mTOR activity is increased after epileptic status. KD reducing the insulin levels [112], is expected to be inhibiting mTOR activity through decreasing the PI3K/Akt signaling pathway. Also, ROS have a role in the efficacy of KD as the production of some mitochondrial uncoupling proteins are increased with KD and this eventuates with a reduction in the mitochondrial membrane potential and an increase in mitochondrial respiration rate [113]. Mitochondrial production of ROS is decreased with ketone bodies via increasing NADH oxidation without affecting endogenous antioxidant glutathione levels [114]. It was shown that in rat neocortical neurons, ketones prevent oxidative injury via decreasing mitochondrial ROS production [115]. Recently, pyruvate seems to be a promising substrate on seizure activity due to its dual action as a scavenger of ROS and a substrate of Krebs cyclus, so as a strategy in treatment, this might be taken into consideration in prolonged seizures [116]. Restricted KD was implied to be an alternative approach in brain cancer management also, with the purpose of changing the metabolic environment of the tumor [117], yet further studies are essential in case the glucose levels of the patients are lowered when simultaneously the ketone levels are elevated, in the lack of radiation or drug toxicity.

Currently, the role of microRNAs (miRNA) is emphasized in the regulation of immune responses. miR-146a, known to be induced via several proinflammatory cytokines such as IL-1β and TNF-α, was shown to be upregulating in experimental epilepsy models [118,119], thereby miRNA is suggested to be a potential target in modulating the inflammatory pathways. Some inflammatory mediators have direct effects on neuronal excitability providing a decrease in seizure threshold which was demonstrated experimentally, so if the activation of inflammatory signalings might be blocked, this may also be appraised as a possible therapeutic approach for epilepsy patients.

Distinctive medications exhibit variable therapeutic approaches for epilepsy patients. Not only improving seizure management but also preventing epilepsy in patients who have high risk should be the main target in the treatment with antiepileptogenics. Future studies are truly required with an acceptable safety profile, especially for herbal and supplemental products as there is an incompetence of relevant clinical results although they are recommended in seizure treatment. Yet, antioxidant compounds, particulary targeting mitochondria, may have beneficial effects on long term consequences of epilepsy.

8. Conclusion

Epileptic seizures are common in patients with brain tumors. The mechanisms laying beneath the pathogenesis of tumor related epilepsy remain substantially unclear. Epileptogenicity might be generated by the tumor itself because of the intrinsic characteristics or the impaired balance between excitation and inhibition arising due to insufficient homeostasis in the peritumoral zone might be the reason where also metabolic, immunological and inflammatory alterations might be contributing. Thereby, clarifying both tumoral and peritumoral pathophysiology would lead in selecting the most convenient medical treatment. Recently, oxidative stress is suggested to be having a crucial role in brain tumor associated epileptic seizures as a means of mitochondrial dysfunction. Yet it should be enlightened with future studies weather treatment with antioxidant compounds would be beneficial on attenuating epileptic seizures. On the other hand, as there are no detectable inflammatory biomarkers with proven significance for epilepsy yet, the challenge should also be defining specific biomarkers which would be helpful in the diagnosis of antiinflammatory or immunomodulatory therapy effects. Apparently, bringing novel concepts out in the treatment strategies for brain tumor related epilepsy should be the main target in the future.

Acknowledgements

We would like to dedicate this chapter to patients having brain tumors suffering from epilepsy seizures.

Author details

Pinar Atukeren[1], Taner Tanriverdi[2] and M. Ramazan Yigitoglu[3]

1 Istanbul University, Cerrahpasa Medical Faculty, Department of Biochemistry, Istanbul, Turkey

2 Istanbul University, Cerrahpasa Medical Faculty, Department of Neurosurgery, Istanbul, Turkey

3 Turgut Ozal University, Faculty of Medicine, Department of Biochemistry, Ankara, Turkey

References

[1] Lote K, Stenwig AE, Skullerud K, Hirschberg H. Prevalence and prognostic significance of epilepsy in patients with gliomas. Eur J Cancer 1998;34 98–102.

[2] You G, Sha Z, Jiang T. The pathogenesis of tumor-related epilepsy and its implications for clinical, treatment. Seizure 2012;21:153–159.

[3] Chao CC, Molitor TW, Hu S. Neuroprotective role of IL-4 against activated microglia. J Immunol. 1993;151:1473–81.

[4] Hulkkonen J, Koskikallio E, Rainesalo S, Keranen T, Hurme, M, Peltola J. The balance of inhibitory and excitatory cytokines is differently regulated in vivo and in vitro among therapy resistant epilepsy patients. Epilepsy Res. 2004;59:199–205.

[5] Vezzani A, French J, Bartfai T, Baram TZ. The role of inflammation in epilepsy. Nat. Rev. Neurol. 2011;7:31–40.

[6] Vezzani A, Maroso M, Balosso S, Sanchez MA, Bartfai T. IL-1 receptor/Toll-like receptor signaling in infection, inflammation, stress and neurodegeneration couples hyperexcitability and seizures. Brain Behav. Immun. 2011;25 (7):1281–1289.

[7] Chernov MF, Kubo O, Hayashi M, Izawa M, Maruyama T, Usukura M, et al. Proton MRS of the peri-tumoral brain. J Neurol Sci 2005;228:137–42.

[8] Norden AD, Blumenfeld H. The role of subcortical structures in human epilepsy. Epilepsy Behav 2002;3:219–31.

[9] Wolf HK, Roos D, Blumcke I, Pietsch T, Wiestler OD. Perilesional neurochemical changes in focal epilepsies. Acta Neuropathol 1996;91:376–84.

[10] Vecht CJ, van Breemen M. Optimizing therapy of seizures in patients with brain tumors. Neurology 2006;67:S10–3.

[11] Liebner S, Fischmann A, Rascher G, Duffner F, Grote EH, Kalbacher H, et al. Claudin-1 and claudin-5 expression and tight junction morphology are altered in blood vessels of human glioblastoma multiforme. Acta Neuropathol 2000;100:323–31.

[12] Chi OZ, Hunter C, Liu X, Tan T, Weiss HR. Effects of VEGF on the blood– brain barrier disruption caused by hyperosmolarity. Pharmacology 2008;82:187–92.

[13] Fidler IJ, Yano S, Zhang RD, Fujimaki T, Bucana CD. The seed and soil hypothesis: vascularization and brain metastasis. Lancet Oncol 2002;3:53–7.

[14] Kempski O, Staub F, Jansen M, Schodel F, Baethmann A. Glial swelling during extracellular acidosis in vitro. Stroke 1988;19:385–92.

[15] Schaller B. Influences of brain tumor-associated pH changes and hypoxia on epileptogenesis. Acta Neurol Scand 2005;111:75–83.

[16] Martinez-Outschoorn UE, Prisco M, Ertel A, Tsirigos A, Lin Z, Pavlides S, et al. Ketones and lactate increase cancer cell stemness, driving recurrence, metastasis and poor clinical outcome in breast cancer. Cell Cycle 2011;10:1271–86.

[17] Hossmann KA, Seo K, Szymas J, Wechsler W. Quantitative analysis of experimental peri-tumoral edema in cats. Adv Neurol 1990;52:449–58.

[18] Avoli M, Louvel J, Pumain R, Kohling R. Cellular and molecular mechanisms of epilepsy in the human brain. Prog Neurobiol 2005;77:166–200.

[19] Badawy RA, Harvey AS, Macdonell RA. Cortical hyperexcitability and epileptogenesis: understanding the mechanisms of epilepsy—part 1. J Clin Neurosci 2009;16:355–65.

[20] Xiao MY, Gustafsson B, Niu YP. Metabotropic glutamate receptors in the trafficking of ionotropic glutamate and GABAA receptors at central synapses. Curr Neuropharmacol 2006;4:77–86.

[21] Bateman DE, Hardy JA, McDermott JR, Parker DS, Edwardson JA. Amino acid transmitter levels in gliomas and their relationship to the incidence of epilepsy. Neurol Res 1988;10:112–4.

[22] Vezzani A, Gramsbergen JB, Speciale C, Schwarcz R. Production of quinolinic acid and kynurenic acid by human gliomas. Adv Exp Med Biol 1991;294: 691–5.

[23] Haglund MM, Berger MS, Kunkel DD, Franck JE, Ghatan S, Ojemann GA. Changes in gamma-aminobutyric acid and somatostatin in epileptic cortex associated with low-grade gliomas. J Neurosurg 1992;77:209–16.

[24] Aronica E, Crino PB. Inflammation in epilepsy: clinical observations. Epilepsia 2011;52 (3):26–32.

[25] Alapirtti T, Rinta S, Hulkkonen J, Makinen R, Keranen T, Peltola J. Interleukin-6, interleukin-1 receptor antagonist and interleukin-1beta production in patients with focal epilepsy: a video-EEG study. J. Neurol. Sci. 2009;280:94–97.

[26] Bauer S, Cepok S, Todorova-Rudolph A, Nowak M, Koller M, Lorenz R, Oertel WH, Rosenow F, Hemmer B, Hamer HM. Etiology and site of temporal lobe epilepsy influence postictal cytokine release. Epilepsy Res. 2009;86:82–88.

[27] Ravizza T, Vezzani A. Status epilepticus induces time-dependent neuronal and astrocytic expression of interleukin-1 receptor type I in the rat limbic system. Neuroscience 2006;137:301–308.

[28] Ravizza T, Gagliardi B, Noé F, Boer K, Aronica E, Vezzani A. Innate andadaptive immunity during epileptogenesis and spontaneous seizures: evidence from experimental models and human temporal lobe epilepsy. Neurobiol. Dis. 2008;29:142–160.

[29] Brenner AV, Butler MA, Wang SS, Ruder AM, Rothman N, Schulte PA, et al. Single-nucleotide polymorphisms in selected cytokine genes and risk of adult glioma. Carcinogenesis 2007;28:2543–7.

[30] Chao CC, Molitor TW, Hu S. Neuroprotective role of IL-4 against activated microglia. J Immunol 1993;151:1473–81.

[31] Block ML, Zecca L, Hong JS. Microglia-mediated neurotoxicity: uncovering the molecular mechanisms. Nat Rev Neurosci 2007;8:57–69.

[32] Hulkkonen J, Koskikallio E, Rainesalo S, Keranen T, Hurme M, Peltola J. The balance of inhibitory and excitatory cytokines is differently regulated in vivo and in vitro among therapy resistant epilepsy patients. Epilepsy Res 2004;59:199–205.

[33] Maroso M, Balosso S, Ravizza T, Liu J, Aronica E, Iyer AM, Rossetti C, Molteni M, Casalgrandi M, Manfredi AA, Bianchi ME, Vezzani A. Toll-like receptor 4 and high-mobility group box-1 are involved in ictogenesis and can be targeted to reduce seizures. Nat. Med. 2010;16:413–419.

[34] Riazi K, Galic MA, Pittman QJ. Contributions of peripheral inflammation to seizure susceptibility: cytokines and brain excitability. Epilepsy Res. 2010;89:34–42.

[35] Zurolo E, Iyer A, Maroso M, Carbonell C, Anink JJ, Ravizza T, Fluiter K, Spliet GWM, van Rijen PC, Vezzani A, Aronica E. Activation of TLR, RAGE and HMGB1 signaling in malformations of cortical development. Brain 2011;134: 1015–1032.

[36] Cacheaux LP, Ivens S, David Y, Lakhter AJ, Bar-Klein G, Shapira M, Heinemann U, Friedman A, Kaufer D. Transcriptome profiling reveals TGF-beta signaling involvement in epileptogenesis. J. Neurosci. 2009;29:8927–8935.

[37] Friedman A, Kaufer D, Heinemann U. Blood–brain barrier breakdown-inducing astrocytic transformation: novel targets for the prevention of epilepsy. Epilepsy Res. 2009;85:142–149.

[38] Shlosberg D, Benifla M, Kaufer D, Friedman A. Blood–brain barrier breakdown as a therapeutic target in traumatic brain injury. Nat. Rev. Neurol. 2010;6:393–403.

[39] Floyd RA. Antioxidants, oxidative stress, and degenerative neurological disorders, Proc Soc Exp Biol Med, Vol. 1999;222(3):236– 45

[40] Halliwell B. Role of free radicals in the neurodegenerative diseases: therapeuti implications for antioxidant treatment, Drugs Aging 2001;18:685-716.

[41] Spitz DS, Sim JE, Ridnour LA, Galoforo SS, Lee YJ. Glucose deprivation-induced oxidative stress in human tumor cells: a fundamental defect in metabolism?, Ann. N. Y. Acad. Sci. 2000;899:349-362.

[42] Vaughn AE, Deshmukh M. Glucose metabolism inhibits apoptosis in neurons and cancer cells by redoxin activation of cytochrome c, Nature Cell Biology 2008;10:1477-1483.

[43] Dajas F. Life or death:Neuroprotective and anti cancer effects of quercetin, Journal of Ethnopharmacology 2012;143(2):383-96.

[44] Oberley LW, Oberley TD, Buettner GR. Cell division in normal and transformed cells: the possible role of superoxide and hydrogen peroxide. Med. Hypoth. 1981;7:21-42.

[45] Atukeren P. The impact of redox balance in brain tumors. In: Garami M. (ed.) Molecular Targets Of CNS Tumors. InTech: 2012. p663– p674.

[46] Atukeren P., Yigitoglu MR. The stance of antioxidants in brain tumors. In: Lichter T. (ed.) Clinical Management And Evolving Novel Therapeutic Strategies For Patients With Brain Tumors. InTech: 2013. p523– p551.

[47] Kudin AP, Zsurka G, Elger CE, Kunz WS. Mitochondrial involvement in temporal lobe epilepsy. Exp. Neurol. 2009;218;326–332.

[48] Waldbaum S, Patel M. Mitochondria, oxidative stress, and temporal lobe epilepsy. Epilepsy Res. 2010;88:23–45.

[49] Schweizer U, Brauer AU, Kohrle J, Nitsch R, Savaskan NE. Selenium and brain function: A poorly recognized liaison. Brain Res Rev 2004;45:164-78.

[50] Savaskan NE, Brauer AU, Kuhbacher M, et al. Selenium deficiency increases susceptibility to glutamate-induced excitotoxicity. FASEB J 2003;17:112-4.

[51] Ashrafi MR, Shabanian R, Abbaskhanian A, Nasirian A, Ghofrani M, Mohammadi M, Zamani GR, Kayhanidoost Z, Ebrahimi S, Pourpak Z. Selenium and intractable epilepsy: is there any correlation? Pediatr Neurol. 2007;36(1):25-9.

[52] Kunz WS, Kudin AP, Vielhaber S, Blümcke I, Zuschratter W, Schramm J, Beck H, Elger CE. Mitochondrial complex I deficiency in the epileptic focus of patients with temporal lobe epilepsy. Ann. Neurol. 2000;48:766–773.

[53] Lee YM, Kang HC, Lee JS, Kim SH, Kim EY, Lee SK, Slama A, Kim HD. Mitochondrial respiratory chain defects: underlying etiology in various epileptic conditions. Epilepsia 2008;49:685–690.

[54] Chuang YCh, Chang AYW, Lin JW, Hsu SP, Chan SHH. Mitochondrial dysfunction and structural damage in the hippocampus during kainic acid-induced status epilepticus in the rat. Epilepsia 2004;45:1202–1209.

[55] Sleven H, Gibbs JE, Heales S, Thom M, Cock HR. Depletion of reduced glutathione precedes inactivation of mitochondrial enzymes following limbic status epilepticus in the rat hippocampus. Neurochem. Int. 2006;48:75–82.

[56] Folbergrová J, Ješina P, Drahota Z, Lisý V, Haugvicová R, Vojtíšková A, Houštěk J. Mitochondrial complex I inhibition in cerebral cortex of immature rats following homocysteic acid-induced seizures. Exp. Neurol. 2007;204: 597–609.

[57] Folbergrová J, Ješina P, Haugvicová R, Lisý V, Houštěk J. Sustained deficiency of mitochondrial complex I activity during long periods of survival after seizures induced in immature rats by homocysteic acid. Neurochem. Int. 2010;56:394–403.

[58] Fato R, Bergamini C, Leoni S, Strocchi P, Lenaz G. Generation of reactive oxygen species by mitochondrial complex I: implications in neurodegeneration. Neurochem. Res. 2008;33:2487–2501.

[59] Kudin AP, Bimpong-Buta NY, Vielhaber S, Elger CE, Kunz WS. Characterization of superoxide-producing sites in isolated brain mitochondria. J. Biol. Chem. 2004;279:4127–4135.

[60] Folbergrová J, Otáhal J, Druga R, Tsenov G, Haugvicová R, Kubová H. Effect of (S)-3,4 dicarboxyphenylglycine on epileptogenesis and cognitive impairment following seizures induced in immature rats by homocysteic acid. Epilepsia 2009;50(10): 335.

[61] Hollenbeck PJ, Saxton WM. The axonal transport of mitochondria. J. Cell Sci. 2005;118:5411–5419.

[62] Mattson MP, Gleichmann M, Cheng A. Mitochondria in neuroplasticity and neurological disorders. Neuron 2008;60:748–766.

[63] Zsurka G, Baron M, Stewart JD, Kornblum C, Bös M, Sassen R, Taylor RW, Elger CE, Chinnery PF, Kunz WS. Clonally expanded mitochondrial DNA mutations in epileptic individuals with mutated DNA polymerase gamma. J. Neuropathol. Exp. Neurol. 2008;67:857–866.

[64] Naviaux RK, Nguyen KV. POLG mutations associated with Alpers' syndrome and mitochondrial DNA depletion. Ann. Neurol. 2004;55:706–712.

[65] Zsurka G, Hampel KG, Nelson I, Jardel C, Mirandola SR, Sassen R, Kornblum C, Marcorelles P, Lavoué S, Lombès A, Kunz WS. Severe epilepsy as the major symptom of new mutations in the mitochondrial tRNA(Phe) gene. Neurology 2010;74:507–512.

[66] Zeviani M, Muntoni F, Savarese N, Serra G, Tiranti V, Carrara F, Mariotti C, DiDonato S. A MERRF/MELAS overlap syndrome associated with a new point mutation in the mitochondrial DNA tRNA(Lys) gene. Eur. J. Hum. Genet. 1993;1:80–87.

[67] Shoffner JM, Lott MT, Lezza AM, Seibel P, Ballinger SW, Wallace DC. Myoclonic epilepsy and ragged-red fiber disease (MERRF) is associated with a mitochondrial DNA tRNA(Lys) mutation. Cell 1990;61:931–937.

[68] Finsterer J, Jarius C, Eichberger H. Phenotype variability in 130 adult patients with respiratory chain disorders. Journal of Inherited Metabolic Disease 2001;224:560–76.

[69] Dale N, Frenguelli BG. Release of adenosine and ATP during ischemia and epilepsy. Curr. Neuropharmacol. 2009;7:160-179.

[70] Kovac S, Domijan AM, Walker MC, Abramov AY. Prolonged seizure activity impairs mitochondrial bioenergetics and induces cell death. J Cell Sci. 2012;1(125):1796-806.

[71] Wasterlain CG, Thompson KW, Suchomelova L, Niquet J. Brain energy metabolism during experimental neonatal seizures. Neurochem. Res. 2010;35:2193-2198.

[72] Astrup J, Sorensen PM, Sorensen HR. Oxygen and glucose consumption related to Na+–K+transport in canine brain. Stroke 1981;12:726–730.

[73] Ames A. CNS energy metabolism as related to function. Brain Res. Rev. 2000;34:42–68.

[74] Tang YG, Zucker RS. Mitochondrial involvement in post-tetanic potentiation of synaptic transmission. Neuron 1997;18:483–491.

[75] Duchen MR. Mitochondria and calcium: from cell signaling to cell death. J. Physiol. (London) 2000;529:57–68.

[76] Bindokas VP, Lee CC, Colmers WF, Miller RJ. Changes in mitochondrial function resulting from synaptic activity in the rat hippocampal slice. J. Neurosci. 1998;18:4570–4587.

[77] Trotti D, Danbolt NC, Voltera A, Glutamate transporters are oxidantvulnerable: a molecular link between oxidative and excitotoxic neurodegeneration? Trends Pharmacol. Sci. 1998;19:328–334.

[78] Kilbride SM, Telford JE, Tipton KF, Davey GP. Partial inhibition of complex I activity increases Ca-independent glutamate release rates from depolarized synaptosomes. J. Neurochem. 2008;106:826–834.

[79] Olivier A, Boling WW, Tanrıverdi T. Surgical Techniques in Epilepsy Surgery: The MNI Approach. Cambridge University Press, UK; 2012.

[80] Rogawski MA, Löscher W. The neurobiology of antiepileptic drugs. Nat. Rev. Neurosci. 2004;5:553–564.

[81] Temkin NR. Antiepileptogenesis and seizure prevention trials with antiepileptic drugs: meta-analysis of controlled trials, Epilepsia 2001;42:515–524.

[82] Loscher W. How to explain multidrug resistance in epilepsy? Epilepsy Curr 2005;5:107–12.

[83] Aldenkamp AP, De Krom M, Reijs R. Newer antiepileptic drugs and cognitive issues. Epilepsia 2003;44:21–29.

[84] Perucca E. An introduction to antiepileptic drugs. Epilepsia 2005;46:31–37.

[85] Wlodarczyk BJ, Palacios AM, George TM, Finnell RH. Antiepileptic drugs and pregnancy outcomes. Am. J. Med. Genet. 2012;58:2071–2090.

[86] Perucca P, Gilliam FG. Adverse effects of antiepileptic drugs. Lancet Neurol. 2012;11:792–802.

[87] Maertens P, Dyken P, Graf W, Pippenger C, Chronister R, Shah A. Free radicals, anticonvulsants, and the neuronal ceroid-lipofuscinoses. Am J Med Genet 1995;57:225-8.

[88] Mori A, Yokoi I, Noda Y, Willmore LJ. Natural antioxidants may prevent posttraumatic epilepsy: a proposal based on experimental animal studies. Acta Med Okayama 2004;58:111–8.

[89] Savaskan NE, Brauer AU, Kuhbacher M, et al. Selenium deficiency increases susceptibility to glutamate-induced excitotoxicity. FASEB J 2003;17:112-4.

[90] Ramaekers VT, Calomme M, Vanden Berghe D, Makropoulos W. Selenium deficiency triggering intractable seizures. Neuropediatrics 1994;25:217-23.

[91] Shetty AK. Promise of resveratrol for easing status epilepticus and epilepsy. Pharmacology Therapeutics 2011;131:269–86.

[92] Wu Z, Xu Q, Zhang L, Kong D, Ma R, Wang L. Protective effect of resveratrol against kainate-induced temporal lobe epilepsy in rats. Neurochemical Research 2009;34:1393–400.

[93] Gupta YK, Chaudhary G, Srivastava AK. Protective effect of resveratrol against pentylenetetrazole-induced seizures and its modulation by an adenosinergic system. Pharmacology 2002;65:170–4.

[94] Akhondian J, Kianifar H, Raoofziaee M, Moayedpour A, Toosi MB, Khajedaluee M. The effect of thymoquinone on intractable pediatric seizures (pilot study). Epilepsy Res 2011;93:39–43.

[95] Khopde SM, Priyadarsini KI, Mukherjee T, Kulkarni PB, Satav JG, Bhattacharya RK. Does beta-carotene protect membrane lipids from nitrogen dioxide? Free Radic Biol Med 1998;25:66–71.

[96] Plummer SM, Holloway KA, Manson MM, et al. Inhibition of cyclo-oxygenase 2 expression in colon cells by the chemopreventive agent curcumin involves inhibition of NF-kB activation via the NIK/IKK signaling complex. Oncogene 1999;18:6013–20.

[97] Wu A, Molteni R, Ying Z, Gomez-Pinilla F. A saturated-fat diet aggravates the outcome of traumatic brain injury on hippocampal plasticity and cognitive function by reducing brain-derived neurotrophic factor. Neuroscience 2003;119:365–75.

[98] Huang X, Zhang H, Yang J, Wu J, McMahon J, Lin Y, Cao Z, Gruenthal M, Huang Y. Pharmacological inhibition of the mammalian target of rapamycin pathway suppresses acquired epilepsy, Neurobiol. Dis. 2010;(40):193–199.

[99] Zeng LH, Xu L, Gutmann DH, Wong M. Rapamycin prevents epilepsy in a mouse model of tuberous sclerosis complex, Ann. Neurol. 2008;63:444–453.

[100] Beevers CS, Chen L, Liu L, Luo Y, Webster NJG, Huang S. Curcumin disrupts the mammalian target of rapamycin-raptor complex, Cancer Res. 2009;69:1000–1008.

[101] Jyoti A, Sethi P, Sharma D. Curcumin protects against electrobehavioral progression of seizures in the iron-induced experimental model of epileptogenesis, Epilepsy Behav. 2009;14:300–308.

[102] Marsh EB, Freeman JM, Kossoff EH, Vining EP, Rubenstein JE, Pyzik PL, Hemingway C. The outcome of children with intractable seizures: a 3-to 6-year follow-up of 67 children who remained on the ketogenic diet less than one year, Epilepsia 2006;47:425–430.

[103] Neal EG, Chaffe H, Schwartz RH, Lawson MS, Edwards N, Fitzsimmons G, Whitney A, Cross JH. The ketogenic diet for the treatment of childhood epilepsy: a randomised controlled trial, Lancet Neurol. 2008;7:500–506.

[104] Patel A, Pyzik PL, Turner Z, Rubenstein JE, Kossoff EH. Long-term outcomes of children treated with the ketogenic diet in the past, Epilepsia 2010;51:1277–1282.

[105] Freeman JM, Kossoff EH. Ketosis and the ketogenic diet, 2010: advances in treating epilepsy and other disorders. Adv. Pediatr. 2010;57:315-329.

[106] Cross JH, McLellan A, Neal EG, Philip S, Williams E, Williams RE. The ketogenic diet in childhood epilepsy: where are we now? Arch. Dis. Child. 2010;95:550-553.

[107] Bough K. Energy metabolism as part of the anticonvulsant mechanism of the ketogenic diet. Epilepsia 2008;49(8):91-93.

[108] Bough KJ, Wetherington J, Hassel B, Pare JF, Gawryluk JW, Greene JG, Shaw R, Smith Y, Geiger JD, Dingledine RJ. Mitochondrial biogenesis in the anticonvulsant mechanism of the ketogenic diet. Ann. Neurol. 2006;60:223-235.

[109] Borges K, Sonnewald U. Triheptanoin-A medium chain triglyceride with odd chain fatty acids: a new anaplerotic anticonvulsant treatment? Epilepsy Res 2011;100(3): 239-44.

[110] Shorvon S, Ferlisi M. The treatment of super-refractory status epilepticus: a critical review of available therapies and a clinical treatment protocol. Brain 201;134:2802-2818.

[111] Samoilova M, Weisspapir M, Abdelmalik P, Velumian, AA, Carlen PL. Chronic in vitro ketosis is neuroprotective but not anti-convulsant, J. Neurochem. 2010;113:826–835.

[112] Thio LL, Erbayat-Altay E, Rensing N, Yamada KA. Leptin contributes to slower weight gain in juvenile rodents on a ketogenic diet, Pediatr. Res. 2006;60:413–417.

[113] Sullivan PG, Rippy NA, Dorenbos K, Concepcion RC, Agarwal AK, Rho JM. The ketogenic diet increases mitochondrial uncoupling protein levels and activity. Ann. Neurol. 2004;55:576—580.

[114] Maalouf M, Sullivan PG, Davis L, Kim DY, Rho JM. Ketones inhibit mitochondrial production of reactive oxygen species production following glutamate excitotoxicity by increasing NADH oxidation. Neuroscience 2007;145:256—264.

[115] Kim DY, Rho JM. The ketogenic diet and epilepsy. Curr. Opin. Clin. Nutr. Metab. Care 2008;11:113—120.

[116] Norwood BA, Bauer S, Wegner S, Hamer HM, Oertel WH, Sloviter RS, Rosenow F. Electrical stimulation-induced seizures in rats: a "doseresponse" study on resultant neurodegeneration. Epilepsia 2011;52:109-112.

[117] Seyfried TN, Kiebish MA, Marsh J, Shelton LM, Huysentruyt LC, Mukherjee P. Metabolic management of brain cancer. Biochim Biophys Acta. 2011;1807(6):577-94.

[118] Aronica E, Fluiter K, Iyer A, Zurolo E, Vreijling J, van Vliet EA, Baayen JC, Gorter JA. Expression pattern of miR-146a, an inflammation-associated microRNA, in experimental and human temporal lobe epilepsy. Eur. J. Neurosci. 2010;31:1100–1107.

[119] Song YJ, Tian XB, Zhang S, Zhang YX, Li X, Li D, Cheng Y, Zhang JN, Kang CS, Zhao W. Temporal lobe epilepsy induces differential expression of hippocampal miRNAs including let-7e and miR-23a/b. Brain Res. 2011;1387:134–140.

Chapter 6

Alterations in *TP53* gene – Implications in Tumorigenesis Process and Prognosis in Central Nervous System Cancer

Igor Andrade Pessôa, Fabio P. Estumano da Silva,
Nilson Praia Anselmo and
Edivaldo Herculano C. de Oliveira

Additional information is available at the end of the chapter

http://dx.doi.org/10.5772/58334

1. Introduction

1.1. *TP53* Mutations and CNS tumors

Central nervous systems (CNS) malignancies, as others cancers, are formed by the uncontrolled cell growth that involves the sequential accumulation of alterations in genes controlling cell proliferation, lifespan, responses to stress, relationships with neighbors, and gene homeostasis. These genetic alterations can be achieved by intragenic mutations, chromosome alterations or epigenetics modifications, all playing important role in the activation or inactivation of key genes, such as oncogenes and tumor suppressor genes. Some of these mutations can be most frequently encountered in specific cancers or group of cancers and correlated with tumor biologic behavior and have implications on diagnosis, prognosis or treatment [1].

Biomarkers are important oncology tools in diagnostic, monitoring disease progression, helping in determining prognosis and predicting therapeutic response. Biomarkers vary from specific proteins and antigens to unique genetic, epigenetic or cytogenetic profiles, but common to all markers is that they provide specific information to a disease process. They function as supplementary and rarely supplanting, the histopathologic examination of tissues that is still the mainstay of traditional oncologic pathology [2, 3]. For this reason, we intend to compile the vast information about the important contribution of *TP53* gene as a biomarker in CNS cancer genesis, progression, stratification, prognosis, treatment and its importance to future targeted therapies.

INTECH
open science | open minds

© 2014 The Author(s). Licensee InTech. This chapter is distributed under the terms of the Creative Commons Attribution License (http://creativecommons.org/licenses/by/3.0), which permits unrestricted use, distribution, and reproduction in any medium, provided the original work is properly cited.

CNS cancers are heterogeneous diseases, arbitrarily grouped by the systems that are affected. The "WHO (World Health Organization) Classification of Tumors of the Central Nervous System" discriminates more than one hundred different diseases derived from different cell types, affecting patients of different ages, with a vast biological behavior and clinical implications. It is not our intention to describe the features of each CNS tumor. Hence, authors will follow the WHO classification for CNS tumors [4].

TP53 tumor suppressor gene is the most frequently mutated gene in human tumors and one of the most studied on different kinds of cancer. It is a large and complex gene located on chromosome site 17p13.1 (Figure 1). It has 11 exons along approximately 20.000bp. This gene codifies a protein with 393 amino acids in which different domains are responsible for diverse functions as exhibited on Figure 1. Genetic variations in this gene contribute to human cancers in many different ways. Firstly, somatic mutations are frequent in most cancers [5]: it is estimated that mutations in this gene are present in half of the human cancers. The antiproliferative role of p53 protein in response to various stresses and during physiological processes such as senescence makes it a primary target for inactivation [6], mainly by a combination of single-base substitution and loss of alleles [7]. Secondly, inheritance of a mutated *TP53* causes predisposition to early-onset cancers including breast carcinomas, sarcomas, brain tumors, and adrenal cortical carcinomas, defining the Li-Fraumeni (LFS) and Li-Fraumeni-like (LFL) syndromes [8, 9]. Thirdly, *TP53* is highly polymorphic in coding and noncoding regions and some of these polymorphisms have been shown to increase cancer susceptibility and to modify cancer phenotypes in *TP53* mutation carriers [10].

Commonly, advanced stage or aggressive behavior cancers have a higher frequency of *TP53* mutations [11, 12]. Moreover, in cancers with low mutation rates, p53 is often inactivated by alternative mechanisms, like protein degradation. *TP53* allelic deletion is also observed in many tumors, resulting in the reduction of expression of tetramers and decreased expression of genes inhibiting cell growth [13]. The cancer-associated somatic mutations in *TP53* are primarily missense substitutions (72.28%) nonrandomly distributed along the molecule, [14]. Over 90% of p53 mutations occur in the central DNA-binding-domain (Figure 1) into exons 4 – 9. These single aminoacid changes affect the transcriptional activity of the gene to various degrees; sometimes missense mutants may even acquire new functions [15, 16]. The *TP53* mutational pattern has proved to be a clinically relevant "molecular sensor" of genotoxic exposure to environmental carcinogens and endogenous mutagens [17].

Among single-base substitutions, about 25% are C:G>T:A substitutions at CpG sites. CpG dinucleotides mutate at a rate 10 times higher than other nucleotides, generating transitions [18]. About 3%–5% of cytosines in the human genome are methylated at position 5′ by a postreplicative mechanism that is restricted to CpG dinucleotides and is catalyzed by DNA methyltransferases. The 5′ methylcytosine (5mC) is less stable than cytosine and undergoes spontaneous deamination into thymine at a rate five times higher than the unmethylated base. This process is enhanced by oxygen and nitrogen radicals, leading to a higher load of CpG transitions in cancers arising from inflammatory precursors such as Barrett's mucosa or ulcerative colitis [19, 20]. Among the 22 CpG of the DNA-binding domain (DBD), three hotspot codons (175, 248, and 273) represent 60% of CpG mutations and another five residues (196, 213,

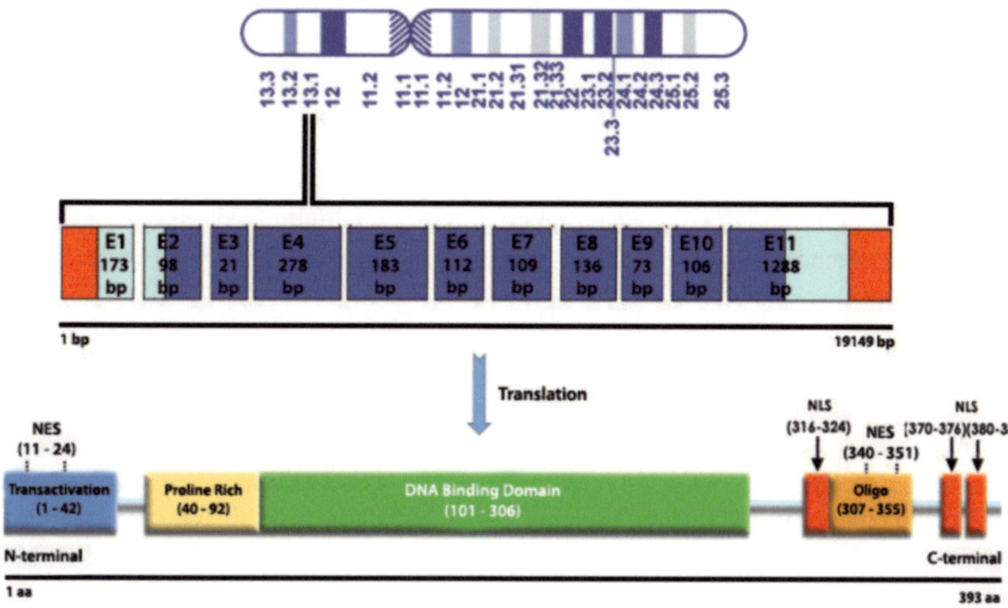

Figure 1. *TP53* gene: Structure, chromosome localization and protein domains distribution. *TP53* is mapped on human chromosome site 17p13.1. It is a long gene, with 19, 149 base pair comprising 11 exons that codify a protein with 393 amino acids long, in which the transactivation, proline-rich, DNA binding and the oligomerization domains are distributed. There are nuclear export/localization signals inside and between some domains (NES/NLS).

245, 282, and 306) account for 26% of these mutations. The lack of mutations at other CpG sites may reflect the fact that substitutions at these residues do not generate a dysfunctional protein. Although the same CpG hotspot mutations occur in many cancer types, other types of mutations tend to show differences among different cancers. Some of these differences have been linked to the effect of specific mutagens. This idea is endorsed by geographic differences which can be related to different environmental exposures [21].

All these mutational information about *TP53* are compiled in the International Agency for Research on Cancer (IARC) *TP53* Database [14], which provides structured data and analysis tools to study *TP53* mutations for specific cancers or investigate the functional and clinical impact of some mutations. The existence of this database, dedicated to annotate *TP53* mutations, polymorphism and respective implications in clinical and pathological behavior of human cancers, demonstrates the importance and the necessity of more knowledge to complete understand its implication on cancer [22].

Several studies have investigated the predictive value of *TP53* mutation status for tumor response to treatment and patient outcome in various cancers. However, different clinical and methodological settings have been used and the results have often been heterogeneous and contradictory [22]. The number and complexity of pathways in which *TP53* participates, the different mutational profiles of each cancer and the diverse environment conditions are variables that can contribute to these heterogeneous results.

The majority of mutations led to protein accumulation in the nucleus of the cells, which can be detected by immunohistochemistry (IHC) assays. Although some studies have shown an association between p53 positive immunostaining and poor outcomes, several studies have produced conflicting results and expectations on the use of p53 as a useful clinical biomarker failed [23]. Therefore, it seems IHC is a poor surrogate for gene mutation detection, as many mutations do not lead to protein accumulation, and because accumulation of wild-type p53 may also occur in the absence of gene mutation, producing a high rate of false negative and positive results. Hence, the use of IHC leads to an unacceptable number of misclassified cases and to a greater inter-study variability [1, 22].

By contrast, the screening for *TP53* mutations by gene sequencing, precisely identifying the mutation, have produced more consistent results, at least for some types of cancers such as breast, head and neck squamous cell carcinoma (HNSCC), and leukemia, in which the presence of a *TP53* mutation is associated with poor outcomes. In other types of cancer such as brain and pancreas, mutations were also found to be associated with both poor and good prognosis, depending on the study and cancer. These results show that the type of tissue and treatment may be important determinants of the prognostic and predictive value of *TP53* mutations [1, 22]. Figure 2 illustrates the use of different techniques in the evaluation of mutational status of *TP53* and expression of p53 protein in gliomas. Fluorescence *in Situ* Hybridization (FISH), sequencing and IHC techniques.

2. *TP53* genetic alterations in CNS tumors

CNS tumors have historically been classified on the basis of morphological and, more recently, immunohistochemical features with less emphasis on their underlying molecular pathogenesis. The past two decades, however, have seen striking advances in basic brain tumor biology, especially with regard to malignant gliomas and medulloblastomas, the most common CNS cancers of adults and children, respectively [24, 25]. Molecular signatures of tumors may play roles as diagnostic, prognostic, and predictive markers and influence the clinical decision making process. A dynamic classification of tumors is critical for the continuous integration of newly established molecular tools. This topic focuses on various genetics and epigenetics *TP53* changes in the CNS tumors which have been integrated into daily practice and gained significance for molecular diagnostic testing. Detailed discussion of neuronal and mixed neuronal-glial tumors, tumors of the pineal region, tumors of cranial and paraspinal nerves, mesenchymal tumors, lymphomas and haematopoietic neoplasms and other tumor entities is beyond the scope of this chapter, especially because there is only limited molecular information used in clinical management available for this types of tumors.

2.1. Gliomas

Gliomas are the most frequent primary brain tumors and include a variety of different histological types and malignancy grades. Although the cellular origin of gliomas is still unknown, experimental data in mice suggest an origin from neoplastically transformed neural

http://dx.doi.org/10.5772/58334

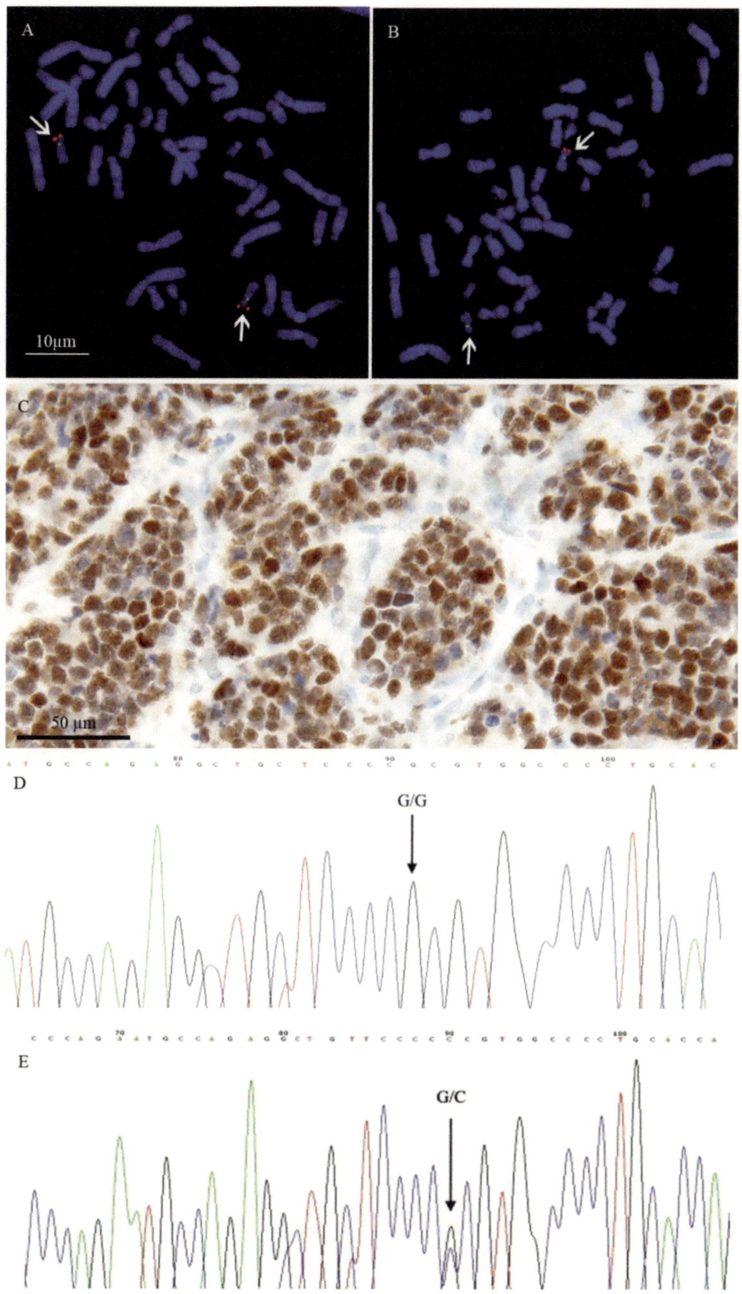

Figure 2. Different approaches used in the analysis of *TP53* gene in gliomas. (A) and (B) FISH experiments using *TP53* locus specific probe (red) and 17 centromeric probe (green) in metaphase chromosomes. A normal pair of chromosome 17 is showed in (A), while a heterozygous deletion of *TP53* can be observed in (B). (C) Immunopositive p53 sample, demonstrated by immunohistochemical staining. (D) Electropherogram of an patient with the wild type sequence (CGC) in the codon 72 while (E) illustrates a base exchange mutation in this position (CCC) predicting de aminoacid substitution arginine → proline.

stem or progenitor cells. However, histological classification of gliomas essentially relies on morphological similarities of the tumor cells with non-neoplastic glial cells and the presence of particular architectural features; thereby, most gliomas can be classified as astrocytic, oligodendroglial, mixed oligoastrocytic or ependymal tumors according to the criteria of the WHO classification of CNS tumors [4]. Clinical experiences derived from the prospective randomized clinical trials have shown that the histomorphological criteria alone might not be sufficient to predict the clinical outcome. Moreover, lately integrated genomic studies and exome sequencing have revealed the existence of multiple distinct molecular subtypes within histologically similar looking tumors [26]. For instance, even gliomas with identical histopathological features differ considerably regarding clinical course or response to therapy.

Knowledge of the genetic alterations in the various types and malignancy grades of gliomas has drastically increased over the past years. The evolution of classical tumor molecular and cytogenetic techniques, as well as the development of newer array-based assays of comparative genomic hybridization and RNA expression, allowed subclasses of gliomas to be identified based on molecular or gene expression patterns, showing substantial genetic and gene-expression heterogeneity within and between histologic grades of different histologic types of gliomas [27]. These approaches have identified point mutations and copy number changes (deletions, amplifications, gains) in several regions; deletions and loss of heterozygosity in tumors might point to genes involved in tumor suppression, whereas amplifications and gains might point to genes involved in initiation or progression processes (e.g. oncogenes) [28].

Numerous molecular abnormalities have been associated to the underlying biology of gliomas. The p53 pathway is nearly invariably altered in sporadic gliomas: loss of p53, through either point mutations that prevent DNA binding or deletion in chromosome 17p, is a frequent and early event in the pathological progression of secondary glioblastoma (GBM) [29, 30]. The importance of p53 in gliomagenesis is also underscored by the increased incidence of gliomas in LFS, a familial cancer-predisposition syndrome associated with germline p53 mutations [31]. This genetic linkage has been reinforced by a glioma-prone condition in mice engineered with a commonly observed Li-Fraumeni p53 mutation [32] as well as in $p19^{ARF}$-null mice, albeit at a low frequency [33]. In human gliomas, p53 mutations are primarily missense mutations and target the evolutionarily conserved domains in exons 5, 7, and 8, thus affecting residues that are crucial to DNA binding [30].

The finding that a second promoter drives an alternatively spliced transcript at the *CDKN2A* locus prompted the discovery of an additional tumor suppressor gene that is inactivated at this locus [34]. The second protein encoded by *CDKN2A*, $p14^{ARF}$, was subsequently shown to be an important accessory to p53 activation under conditions of oncogenic stress due to its neutralization of the p53 ubiquitin ligase, *MDM2* [35, 36], an oncogene originally discovered amplified as double minute chromosomes in a spontaneously transformed murine cell line, and then later found to be a key negative regulator of p53 during normal development and in tumorigenesis [37-39]. Concordantly, the chromosomal region containing *MDM2*, 12q14-15, is amplified in ~10% of primary GBM, the majority of which contain intact p53 [40]. The discovery of the *MDM2*-related gene, *MDM4* (chromosome 1q32), which inhibits p53 transcription and enhances the ubiquitin ligase activity of MDM2, prompted the finding that the p53 pathway is also inactivated by the amplification of *MDM4* in 4% of GBM with neither *TP53* mutation nor *MDM2* amplification [41, 42]. Additionally, the recently discovered tumor suppressor gene *CHD5* (chromodomain helicase DNA-binding domain 5), which maps to chromosome 1p36 and is therefore frequently hemizygously deleted in those human gliomas with loss of 1p, has been shown to maintain p53 levels by facilitating expression of p19 ^{Arf} (mouse p14^{ARF} ortholog), and thus presents an additional mechanism for inactivation of this critical pathway [43].

2.1.1. Astrocytic tumors

The incidence of *TP53* mutations in pilocytic astrocytomas is controversial, with some authors reporting only infrequent mutations [44-47], while more common mutations are rare [48]. Hayes *et al.* [48], were the first to find a higher rate of *TP53* mutations in an analysis of 20 pilocytic astrocytomas in children, based on a comprehensive denaturing gradient gel electrophoresis mutation detection assay of the entire coding region, including all splice site junctions of *TP53*, showed mutations considered as causative in 7 of the 20 (35%) pilocytic astrocytomas. Few Cytogenetic studies have been carried out, showing allelic losses on both 17p and 17q including the *TP53* and *NF1* loci in pilocytic astrocytomas [49]. These results suggest that *TP53* mutations may well play a role in the development of these tumors.

TP53 mutations are a genetic hallmark of low-grade diffuse astrocytomas, for > 60% of these tumors carrying mutations in this gene [47, 50], mainly in gemistocytic astrocytomas with *TP53* mutations in up to 80% of the cases [51, 52]. In most cases, *TP53* mutation is accompanied by loss of heterozygosity (LOH) on 17p resulting in the complete absence of the wild-type *TP53* gene. Those diffuse astrocytomas with no *TP53* mutations may have altered the p53-dependent growth control by alternative mechanisms, for example, promotor methylation of the *p14* ^{ARF} gene at 9p21. Nakamura *et al.* [53] found hypermethylation of *p14*^{ARF} in one third of low-grade diffuse astrocytomas samples. These results suggest that aberrant *p14*^{ARF} expression due to homozygous deletion or promoter hypermethylation is associated with the evolution of both primary and secondary GBMs, and that *p14*^{ARF} promoter methylation is an early event in subset of astrocytomas that undergo malignant progression to secondary GBM.

Studies assessing the presence of *TP53* mutations as predictor of clinical outcome in diffuse astrocytomas have been made and the results are controversial. However most of them associated the presence of *TP53* mutations to a poor prognosis [51, 54, 55]. Peraud *et al.* [54] analyzed retrospectively timing, frequency, and prognostic impact of *TP53* mutations and p53 protein accumulation in 159 patients consecutively treated at a single neurosurgical clinic. *TP53* mutations were frequently found and univariate analysis found that gemistocytic subtype and *TP53* mutation were associated with worse prognosis, with only the gemistocytic subtype remaining an unfavourable prognostic factor on multivariate analysis. In non-gemistocytic astrocytomas, a mutation in *TP53* hot spot codon 175 indicated a worse prognosis in terms of time to progression and malignancy.

Xanthoastrocytoma pleomorphic (PXAs) are rare astrocytic malignancies classified as grade II lesions by the WHO. Because of the relative rarity of this lesion, the molecular background is still unclear. Among the abnormalities frequently observed in astrocytic tumors, PXA shares only *TP53* mutations, and, although *TP53* mutations in anaplastic PXA have previously been reported, the significance of this alteration for tumor malignant progression is not clear [56, 57].The high frequency of *TP53* mutations in low-grade astrocytomas raises the question of whether these alterations play an important role in the tumorigenesis of PXA. Paulus and coworkers [58] reported the highest frequency of TP53 mutations, around 25%. However, in contrast, Giannini *et al.* [59] identified mutation in only 1 of 47 samples, all of which were nonrecurrent lesions and all lacked anaplastic transformation, while Bettegowda *et al.* [60] sequenced the exomes of 12 PXAs and identified mutation in only 2 cases.

Anaplastic astrocytomas, from a clinical, morphologic and genetic point of view, represents an intermediate stage on the route of progression to GBM. They exhibit high *TP53* mutation rate (40-70%) similar to diffuse astrocytomas and high frequency of LOH at 17p [61, 62]. In a study of almost 200 astrocytomas of grades II-IV, 72% of anaplastic astrocytomas were found to have a disruption in the p53 pathway [63].

An important clue to pathways involved in gliomagenesis may lie in the two GBM subtypes that have been clinically identified [50]. Primary GBM is typically present in older patients as aggressive, highly invasive tumor, usually without any evidence of prior clinical disease. Secondary GBM have a very different clinical history, being usually observed in younger patients who initially presented low-grade astrocytoma that transformed in GBM within 5–10 years of the initial diagnosis, regardless of prior therapy. The cataloging of genetic lesions in these GBM subtypes has identified differences in their genetic profiles, predominantly in the penetrance of specific genetic mutations. As a result, it has been proposed that primary and secondary GBMs represent two distinct clinical entities, each developing along distinct genetic pathways [50].

TP53 mutations are a genetic hallmark of secondary GBM, because these tumors have a high incidence of mutations in this gene (>65%), suggesting that p53 pathway plays a crucial role in their development tumors [62, 64-66]. *TP53* mutations are the first detectable genetic alteration in > 60% of precursor low-grade diffuse astrocytomas or in anaplastic astrocytomas in a similar frequency, and secondary GMBs derived thereof [64, 67]. *TP53* mutations also is present in primary GMBs, but with significantly lesser frequency (25-30% of cases) [47, 67]. Giant cell glioblastoma, a histological variant of GBM, carry *TP53* mutations in high frequency (75 – 90%) [68, 69], while gliosarcoma, another GBM variant characterized by a biphasic tissue pattern, has a lower *TP53* mutation rate (23–24%) [70, 71], and identical *TP53* mutations in both gliomatous and sarcomatous components [70].

In secondary GBMs, 57% of mutations have been reported to be located in the two hotspot codons 248 and 273; however, in primary GBMs, mutations were more equally distributed through all exons, with only 17% occurring in codons 248 and 273 [67]. Furthermore, G:C > A:T transitions at CpG sites were significantly more frequent in secondary than in primary GBMs [67]. The less specific pattern of *TP53* mutations in primary GBMs suggests a different molecular mechanism underlying the acquisition of *TP53* mutations in these subtypes.

Amplification of *MDM2* is present in < 10% of GBMs, and this event appears to be associated to primary GBMs with no *TP53* mutations [72]. Loss of p14 ^{ARF} expression has been observed frequently in GBMs (76%), and correlated with homozygous deletion or promoter methylation of the p14 ^{ARF} gene [53]. Comparing the overall frequency of p14 ^{ARF} alterations between primary and secondary GBMs, no significant difference was observed, while p14 ^{ARF} promoter methylation was more frequent in secondary than primary GBMs [53]. The analysis of multiple biopsies from the same patients revealed p14 ^{ARF} methylation already in one-third of low-grade astrocytomas [53].

But, have all these data any prognostic value for GBMs? Although there is some discordance among different studies, promising data have already been gained. Hence, some studies showed no association between *TP53* status and outcome of GBM patients [73, 74] or between p53 score analyzed by IHC and patient survival [75]. Schmidt *et al.* [76] analyzed 97 GBM cases and found that the presence of *TP53* mutations was a favorable prognostic factor. In the same way, Ohgaki *et al.* [67] showed that the presence of *TP53* mutations was a favorable prognostic factor, and at the population level, univariate analysis revealed that the presence of these mutations was predictive of longer survival; however, age-adjusted multivariate analysis revealed no difference in survival between patients with and without *TP53* alterations.

El Hallani *et al.* [77] showed that the Pro/Pro genotype (a functional single nucleotide polymorphism at codon 72 of *TP53* gene results in the presence of either proline (Pro) or arginine (Arg) in the amino acid sequence) is significantly over-represented in young patients with GBM (<45 years) (7 of 43 cases, 16.3%) compared to older patients (>45 years) (14 of 217, 6.5%) (P=0.05), whereas no difference of frequencies for Arg/Arg versus Arg/Pro between the two groups were observed. These data suggest a recessive effect of the Pro allele on the oncogenesis of GBM in young patients. This result is in line with previous reports showing consistent associations between the codon 72 polymorphism with age of onset in oral cancer, head and neck carcinomas, hereditary nonpolyposis colorectal cancer, and prostate cancer [78, 79]. The polymorphism described by El Hallani *et al.* [77] at *TP53* codon 72 is associated with age at onset of glioblastoma. In a study in 2009, Zawlik et al. (66) revealed that *TP53* codon 72 Pro allele was significantly associated with shorter survival among patients with GBMs carrying a *TP53* mutation (Arg/Pro or Pro/Pro), and among those treated with surgery plus radiotherapy (Arg/Pro).

Considering the association between mutations and treatments, recent studies have shown that the status of the *TP53* gene interferes with the effectiveness of treatment by DNA alkylating agent temozolomide (TMZ), the most effective chemotherapeutic for GBM. Blough *et al.* [80] related that GBM cell lines that did not express a functional p53 were significantly more sensitive to TMZ than cell lines with functionally intact wild-type p53 expression, while altered p53 expression or function had only minor effects on TMZ sensitivity in brain tumor initiating cells and tended to decrease sensitivity to TMZ.

2.1.2. Oligodendroglial and oligoastrocytic tumors

In contrast to diffuse astrocytomas, loss of 17p and *TP53* mutations are rare in oligodendroglial tumors (~10%) and mutually exclusive to 1p/19q deletion, a hallmark alteration in oligodendrogliomas (~ 70%), while oligoastrocytomas frequently carry either *TP53* mutations (~40%)

or loss of 1p/19q (~45%), indicating that oligoastrocytomas are genetically monoclonal, and carry genetic alterations similar to either diffuse astrocytomas or oligodendrogliomas. Furthermore, G:C > A:T transitions at CpG sites are the most frequent *TP53* mutations in these tumors [81-83]. According to Muller *et al.* [84] oligoastrocytomas in the temporal lobe showed LOH on 1p and 19q less frequently (33%) than *TP53* mutations (45%). In contrast, oligoastrocytomas arising outside the temporal lobe demonstrated LOH on 1p and 19q in nearly 75% of the cases while *TP53* mutations were found in less than 20% [85].

Watanabe *et al.* [86] reported that genetic alterations in the p53 pathway are more frequent in anaplastic oligodendroglioma (50%) than in oligodendroglioma WHO grade II (21%), and showed that simultaneous disruption of the *RB1/CDK4/p16* ^{INK4a} */p15* ^{INK4b} and the *TP53/p14* ^{ARF} */MDM2* pathways occurs in 45% (9/20) of anaplastic oligodendrogliomas, suggesting that these phenomena contribute to their malignant phenotype. Anaplastic oligoastrocytoma typically exhibits the type and distribution of molecular lesions observed in oligoastrocytoma: loss of 1p/19q or *TP53* mutations [84].

A number of genetic alterations have been correlated with poorer response to chemotherapy or worse overall survival in anaplastic oligodendrogliomas. Ino *et al.* [87] suggested that a variety of relatively infrequent genetic alterations (*EGFR* gene amplification, 10q loss, *CDKN2A* homozygous deletion, *PTEN* mutation, and *TP53* mutation) were associated with worse prognosis. Interestingly, *TP53* mutation was associated with an improved likelihood of chemotherapeutic response but with a poor overall prognosis, since responses were not durable in the setting of *TP53* mutation.

Kim *et al.* [83] evaluated 413 tumors confirmed as low-grade diffuse gliomas WHO grade II (206 diffuse astrocytomas, 73 oligoastrocytomas, and 134 oligodendrogliomas) and observed that the median survival of patients with *TP53* mutation combined with *IDH1/2* mutation was significantly shorter than the observed in patients with 1p/19q loss combined with *IDH1/2* mutation (51.8 months vs. 58.7 months, respectively; P=0.0037). A Multivariate analysis with adjustment for age and treatment confirmed these results (P=0.0087) and also revealed that *TP53* mutation is a significant prognostic marker for shorter survival (P=0.0005) and 1p/19q loss for longer survival (P=0.0002).

2.1.3. Ependymal tumors

TP53 mutations were rarely reported in ependymal tumors by molecular analysis [88, 89]. However, p53 protein is identified in about 60% of ependymal tumors [90]. Shuangshoti *et al.* [91] suggested that the discrepancy may be due to expression of wild type p53 gene in tumor cells, alternative mechanisms of p53 gene inactivation or simply a cross-reaction of the antigen-antibody complex.

A number of studies have documented a correlation between p53 expression and tumor grade in ependymomas [90, 92, 93]. Sharma *et al.* [94] analyzed p53 protein expression in 119 ependymomas tumors (17 cases were of grade I, 54 of grade II and 48 of grade III) and observed its expression in only two cases of grade I tumors (11.5% and 6.4%). Five cases of grade II tumors showed p53 protein expression and this percentage of nuclear positivity was very low

(< 1.0%), while eighteen of 48 grade III tumors (37.5%) showed expression of p53 and mean positivity was 5.5%. Manasa *et al.* [95] reported 66% p53 positivity, performing p53 immunohistochemical analysis in 54 samples of different grades and subtypes of ependymomas and observed that p53 indices were higher in grade II and grade III tumors (26.27 % and 26.08% respectively) as compared to subependymomas (grade I) (7.25%). However, p53 index of myxopapillary ependymoma (grade I) (26%) was similar to grade II and grade III tumors. But these values did not show statistical significance (P=0.2). Papillary ependymoma (grade II) showed p53 expression in 24% cells.

Some authors have advocated that p53 immunolabeling are important prognostic markers in ependymomas. Zamecnik *et al.* [96] found that p53 immunopositivity is the strongest indicator of aggressive tumor behavior and poor prognosis. Gaspar *et al.*, [88] studied the p53 pathway in primary intracranial childhood ependymomas and p53-mediated response to DNA-damage in two newly described ependymoma xenograft models. Their findings do not suggest a role of p53 genetic/epigenetic alterations in the tumorigenesis or progression of childhood ependymomas; however, radioresistance of these tumors might be due to alterations in p53-mediated growth arrest. Despite the lack of *TP53* mutations, immunocytochemical accumulation of p53 occurs, particularly in tumors with poor outcome. Moreover, the data concerning immunoexpression of the p53 protein indicate its usefulness in identification of more aggressive clones in ependymomas and its superior predictive value [94].

2.2. Embryonal tumors

2.2.1. Medulloblastoma

The genetic and genomic understanding of medulloblastoma (MB) has evolved dramatically in the past few years, but the role of p53 in MB pathogenesis has only initiated to be elucidated. Patients with LFS, caused by a germline mutation in p53, develop MB at a higher incidence than the general population [97, 98]. Similarly, p53 deficiency in mice in combination with mutations in other genes, including poly (ADP-ribose) polymerase (PARP), the cell cycle regulatory protein retinoblastoma (Rb), or the Sonic hedgehog (Shh) receptor Patched1 (Ptch1), greatly increases tumor incidence [99, 100], indicating that loss of p53 can promote MB tumorigenesis. However, in contrast with the high incidence of p53 mutations in most human tumors, the *TP53* gene is altered in <10% of sporadic human MB. Chromosome 17p, where *TP53* is located, is lost in 40% to 50% of sporadic MB tumors. However, it has been found that losses of 17p and p53 status are unrelated in MB [101, 102].

New support for a role for p53 in MB tumorigenesis came from a better understanding of heterogeneity underlying MB tumors. Recently, several groups were able to demonstrate that although morphologically similar, MBs could be divided into several subgroups on the basis of expression profiling [103, 104]. A consensus meeting resulted in the current molecular subclassification of MB into four subgroups: wingless (WNT), sonic hedgehog (SHH), group 3, and group 4 [105]. Hopefully, in the near future, this subclassification will be used to select targeted therapies and improve understanding of the behavior of this disease.

As observed for other CNS, reports detailing the prognostic impact of *TP53* mutations in MB offer conflicting conclusions. Pfaff *et al.* [106] reported that *TP53* mutations occur at low frequency in MBs but are overrepresented in the prognostically favorable subgroup featuring alterations in the Wnt pathway. In addition, because no correlation between *TP53* mutation status and patient outcome was observed in more than 300 patients, these authors concluded that *TP53* mutation is not a universal prognostic marker for MB. These results were supported by Lindsey *et al.* [107] in an independent and representative series of all major established clinical and molecular subtypes of MBs. Nevertheless, Gessi *et al.* [108] reported that *TP53* expression is associated with rapid disease progression and poor prognosis in patients with metastatic MB, with a statistically significant inverse correlation between *TP53* expression and patient survival.

A large whole-genome and exome sequencing efforts recently published by different groups revealed an additional, albeit small number, of *TP53* mutations in MB [109, 110]. These independent groups found *TP53* mutations enriched in the SHH group and associated with poor survival. Zhukova *et al.* [111] evaluated the association of *TP53* mutations, molecular groups, and survival in MBs patients and confirmed that *TP53* mutations are enriched among SHH MBs, in which they portend poor outcome and account for a large proportion of treatment failures in these patients.

Carvalho *et al.* [112] were the first to investigate the role of the *TP53* Arg72Pro SNP as a potential risk factor and/or prognostic marker of MB by performing a case–control analysis using a polymerase chain reaction-restriction fragment length polymorphism approach. The date suggested that, although there is no association between the *TP53* Arg72Pro SNP and MB risk, the Pro/Pro genotype is associated with shorter overall survival of patients submitted to adjuvant therapy.

Some researchers justify the p53 inactivation in MB tumors lacking *TP53* gene mutations through alternative mechanisms. Mendrysa *et al.* [113] supported MDM2 as an important contributor to the inhibition of p53 in SHH-driven MB tumorigenesis. In cerebellar development, *MDM2* is required to inhibit p53-mediated apoptosis in granular neuronal precursors, the presumed cell of origin for MB tumors of the Shh subgroup, and *MDM2* deficiency potently restricts cerebellar tumorigenesis in Ptch1+/– mice, a model of human Shh-induced MB.

2.2.2. *CNS primitive neuroectodermal tumors*

The presence of *TP53* mutations have been identified in CNS primitive neuroectodermal tumors (PNETs), mainly in adult patients [114]. However, *TP53* mutations in PNET have also been occasionally reported in children [115, 116], but the overall incidence of somatic *TP53* mutation in pediatric CNS-PNET seems to be very low [115]. Gessi *et al.* [117] analyzed the clinicopathologic and molecular features of 12 cases of PNETs in adult patients. The p53 staining showed strong nuclear positivity (>20% of stained nuclei) in 9 cases, evidencing the presence of *TP53* mutations in these tumors. The use of single strand conformation polymorphism (SSCP) followed by sequencing of the *TP53* gene showed point mutations of this gene in 4 of these 9 cases, identifying 5 mutations in exons 4, 5, 7, and 8.

Although the presence of *TP53* mutations seems to mainly occur in adult s-PNETs, nuclear accumulation of p53 has been described to be frequent not only in adults but also in pediatric CNS-PNETs [118]. This observation led to the hypothesis that the p53 pathway is pivotal in CNS-PNET biology and can also be activated by mechanisms other than mutation.

Immunohistochemical staining for the p53 gene product is a good predictor of poor outcome in PNETs. Robert *et al.* [119] observed stained intensely for the p53 protein in 10 patients (n=40) with PNETs and 11 had weakly staining nuclei, while 19 specimens had no staining. The patients with specimens that stained intensely had a statistically significant decreased disease free survival (P=0. 03). Intense p53 immunostaining may predict a poor prognosis in PNETs of childhood [120], however, the significance of p53 in recurrent CNS PNETs is unknown.

2.2.3. *Atypical teratoid/ Rhabdoid tumor*

The role of p53 in atypical teratoid/ rhabdoid tumor (AT/RT) is also poorly understood. Cell lines established from malignant rhabdoid tumor (MRT) show overexpression of p53, without associated *TP53* gene mutations [120]. On the other hand, missense mutations in *TP53* were reported in 3/6 cases of non-CNS MRT [121]. Knockdown of *SMARCB1* in cell lines and animal models results in activation of p53 [122, 123]. Intriguingly, combined inactivation of *Smarcb1* and *TP53*, but not *Rb* or $p16^{ink4a}$, leads to accelerated development of MRT in mouse models [122, 124]. These data have led to the hypothesis that two successive hits involving *SMARCB1* and *TP53* may contribute to malignant transformation and tumor development. Venneti *et al.* [125] studied the expression of p53 and determined *TP53* mutational status in 36 AT/RT and 16 non-CNS MRT patients. They also studied the relationship of p53 expression with its regulators $p14^{ARF}$/*MDM2* in AT/RT and non-CNS MRT. p14 ^{ARF} expression was seen in many cases, which correlated positively with p53 and inversely with Mdm2 immunostaining in AT/RT, while *TP53* mutational analysis in 19/25 AT/RT and 8 in 11 non-CNS MRT cases showed point mutations in only 3 AT/RT cases, suggesting that p53 expression was driven mainly by p14 ^{ARF}.

2.3. Choroid plexus tumors

Choroid plexus tumors (CPT) are rare tumors, often occurring during childhood. Previous studies have shown high frequencies of germline *TP53* mutations in patients with CPT (44–100%) irrespective of family history [126, 127]. According to the latest clinical criteria for LFS, it is suggested that patients with CPT should be considered for *TP53* testing [128, 129]. In addition, somatic mutations of the *TP53* gene and subsequent accumulation of p53 protein have been described in up to 50 % of choroid plexus carcinomas (CPC) [130, 131].

The prognostic role of p53 in choroid plexus carcinomas has been recently demonstrated. Tabori *et al.* [131] studied 54 patients with CPTs, including CPC (n=36) and choroid plexus papilloma (CPP) (n=18), and demonstrated that patients with CPC who have low tumor total structural variation and absence of *TP53* dysfunction had a favorable prognosis and could be successfully treated without radiation therapy. Krzyzankova *et al.*, [132], investigated the role of p53 in the growth-inhibitory potential of a variety of anticancer agents in the immortalized rodent choroid plexus epithelial cell line Z310 and observed that growth-inhibitory activity of vincristine, doxorubicin, carboplatin, etoposide, and TMZ was significantly impaired by silencing of *TP53*, showing the potential predictive role of p53 in choroid plexus carcinomas.

2.4. Meningiomas

Few studies have examined the *TP53* gene directly for mutations in meningiomas, [133-135], and these studies typically have not observed mutations in this gene, although rare mutants have been described, mainly associated with malignant histology [134, 136]. One group working on specimens from Korean patients has documented a rate of nearly 40% of p53 over-expressing meningiomas as having mutations, and observed that the mutation rate was associated with both histological grade and recurrence [137].

In contrast the low frequency of *TP53* point mutations, expression of p53 was found in 10% to 90% of meningiomas [138], but their role in pathogenesis is still uncertain. Studies suggested the involvement of the p53 pathway in meningioma development: the correlation of p53 protein expression with histological tumor grade and meningioma recurrence [139]; methylation of the $p14^{ARF}$ gene in 8.6% of benign, 20% of atypical and in 50% of anaplastic meningiomas and loss of detectable Mdm2 protein in high grade meningiomas [140]; defective p53 response to gamma ray stress in meningioma cells [141]. In addition, the *NF2* protein product was reported to increase p53 stability through downregulation of Mdm2 levels in mouse fibroblast [142]. It follows that loss of NF2 may increase the likelihood of p53 suppression, thus decreasing tumor suppression activity and providing a possible mechanism for the involvement of the p53 pathway in meningiomas.

Many studies have examined benign and atypical/malignant meningiomas for over-expression of the p53 protein with diverse results: p53 over-expression has been reported in 0–10% of benign, 50–72.7% of atypical and 77–88.9% of anaplastic or malignant meningiomas [143]. Despite the differing rates, all of the studies are consistent, with atypical/malignant tumors showing higher rates of over-expression than benign meningiomas. However, studies on the biological significance of p53 over-expression are highly contradictory. While over-expression of p53 has been associated with recurrence in some studies [139, 144], no association has been found in others [133, 145]; and still other studies have suggested that expression of high levels of p53 may be protective against recurrence [146].

Terzi *et al.* [147] analyzed the immunohistochemical expression of Ki-67, p53, p21, p16, and *PTEN* proteins in 130 meningiomas (64 benign, 39 atypical, and 27 malignant meningiomas) using tissue microarray and demonstrated that Histological grade, p53, Ki-67 labeling indices, and overexpression of p16 were strongly associated with decreased event-free survival in univariate analysis and Ki-67 and p53 labeling indices are useful additional tools in discriminating atypical from benign or anaplastic meningiomas.

3. Epigenetic mechanisms in CNS tumors

Epigenetics is defined as mitotically heritable changes in gene expression that are not due to changes in the primary DNA sequence. The coordinated interaction of these changes regulates gene expression activity and several types of epigenetic marks work in concert to drive appropriate gene expression, like DNA methylation at CpG dinucleotides, covalent modifications of histone proteins, non-coding RNAs, and other complementary mechanisms controlling higher order chromatin organization within the cell nucleus. Epigenetic alterations have been recognized as important mechanisms in neoplastic transformation, malignant progression of cancer, and although epigenetic changes are somatically inheritable, they are reversible and hence may represent actionable targets for novel therapies [148, 149]

Epigenetic changes are often observed at the earliest stages of neoplasia within the altered tissue stem and progenitor cells. These observations have led to the epigenetic progenitor model [149]. This model explains that transformation to a malignant state occurs in three steps. First, there is an expansion of an epigenetically permissive population due to an essential early epigenetic disruption of stem/progenitor cells. Second, an initiating genetic alteration in an oncogene or tumor suppressor gene occurs. Finally, genetic and epigenetic plasticity resulting in an enhanced ability to stably evolve the phenotype is observed. An important difference to the clonal genetic model is that the epigenetic 'hits' occur early, and are necessary to create an appropriate expansion of a polyclonal population, that is the cellular substrate for subsequent genetic alterations and transformation [150].

To better understand the multiple cellular pathways involved in their development, establishment markers of resistance to traditional therapies, and contribution to the development of targeted therapies, a comprehensive appreciation of the integrated genomics and epigenomics of CNS tumors is needed [151].

3.1. DNA methylation of gene *TP53*

Hypermethylation of promoters usually occurs at CpG islands. Methylation of *TP53* was reported as a mechanism for its inactivation in neoplasias, such as acute lymphoblastic leukemia, multiple myeloma, malignant glioma cells, and brain metastases of solid tumors [152]. Since the promoter region of *TP53* does not contain a classic CpG island, methylation of one or two sites may produce a proportionately greater effect in downregulation of transcription compared to a tumor suppressor gene with a classic CpG island in the promoter [153]. The *TP53* promoter region has been sequenced and basal promoter activity localized to an 85 bp region (nucleotide 760–844) that is indispensable for full promoter activity and the *TP53* promoter has putative binding sites for transcriptional factors [154]. Schroeder and Mass [155] have shown that methylation in the promoter region of the p53 gene reduces reporter gene activity. They found down-regulation of p53 in cultured cells transfected with a plasmid incorporating a *TP53* promoter containing methylated CpG dinucleotides. Furthermore, this region has been shown to be methylated in several cancers [156].

Analyses of methylation of *TP53* promoter region are controversial. While some researchers reported low frequencies of *TP53* methylation in neuroblastic tumors (0/44), astrocytomas (2/24, 8%), GBM (1/43, 2%) [157], oligodendroglial tumors (0/41) and ependymomas (0/7) [158], other authors observed a higher frequency [159, 160]. The reason for this discrepancy remains to be clarified.

Amatya *et al.* [159] assessed whether promoter methylation was present in cells of six malignant gliomas and whether there is an association with reduced expression of *TP53* mRNA and protein. They also assessed the frequencies of disruption of the p53/p14 ^{ARF} pathway in 49 low-grade astrocytomas (40 fibrillary astrocytomas and 9 gemistocytic astrocytomas), 42 oligodendrogliomas and 18 oligoastrocytomas. The Methylation-specific PCR (MS-PCR) revealed methylation of the promoter region of the *TP53* gene in three (U87MG, LNT-229, T98G) out of six malignant glioma cell lines. Real time RT-PCR revealed that two malignant glioma cell lines (U87MG and T98G) led to up-regulated expression of *TP53* mRNA and protein after treatment with 5-aza-2′-deoxycytidine (5-aza-dC, an epigenetic modifier that results in DNA demethylation), suggesting that promoter methylation is associated with reduced expression in some malignant glioma cells. *TP53* promoter methylation in primary tissue of low-grade gliomas was observed in 29/48 (60%) low-grade astrocytomas, 11/18 (61%) oligoastrocytomas, and 31/42 (74%) oligodendrogliomas, while promoter methylation of the p14 ^{ARF} was detected by MS-PCR in 5/49 (10%) low-grade astrocytomas, 7/18 (39%) oligoastrocytomas, and 15/41 (37%) oligodendrogliomas. Briefly, alterations of at least one of *TP53* promoter methylation, p14 ^{ARF} promoter methylation, and *TP53* mutations were found in 43/49 (88%) of low-grade astrocytomas, 15/18 (83%) of oligoastrocytomas, and 35/42 (83%) oligodendrogliomas, suggesting that disruption of the p53/p14 ^{ARF} pathway is frequent in all histological types of low-grade glioma.

Almeida *et al.* [160] evaluated the promoter hypermethylation profile of the *TP53* gene in 90 extra-axial brain tumors (48 meningiomas, 23 schwannomas and 19 metastases) using MS-PCR and sequencing. The group showed that the methylation of the *TP53* gene is an important event associated with extra-axial brain tumors, since 37.5% of meningiomas, 30% of schwannomas and 52.6% of metastases were hypermethylated. When tumor grade was compared, 35.3% of benign tumors and 48% of malignant tumors were methylated, and these results suggested that *TP53* methylation can be involved in the progression of these tumors.

3.2. The new insights of MicroRNAs/*TP53* in cancer

MicroRNAs (miRNA) are a large class of small, non-coding RNAs, 21 – 28 nucleotides long, produced naturally in cells after being cut into segments from larger strands of RNA by the enzyme Dicer. They function by binding to complementary sites on the 3′-untranslated region (3′-UTR) of genes and promoting the recruitment of protein complexes responsible for impairing translation and/or decreasing the stability of mRNA [161, 162]. A specific miRNA may simultaneously regulate multiple targets, thereby enabling complex changes in protein expression profiles. Furthermore, a single target can be regulated by multiple miRNAs, and upstream regulation of a given miRNA can involve multiple regulators at different steps of miRNA biogenesis. Thus, miRNAs take part in complex regulatory networks that may influence almost every cellular process [163]. Currently, 1, 048 human microRNAs are known to modulate approximately 3 % of all genes and up to 30 % of protein-coding genes. Vital for protein expression, microRNAs are integrally associated with both normal and abnormal biological processes [164].

miRNAs play important roles in the regulation of normal gene expression at developmental timing, cell proliferation and apoptosis [165]. As these processes are altered in cancer cells, there are in literature several studies that were undertaken to provide evidence for an involvement of miRNAs in cancer formation. miRNA-encoding genes as well as mRNA-encoding genes have been meanwhile classified as oncogenic or tumor suppressive genes according to their function in cellular transformation and expression in tumors [166, 167]. Furthermore, tumor cells seem to undergo a general loss of miRNA expression, and forced reduction of global miRNA expression promotes transformation [168]. Interestingly, miRNAs cluster within fragiles sites and other genomic regions frequently altered in cancers [169]. Because of their role in tumor formation, miRNAs may be very useful for the classification, diagnosis, prognosis, and therapy of malignancies [166, 167].

Profiling miRNA provides an attractive, novel, and non-invasive biomarker for tumor diagnosis and prognosis. Molecular biology techniques, such as Northern blot, RNase protection assay, and primer extension assay can measure expression of a miRNA. The small size of miRNAs initially hampered polymerase chain reaction-based methods. However, PCR-based techniques have become very popular since the development of adaptor-mediated quantitative real-time PCR (qRT-PCR) due to their high sensitivity [170]. Microarray techniques are widely used to comprehensively assay the entire miRNome (the global miRNA expression profile) in tissues or in cell lines [171]. In addition to microarray and qRT-PCR, miRNomes are obtained by *in situ* hybridization [172] and serial analysis of gene expression adapted for small RNAs [173]. Overall, these technical improvements are expected to greatly widen the repertoire of miRNAs in a variety of biological systems.

p53 is a transcription factor, so transactivates or represses many protein-encoding genes and this underlies much of its tumor suppressor function. Recently, it has been reported that p53 directly transactivates specifics miRNAs [174]. miRNA have also been shown to target p53 and/or components of p53 regulatory pathways affecting its activities directly and/or indirectly [175, 176].

Several reports shed light on the involvement of miRNAs in the p53 pathway. He *et al.* [177] profiled miRNA gene expression in wild-type (wt) and p53-deficient cells and found that the miR34s (miR-34 gene family, including miR-34a, b and c) was among the most upregulated in wt p53 cells. In addition, Luan *et al.* [178] analyzed the expression levels of miR-34a in human glioma cell lines (U251, A172 and SHG-44) using real time quantitative PCR and compared with that observed in normal brain and determined its role in cell proliferation, cycle distribution, apoptosis and capabilities of in vitro migration and invasion of p53-mutant glioma cells. The results showed that miR-34a is remarkably reduced in p53-mutant glioma cell line U251, that had a mutation of codon 273 (CGT/CAT; Arg/His) in exon 8 than other p53-wild glioma cell lines A172, SHG-44 and normal brains.

miR34s are induced after genotoxic stress in a p53-dependent manner *in vitro* and *in vivo*. miR-34b and-34c are clustered at chromosome 11, whereas miR-34a is located in a separate genomic locus. p53 directly activates both pri-miRNAs. The miR-34s seem to be critical downstream effectors of p53, as ectopic expression of the miR-34s recapitulate the phenotype of p53 activation. The miR-34s promotes repression of several direct targets, such as Bcl-2, Cdk4, hepatocyte growth factor receptor (MET), and other, resulting in cell cycle arrest, apoptosis, and senescence [179] (Figure 3). Several other laboratories corroborated the finding that miR-34s are critical components of the p53 network [180-182]. Taken together, these results support a pivotal downstream role of miRNAs in the regulation of the p53 pathway.

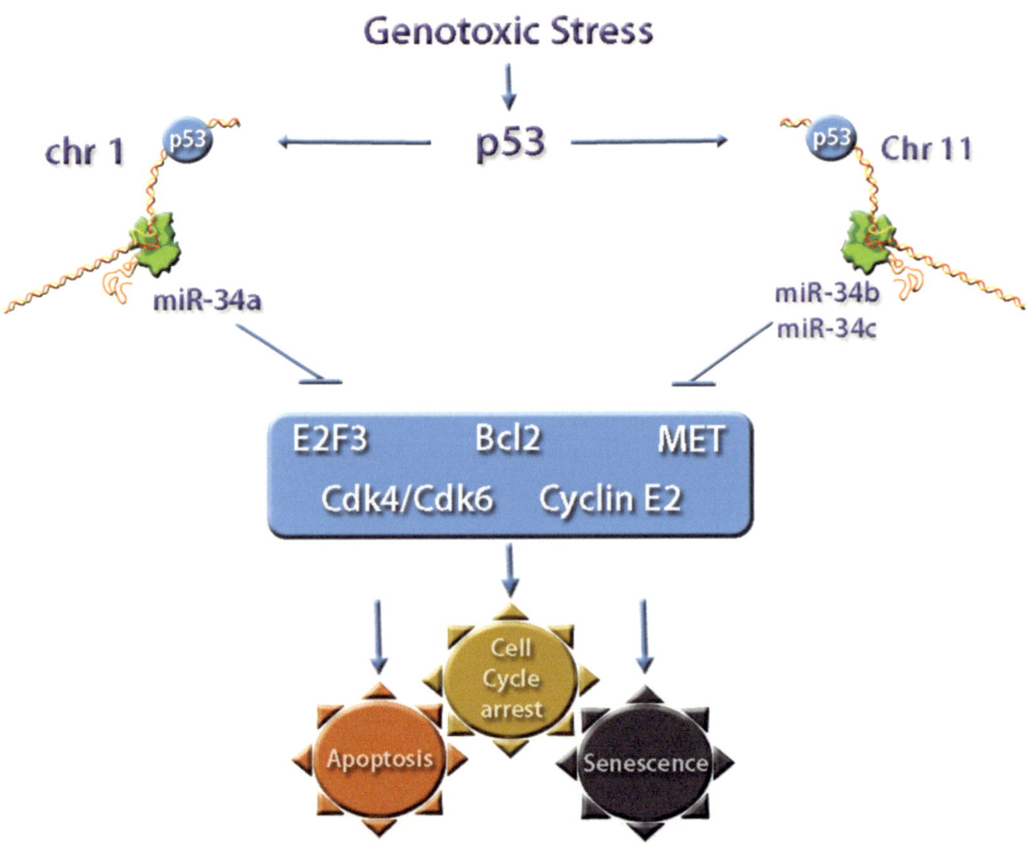

Figure 3. Representation of p53 and the miR-34 family interactions. The p53 protein stimulates the transcription of miR34s, which inhibits oncoproteins and leads to cell senescence, apoptosis and cell cycle arrest.

As cell cycle arrest, senescence, and apoptosis are tumor suppressive mechanisms, the inactivation of members of the miR-34 family, which induce these cellular responses, may be a selective advantage for cancer cells. Besides decreased expression of MiR-34 due to inactivating mutations of p53, the miR-34 encoding genes themselves may be targets for mutational or epigenetic inactivation in cancer. For example, loss of miR34a expression was observed in neuroblastoma, which may be due to the relatively common deletion of a region on chromosome 1p36, which encompasses miR-34a [183]. However, the mechanisms leading to decreased expression of miR-34s require further exploration.

Other miRNAs may be important in the p53 network. miR-30c, -103, -26a, -107, and-182 were induced clearly, although less robustly, upon DNA damage in a p53-dependent manner [181]. In another approach, the searching for p53-binding elements in DNA sequences near miRNAs identified miR-129 as a good candidate for regulation by p53 [184]. miR-125b, a brain-enriched microRNA, was identified as a bona fide negative regulator of p53 in both zebrafish and humans [185]. Recently, Hu *et al.* [186] showed that miR-504 directly represses p53 expression and function in human cell lines.

Since recent studies have indicated that p53 enters into miRNA world [187], some researchers provided important insights into the central roles of miRNAs in a well-known tumor suppressor network, the p53 pathway, which may provide a route to therapeutic miRNA intervention in CNS tumors. Shyamal *et al.* [188] were the first to demonstrate that miR-34a directly targets the *MAGE-A* family of oncogenes, disengaging p53 from *MAGE-A*–mediated repression. The group demonstrated that miR-34a directly targets the 3 ′ UTR of *MAGE-A* genes and decreases MAGE-A protein levels in medulloblastoma cell lines. This decreasing in *MAGE-A* results in a concomitant increasing in p53 and its associated transcriptional targets, p21/WAF1/CIP1 and, importantly, miR-34a. This establishes a positive feedback loop where miR-34a is not only induced by p53 but increases p53 mRNA and protein levels through the modulation of *MAGE-A* genes and a consequence of this mechanism is that sensitizes medulloblastoma cells to chemotherapeutic agents via delayed G2/M progression and increased apoptosis.

Recently, Suh *et al.* [189] identified two miRNAs (miR-25 and-32) as p53-repressed miRNAs in glioblastoma multiforme cells through p53-dependent negative regulation of their transcriptional regulators, E2F1 and MYC. The study provided compelling evidence that expression of these miRNAs causes tumor suppression through mechanisms that lead to accumulation of p53 protein, by directly targeting Mdm2 and TSC1, leading to inhibition of cellular proliferation through cell cycle arrest. Thus, there is a recurrent autoregulatory circuit involving expression of p53, E2F1, and MYC to regulate the expression of miR-25 and-32, which are miRNAs that, in turn, control p53 accumulation. Significantly, overexpression of transfected miR-25 and-32 in cells of GBM inhibited growth of these cells in mouse brain *in vivo*. The results define miR-25 and-32 as positive regulators of p53, underscoring their role in tumorigenesis in glioblastoma.

4. The cancer stem cell model

Until a few years ago, the brain was thought to lack a stem cell population, but actually, it is now known that there are two regions of the adult human brain that contain neural stem cells (NSCs) (a group of self-renewing cells in the nervous system that can generate both neurons and glia): the dentate gyrus of the hippocampus and the subventricular zone. NSCs can form neurons, astrocytes and oligodendrocytes *in vitro*, although their normal physiological role in the adult human brain is disputed [190].

With the accumulation of knowledge concerning the stem cell and the mechanisms regulating their behaviour, it was noted that many of the characteristics of stem cells were also present in cancer. These findings reinforce the "cancer stem cell model", which states that the cellular heterogeneity within the tumor is ascribed entirely to the differentiating tumor cells that derive from the cancer stem cells (CSCs), that can be defined as cells that possesses the capacity to self-renew and to originate the heterogeneous lineages of cancer cells that comprise the tumor. The term "tumor-initiating cell" also has been used to describe a cell with the potential to initiate a tumor. This term are essentially functionally equivalent to CSCs if it is used to refer to the subclones of cells within an established tumor that gives rise to a new tumor when transplanted [190-192].

CSCs were first observed by John Dick's group in acute myeloid leukemia and posteriorly other researchers reported CSCs in solid tumors, including those formed by breast, colon, prostate, pancreatic, lung, liver and brain [193-196], Subsequently there has been a large amount of work to identify the cancer stem cell population, and to study its role in progression of disease and resistance to treatment, allowing many experimental therapies targeting cancer stem cells can be developed and tested in preclinical models [190, 195, 196].

CSCs have been isolated from a wide range of CNS neoplasms, including adult and pediatric, anaplastic oligodendrogliomas and malignant medulloblastomas [197]. For gliomas, several researchers isolated brain tumor stem cells (BTSC) from primary tumors based in the ability to form neurospheres NSCs do and other criteria: ability to be serially transplanted; unique ability to engraft; ability to recapitulate the tumor of origin morphologically and immunophenotypically in xenografts [198].

4.1. P53 role in neuronal and brain tumor stem cell

In the ependymal cell lining of the lateral ventricle wall as well as most cells of the subventricular zone, including astrocytes and progenitors, abundance of nuclear p53 is evident and in agreement with the down-regulation of p53 in differentiating cells observed during embryogenesis. The nuclear p53 immunoreactivity is absent or found at low levels in the majority of the mature brain, including differentiating cells in the rostral migratory stream, suggesting that p53 is preferentially expressed in neural precursors [113]. Several studies show the important role(s) of p53 in the regulation of mammary [199], hematopoietic [200], embryonic and neuronal stem cells [201] by regulating self-renewal, symmetric division, quiescence, survival, and proliferation.

Meletis *et al.* [202] demonstrated that *TP53* is expressed in the neural stem cell lineage in the adult brain and negatively regulates proliferation and survival, and thereby self-renewal, of neural stem cells. Analyses of the neural stem cell transcriptome identified the dysregulation of several cell cycle regulators in the absence of p53, most notably a pronounced downregulation of p21 expression. These data reinforce the p53 role as a suppressor of tissue and cancer stem cell self-renewal.

Armesilla-Diaz *et al.* [203] demonstrated that p53 controls the chromosomal stability, proliferation and differentiation patterns of embryonic mouse olfactory bulb stem cells. The group reported that the absence of this protein increases the number of neurosphere-forming cells and the proliferation of these stem cells, and observed that differentiation of p53 knockout-derived neurospheres was biased toward neuronal precursors. Moreover, the relevance of p53 in maintaining chromosomal stability in response to genotoxic insult was demonstrated, and additionally, the results showed that neurosphere stem cells are highly resistant to long-term epidermal growth factor (EGF) and basic fibroblast growth factor (bFGF) deprivation in a p53-independent fashion, and they preserve their differentiation potential.

While the role of p53 in apoptosis of neuronal cells was well elucidated [202, 204, 205], its function in astrocytes, oligodendrocytes and their precursors is poorly understood. Oligodendrocyte precursors cultured *in vitro* can undergo p53-dependent differentiation although the cells appear to have a low basal level of p53 expression [206]. Both oligodendrocytes and astrocytes can undergo apoptosis following infection with an adenovirus expressing p53 [207].

CSCs exhibit genetic or chromosomal alterations in addition to aberrant differentiation properties, unlike the normal stem cells [208]. It is important to highlight the fundamental differences between normal stem cells and CSCs. The first are known for the vigilance with which their proliferation is controlled and for the care with which their genomic integrity is maintained, while CSCs lack such ability [209]. The cell-of-origin of CSCs remains elusive, however evidences indicate that CSCs may originate from malignant transformation of normal stem cells, because of the perennial nature and high proliferative potential characteristics of stem cells. Some studies have shown that oncogene activation or tumor suppressor gene inactivation increased the frequency of tumor formation in primitive nestin-expressing cells but not in the more differentiated glial fibrillary acidic protein (GFAP)-expressing astrocytes [210, 211] while other researches indicate that differentiated astrocytes and NSCs may be equally permissive to transformation when genomic alterations are introduced [212].

The role of p53 in BTSC has not been well established, however based on current understanding of its function in neural precursors available in the literature, several hypotheses may be develop. First, loss of p53 may increase the self-renewal and proliferation of neural stem and/or lineage-restricted progenitors, thereby expanding the pool of cells available for additional mutations in specifics oncogenes. Another hypothesis is that, depending on cellular context, p53 can both inhibit or promote cell differentiation, as well as influence cell fate decisions, so the differentiation program of neural precursors can be changed by p53 mutation. Lastly, accumulated evidences support a role for p53 in the suppression of cell migration, although much focus on p53 is directed at its growth inhibitory properties [213]. The neurogenic niche has been shown to be important for the maintenance of stem cells in an undifferentiated state, and the premature exit of NSCs from the neurogenic niche may alter their capacity for tissue invasion or differentiation program in the absence of p53 [214].

The number of studies concerning the cellular, molecular, and environmental factors that regulate p53 function in NSCs has increased drastically and brought a better understanding of these factors, and together with the advances in molecular biology techniques, provided much valuable information about the role of p53 in BTSCs. This scenario stimulates future studies exploring the significance of p53 alterations for prognosis and prediction of treatment response that would help development of individual treatment strategies as well as help clarifying the clinical importance of cancer stem cell biology.

5. p53-based gene therapy: GBMs as an example

Malignant tumors within the brain remain a therapeutic challenge, but current strategies tested in animal models as well as in the clinics have shown promising results. The rapid progress in knowledge of the p53 pathway have led to many different approaches to p53 based cancer therapy as mentioned previously and the field has excited great interest both academically and commercially [215]. The long awaited molecular treatment of GBM and other CNS tumors and utilization of knowledge surrounding p53 may then be foreseeable goals in the future. It will also be important and likely therapeutically be effective to combine gene therapy with other therapeutic modalities, including the standards-of-care [216].

Standard treatment of care for GBM, for example, consists of surgical resection, followed by radiotherapy and chemotherapy [217, 218]. Despite significant advances in current treatment approaches, including the gamma knife (radiation) and TMZ (chemotherapy) [217, 219], GBM continues to present a poor prognosis, with median survival still remains less than 15 months. It is important to remember that GBMs are the most common and least curable among CNS tumors [220]. Moreover, for this type of tumor, complete resection is practically impossible due to its diffuse nature and the proximity of the tumor to vital brain structures. Moreover, it often recurs in an area close to the original resection cavity [221]. The intrinsic resistance of glioblastoma cells to radiotherapy and chemotherapy confers another therapeutic challenge of this disease [222]. On the other hand it has been reported that invading GBM cells, which give rise to recurrences, are resistant to cytotoxic therapies due to the constitutive activation of antiapoptotic signaling pathways [221]. Novel therapeutic approaches and adjuvants to be employed in combination with standard therapeutic strategies are sorely needed for GBM patients, because although isolated traditional therapies allow an increase in the quality of life and survival of these patients, they are not curative and long-term survival is very rare [221, 223, 224].

Gene therapy for CNS tumors is evolving every year, especially for GBM, with the ultimate goal being specific delivery of therapeutic genes or oncolytic viruses to eliminate the tumor. Besides results in cell death, also enhanced immune responses to tumor antigens and disruption of the tumor microenvironment [216]. A variety of gene therapy strategies has been examined in GBM preclinical models and clinical trials and includes the use of selective replication-competent oncolytic viruses, non-replicating viral vectors or normal adult stem/

progenitor cells for the delivery of immunostimulatory genes, cytotoxic genes and genes modulating the tumor microenvironment [216].

The fact that p53 pathway is activated in tumor cells, but not in normal cells, provides a potentially important therapeutic selectivity, indifferent of which signal in the tumor cells activates p53 following its restoration [225]. In this context, the evidences that tumor cells, but not normal cells, have a cellular environment that activates the p53 pathway would create a setting of an advantageous therapeutic index, whose main objective is the development of interventions that selectively kill tumor cells instead normal cells [225].

Different approaches to achieve this goal are already in various stages of development and a diversity of small druglike molecules targeting the p53 system have been developed and several are now in clinical trials. Of critical importance has been the development of: agents which can increase active p53 in tumor cells by interfering with the p53–MDM2 interaction are therefore considered to have therapeutic utility in sensitizing tumor cells for chemo-or radiotherapy, such as the Nutlins [226, 227]; molecules that activate p53 via direct interaction with p53 itself, as PRIMA-1, of which there is evidence of induction of expression of mediators of p53-dependent apoptosis such as Puma, Noxa, and Bax in cells with mutant p53 [228, 229]; small molecules activating p53 family members in a p53 mutant or deficient background; molecules activating p53 by inhibiting class III histone deacetylases, nuclear export, transcriptional and nucleolar distuption. These screens in combination with RNAi based approaches are of utmost importance for the discovery of new targets for therapy in the p53 pathway [215].

Transfection of wild-type p53 in order to normalize function in mutant p53-containing tumors has been a long-pursued goal of gene therapy. Mercer *et al.* [230] initially demonstrated that plasmid-mediated transfection of the p53 gene is capable of suppressing cell growth in gliomas by inhibition of G0/G1 progression into S phase. Kock *et al.* [231] and Gomez-Manzano *et al.* [232] were among the first to demonstrate that delivering the p53 gene using an adenovirus vector (Ad-p53) resulted in high levels of apoptosis in glioma cell lines, by elevation of the levels of the p21 (cell cycle-related) and Bax (apoptosis-related) proteins. Frederick *et al.*[233] undertook a phase I trial of Ad-p53 in the treatment of patients with recurrent malignant gliomas with the purpose of determine the clinical toxicity of Ad-p53 and obtain molecular information regarding the expression and distribution of the p53 protein after intratumoral treatment of human gliomas with Ad-p53. Thus, their results conclude that Intratumoral injection of Ad-p53 allowed the exogenous transfer of the p53 gene and expression of functional p53 protein, with minimaltoxicity observed.

To the generation of an effective systemic anti-tumor immune response, it is necessary the development of strategies that promote the GBM tumor cell death, which is essential not only to kill tumor cells and reduce tumor burden, but also to induce the release of inflammatory molecules from dying tumor cells [234]. Drug combinations have been developed to selectively kill cancer cells that lack p53 function while protecting normal cells. The potential to explore the defective checkpoint status of cells with inactive *TP53* genes has also been largely recognized and in part stimulated the search of drugs that can inhibit PLK1, AURKB, and other proteins that regulate the G 2 /M checkpoint [235]. Shchors et al. [236] used a preclinical model of GBM in combination with a switchable p53 allele to model the therapeutic effect of p53 pathway restoration. It was observed that the therapeutic efficacy of p53 pathway restoration was greatly influenced by both the initial mechanism of p53 pathway-inactivating mutation and the temporal manner in which the selective pressure elicited by p53 pathway restoration was applied. Their results suggested that intermittent dosing regimens of drugs that restore wild-type tumor-suppressor function onto mutant, inactive p53 proteins will prove to be more efficacious than traditional chronic dosing by similarly reducing adaptive resistance.

This topic focused on GBM because of its poor prognosis and the target for most clinical trials. However, it is important to recognize that there are many other brain tumors which are also targets for gene therapy. Recently, Kunkele *et al.* [227] observed that targeting the p53-MDM2 complex using nutlin-3 significantly reduced cell viability and induced either apoptosis or cell cycle arrest and expression of the p53 target gene p21 in 4 of 6 human medulloblastomas cell lines. However, UW-228 and DAOY cells harboring *TP53* mutations were almost unaffected by nutlin-3, showing that the mutational status of the gene interfere in the efficacy of the treatment. MDM2 knockdown in medulloblastoma cells by siRNA mimicked nutlin-3 treatment, whereas expression of dominant negative p53 abrogated nutlin-3 effects. Oral nutlin-3 treatment of mice with established medulloblastoma xenografts inhibited tumor growth and significantly increased survival. Hence, the authors suggested that inhibition of the MDM2-p53 interaction with nutlin-3 is a promising therapeutic option for medulloblastomas with functional p53 that should be further evaluated in clinical trials.

6. Conclusion

After a detailed review of the literature about the role of the *TP53* gene in the genesis and development of CNS tumors we can conclude that both genetic and epigenetic alterations that inactivate this gene are directly related to these phenomena in specific histopathological tumors. In addition, several studies have investigated the predictive value of *TP53* mutation status and have shown that specific types of genetic mutations can alter the function and expression of p53, influencing tumor response to treatment and patient outcome, revealing thus to be a useful prognostic tool. Genetic alterations in the p53 pathway are early events in the molecular pathogenesis of diffuse astrocytoma and the highest frequencies of allelic loss and/or mutation of *TP53* gene are mostly seen in gliomas, and are a genetic hallmark of: low-grade diffuse astrocytomas (> 60%), mainly in gemistocytic astrocytomas that carry *TP53* mutations in up to 80% of the cases; anaplastic astrocytomas (40-70%); secondary glioblastoma (>65%); oligoastrocytomas (~40%). Genetic *TP53* mutations are rarely found or seen less frequently in other CNS tumors, however, some studies have shown that some changes have found important prognostic value. Recently, our group investigated the presence of numerical aberrations of chromosome 17 and *TP53* in 5 subjects with brain metastasis from breast cancer using dual-color fluorescence in situ hybridization experiments. Deletion of *TP53* was the most frequent alteration observed, suggesting that if this alteration is present in the primary tumors, breast tumors with loss of *TP53* copies have a poorer prognosis and a higher chance for metastasis [237].

http://dx.doi.org/10.5772/58334

Epigenetic events in *TP53* gene has been increasingly recognized as an alternative mechanism for inactivation of function of a tumor suppressor gene. Although less frequently, *TP53* epigenetic abnormalities has been found in CNS tumors and several reports shed light on the involvement of mainly DNA methylation and miRNAs in the p53 pathway, suggesting that this process can be involved in the genesis and progression of these tumors. Clearly, additional studies can provide important insights into the central roles of miRNAs in the p53 pathway, as well as *TP53* promoter methylation, which may provide a route to therapeutic intervention in CNS tumors.

Due the difficulty to the use of traditional therapeutic modalities such as chemotherapy and radiotherapy in the CNS tumors, especially in high grade tumors, such as glioblastomas, , it is expected that in a near future molecular treatment that could be obtain more effective control of disease progression will be used, resulting in an improved clinical course of these patients. Over the years, with the increasing advances of molecular biology techniques, much information has been obtained on the role of p53 in carcinogenesis. Because of the critical role p53 plays in a variety of cancers, a diversity of approaches have been undertaken to target p53 and its altered signaling pathways. Different drugs targeting the p53 system in order to activate the p53 pathway have been developed and several are now in clinical trials, and have shown promising results.

Nomenclature

AT/RT	Atypical Teratoid/ Rhabdoid Tumor
bFGF	Basic fibroblast growth factor
BCL2	B-cell CLL/Lymphoma 2
BTSC	Brain tumor stem cells
CSC	Cancer stem cells
CDK4	Cyclin-dependent kinase 4
CDKN2A	Cyclin-dependent kinase inhibitor 2A
CNS	Central nervous systems
CHD5	Chromodomain helicase DNA binding protein 5
CPC	Choroid plexus carcinomas
CPP	Choroid plexus papilloma
CPT	Choroid plexus tumors
EGF	Epidermal growth factor
FISH	Fluorescence in Situ Hybridization
GFAP	Glial fibrillary acidic protein
GBM	Glioblastoma

IDH1	Isocitrate dehydrogenase 1 (NADP+)
IDH2	Iisocitrate dehydrogenase 2 (NADP+)
IHC	Immunohistochemistry
IARC	International Agency for Research on Cancer
LFS	Li-Fraumeni syndromes
LFL	Li-Fraumeni-like syndromes
LOH	Loss of heterozygosity
MRT	Malignant Rhabdoid Tumor
MDM2	MDM2 oncogene, E3 ubiquitin protein ligase
MDM4	Mdm4 p53 binding protein homolog
MB	Medulloblastoma
MET	Met proto-oncogene
MS-PCR	Methylation-specific PCR
miRNA	MicroRNAs
MYC	v-myc avian myelocytomatosis viral oncogene homolog
HNSCC	Head and Neck squamous cell carcinoma
NES	Nuclear Exclusion Domain
NLS	Nuclear Localization Domain
NSC	Neural stem cell
NF1	Neurofibromin 1
$P14^{ARF}$	Cyclin-dependent kinase inhibitor 2A (encoding p14)
$P19^{ARF}$	Cyclin-dependent kinase inhibitor 2A (encoding p19)
$p15^{INK4b}$	Cyclin-dependent kinase inhibitor 2A (encoding p15)
$p16^{INK4a}$	Cyclin-dependent kinase inhibitor 2A (encoding p16)
PTCH1	Patched homolog 1
PNET	Primitive neuroectodermal tumor
PTEN	Phosphatase and tensin homolog
qRT-PCR	Quantitative real-time PCR
RB1	Retinoblastoma 1
siRNA	small interfering RNA
SMARCB1	SWI/SNF-related matrix-associated actin-dependent regulator of chromatin subfamily B member 1
SSCP	Single strand conformation polymorphism
SHH	Sonic hedgehog
TMZ	Temozolomide

TP53	Tumor protein p53
TSC1	Tuberous Sclerosis 1
WHO	World Health Organization
WT	Wild-type
WNT	Wingless
PXA	Xanthoastrocytoma pleomorphic

Acknowledgements

Authors would like to thank PPGGBM-UFPA, IFPA and IEC for support. We also would like to thank the staffs at Francisco Mauro Salzano Laboratory (UFPA) and Laboratory of Tissue Culture and Cytogenetics (SAMAM, IEC). We are especially grateful to Dr. Cynthia Hawkins (Dept. of Paediatric Laboratory Medicine, The Hospital for Sick Children, Toronto, Canada) for her important contribution.

Author details

Igor Andrade Pessôa[1], Fabio P. Estumano da Silva[1,2], Nilson Praia Anselmo[3] and Edivaldo Herculano C. de Oliveira[1,4,5]

1 Programa de Pós Graduação em Genética e Biologia Molecular, ICB, Universidade Federal do Pará, Belém, PA, Brazil

2 Laboratório de Biociências e Comportamento, Instituto Federal do Pará, Tucuruí, PA, Brazil

3 Laboratório de Biologia Molecular Francisco Mauro Salzano, ICB, Universidade Federal do Pará, Belém, PA, Brazil

4 Faculdade de Ciências Naturais, ICEN, Universidade Federal do Pará, Belém, PA, Brazil

5 Laboratório de Cultura de Tecidos e Citogenética, SAMAM, Instituto Evandro Chagas, Ananindeua, PA, Brazil

References

[1] Olivier M, Taniere P. Somatic mutations in cancer prognosis and prediction: lessons from TP53 and EGFR genes. Current Opinion in Oncology 2011; 23(1):88-92.

[2] Schmitt M, Harbeck N, Daidone MG, Brynner N, Duffy MJ, Foekens JA, Sweep FC. Identification, validation, and clinical implementation of tumor-associated biomarkers to improve therapy concepts, survival, and quality of life of cancer patients: Tasks of the Receptor and Biomarker Group of the European Organization for Research and Treatment of Cancer. International Journal of Oncology 2004; 25(5):1397-406.

[3] Ludwig JA, Weinstein JN. Biomarkers in cancer staging, prognosis and treatment selection. Nature Reviews Cancer 2005; 5(11):845-56.

[4] Louis DN, Ohgaki H, Wiestler OD, Cavenee WK. WHO Classification of Tumours of the Central Nervous System. Lyon: IARC; 2007.

[5] Hollstein M, Sidransky D, Vogelstein B, Harris CC. p53 mutations in human cancers. Science 1991; 253: 49–53.

[6] Levine AJ. p53, the cellular gatekeeper for growth and division. Cell 1997; 88(3): 323-31.

[7] Tommasino M, Accardi R, Caldeira S, Dong W, Malanchi I, Smet A, Zehbe I. The role of TP53 in Cervical carcinogenesis. Human Mutation 2003; 21(3):307-12.

[8] Li FP, Fraumeni JF Jr, Mulvihill JJ, Blattner WA, Dreyfus MG, Tucker MA, Miller RW. A cancer family syndrome in twenty-four kindreds. Cancer Research 1988; 48(18):5358-62.

[9] Olivier M, Goldgar DE, Sodha N, Ohgaki H, Kleihues P, Hainaut P, Eeles RA. Li-Fraumeni and related syndromes: Correlation between tumor type, family structure, and TP53 genotype. Cancer Res 2003; 63(20):6643-50.

[10] Whibley C, Pharoah PD, Hollstein M. p53 polymorphisms: cancer implications. Nature Reviews Cancer 2009; 9: 95–107.

[11] Wang Y, Kringen P, Kristensen GB, Holm R, Baekelandt MM, Olivier M, Skomedal H, Hainaut P, Tropé CG, Abeler VM, Nesland JM, Borresen-Dale AL, Helland A. Effect of the codon 72 polymorphism (c.215G.C, p.Arg72Pro) in combination with somatic sequence variants in the TP53 gene on survival in patients with advanced ovarian carcinoma. Human Mutation 2004; 24(1):21-34.

[12] Langerod A, Zhao H, Borgan O, Nesland JM, Bukholm IR, Ikdahl T, Karesen R, Borresen-Dale AL, Jeffrey SS. TP53 mutation status and gene expression profiles are powerful prognostic markers of breast cancer. Breast Cancer Research 2007; 9(3):R30.

[13] Snustad DP, Simmons MJ. Principles of Genetics. Minessota: Wiley & Sons, Inc; 2012.

[14] International Agency for Research on Cancer. World Health Organization. IARC TP53 Database. http://www-p53.iarc.fr (accessed 15 October 2013).

[15] Weisz L, Oren M, Rotter V. Transcription regulation by mutant p53. Oncogene 2007; 26: 2202–2211.

[16] Brosh R, Rotter V. When mutants gain new powers: news from the mutant p53 field. Nature Reviews Cancer 2009; 9: 701–713.

[17] Hussain SP, Harris CC. p53 mutation spectrum and load: The generation of hypotheses linking the exposure of endogenous or exogenous carcinogens to human cancer. Mutation Research 1999; 428: 23–32.

[18] Jones PA, Rideout WM, Shen JC, Spruck CH, Tsai YC. Methylation, mutation and cancer. Bioessays 1992; 14: 33–36.

[19] Ambs S, Hussain SP, Marrogi AJ, Harris CC. Cancer-prone oxyradical overload disease. IARC Scientific Publication 1999; 150: 295–302.

[20] Vaninetti NM, Geldenhuys L, Porter GA, Risch H, Hainaut P, Guernsey DL, Casson AG. Inducible nitric oxide synthase, nitrotyrosine and p53 mutations in the molecular pathogenesis of Barrett's esophagus and esophageal adenocarcinoma. Molecular Carcinogenesis 2008; 47(4):275-85.

[21] Olivier M, Hollstein M, Hainaut P. TP53 Mutations in Human Cancers: Origins, Consequences, and Clinical Use. Cold Spring Harbor Perspectives Biology 2010; 2:a001008.

[22] Petitjean A, Achatz MIW, Borresen-Dale AL, Hainaut P, M Olivier. TP53 mutations in human cancers: functional selection and impact on cancer prognosis and outcomes. Oncogene 2007; 26, 2157–2165.

[23] Olivier M, Hainaut P, Borresen-Dale AL. Prognostic and predictive value of TP53 mutations in human cancer. In: Hainaut P, Wiman K.(ed). 25 years of p53 research. Dordrecht: Springer; 2005.

[24] Huse JT, Holland EC. Targeting brain cancer: advances in the molecular pathology of malignant glioma and medulloblastoma. Nature Reviews Cancer 2010; 10: 319-331.

[25] Huttner A. Overview of Primary Brain Tumors Pathologic Classification, Epidemiology, Molecular Biology, and Prognostic Markers. Hematology Oncology Clinics of North America 2012; 26(4):715-32

[26] Verhaak RG, Hoadley KA, Purdom E, Wang V, Qi Y, Wilkerson MD, Miller CR, Ding L, Golub T, Mesirov JP, Alexe G, Lawrence M, O'Kelly M, Tamayo P, Weir BA, Gabriel S, Winckler W, Gupta S, Jakkula L, Feiler HS, Hodgson JG, James CD, Sarkaria JN, Brennan C, Kahn A, Spellman PT, Wilson RK, Speed TP, Gray JW, Meyerson M, Getz G, Perou CM, Hayes DN; Cancer Genome Atlas Research Network. Integrated genomic analysis identifies clinically relevant subtypes of glioblastoma characterized by abnormalities in PDGFRA, IDH1, EGFR, and NF1. Cancer Cell 2010; 17(1):98-110.

[27] Schwartzbaum JA, Fisher JL, Aldape KD, Wrensch M. Epidemiology and molecular pathology of glioma. Nature Clinical Practice Neurol. 2006; 2(9):494-503.

[28] Westphal M, Lamszus K. Louis, D.N. The neurobiology of gliomas: from cell biology to the development of therapeutic approaches. Nature Reviews Neuroscience 2011; 12(9):495-508.

[29] Louis DN. The p53 gene and protein in human brain tumors. Journal of Neuropathology and Experimental Neurology 1994; 53: 11–21.

[30] Louis DN, Cavenee W. Molecular biology of central nervous system neoplasms. In Cancer: Principles and practice of oncology. Philadelphia: Lippincott-Raven; 1997.

[31] Srivastava S, Zou ZQ, Pirollo K, Blattner W, Chang EH. Germ-line transmission of a mutated p53 gene in a cancer-prone family with Li-Fraumeni syndrome. Nature 1990; 348: 747–749.

[32] Olive KP, Tuveson DA, Ruhe ZC, Yin B, Willis NA, Bronson RT, Crowley D, Jacks T. Mutant p53 gain of function in two mouse models of Li-Fraumeni syndrome. Cell 2004; 119(6):847-60.

[33] Kamijo T, Bodner S, van de Kamp E, Randle DH, Sherr, CJ. Tumor spectrum in ARF-deficient mice. Cancer Research 1999; 59: 2217–2222.

[34] Quelle DE, Zindy F, Ashmun, RA, Sherr, CJ. Alternative reading frames of the INK4a tumor suppressor gene encode two unrelated proteins capable of inducing cell cycle arrest. Cell 1995; 83: 993–1000.

[35] Stott FJ, Bates S, James MC, McConnell BB, Starborg M, Brookes S, Palmero I, Ryan K, Hara E, Vousden KH, Peters G. The alternative product from the human CDKN2A locus, p14 (ARF), participates in a regulatory feedback loop with p53 and MDM2. The EMBO Journal 1998; 17(17):5001-14.

[36] Honda R, Yasuda H. Association of p19 (ARF) with Mdm2 inhibits ubiquitin ligase activity of Mdm2 for tumor suppressor p53. The EMBO Journal 1999; 18: 22–27.

[37] Honda R, Tanaka H, Yasuda H. Oncoprotein MDM2 is a ubiquitin ligase E3 for tumor suppressor p53. FEBS Letters 1997; 420: 25–27.

[38] Fang S, Jensen JP, Ludwig RL, Vousden KH, Weissman, AM. Mdm2 is a RING finger-dependent ubiquitin protein ligase for itself and p53. The Journal of Biological Chemistry 2000; 275: 8945–8951.

[39] Honda R, Yasuda H. Activity of MDM2, a ubiquitin ligase, toward p53 or itself is dependent on the RING finger domain of the ligase. Oncogene 2000; 19: 1473–1476.

[40] Reifenberger G, Reifenberger J, Ichimura K, Meltzer PS, Collins VP. Amplification of multiple genes from chromosomal region 12q13-14 in human malignant gliomas: Preliminary mapping of the amplicons shows preferential involvement of CDK4, SAS, and MDM2. Cancer Research 1994; 54: 4299–4303.

[41] Gu J, Kawai H, Nie L, Kitao H, Wiederschain D, Jochemsen AG, Parant J, Lozano G, Yuan ZM. Mutual dependence of MDM2 and MDMX in their functional inactivation of p53. The Journal of Biological Chemistry 2002; 277(22):19251-4.

[42] Linares LK, Hengstermann A, Ciechanover A, Muller S, Scheffner M. HdmX stimulates Hdm2-mediated ubiquitination and degradation of p53. Proceedings of the National Academy of Science of USA 2003; 100: 12009–12014.

[43] Bagchi A, Papazoglu C, Wu Y, Capurso D, Brodt M, Francis D, Bredel M, Vogel H, Mills AA. CHD5 is a tumor suppressor at human 1p36. Cell 2007; 128(3):459-75.

[44] Ishii N, Sawamura Y, Tada M, Daub DM, Janzer RC, Meagher-Villemure M, de Tribolet N, Van Meir EG. Absence of p53 gene mutations in a tumor panel representative of pilocytic astrocytoma diversity using a p53 functional assay. International Journal of Cancer. 1998;76(6):797-800.

[45] Cheng Y, Pang JC, Ng HK, Ding M, Zhang SF, Zheng J, Liu DG, Poon WS. Pilocytic astrocytomas do not show most of the genetic changes commonly seen in diffuseastrocytomas. Histopathology 2000; 37(5):437-44.

[46] Tada K, Kochi M, Saya H, Kuratsu J, Shiraishi S, Kamiryo T, Shinojima N, Ushio Y. Preliminary observations on genetic alterations in pilocytic astrocytomas associated with neurofibromatosis 1. Neuro-Oncoly. 2003; 5(4):228-34.

[47] Mellai M, Monzeglio O, Piazzi A, Caldera V, Annovazzi L, Cassoni P, Valente G, Cordera S, Mocellini C, Schiffer D. MGMT promoter hypermethylation and its associations with genetic alterations in a series of 350 brain tumors. Journal of Neuro-oncology 2012; 107(3): 617-31.

[48] Hayes VM, Dirven CM, Dam A, Verlind E, Molenaar WM, Mooij JJ, Hofstra RM, Buys CH. High frequency of TP53 mutations in juvenile pilocytic astrocytomas indicates role of TP53 in the development of these tumors. Brain Pathology 1999; 9(3): 463-7.

[49] Phelan CM, Liu L, Ruttledge MH, Müntzning K, Ridderheim PA, Collins VP. Chromosome 17 abnormal-ities and lack of TP53 mutations in paediatric central nervous system tumours. Human Genetics 1995; 96(6):684-90.

[50] Kleihues P, Davis RL, Ohgaki H, Burger PC, Westphal MM, Cavenee WK. Diffuse astrocytoma. In: Kleihues P, Cavenee WK (eds) Pathology and Genetics of Tumours of the Nervous System. Lyon: IARC; 2000.

[51] Watanabe K, Peraud A, Gratas C, Wakai S, Kleihues P, Ohgaki H. p53 and PTEN gene mutations in gemistocytic astrocytomas. Acta Neuropathologica 1998; 95(6): 559-64.

[52] Okamoto Y, Di Patre PL, Burkhard C, Horstmann S, Jourde B, Fahey M, Schüler D, Probst-Hensch NM, Yasargil MG, Yonekawa Y, Lütolf UM, Kleihues P, Ohgaki H. Population-based study on incidence, survival rates, and genetic alterations of low-

grade diffuse astrocytomas and oligodendrogliomas. Acta Neuropathologica 2004; 108(1):49-56.

[53] Nakamura M, Watanabe T, Klangby U, Asker C, Wiman K, Yonekawa Y, Kleihues P, Ohgaki H. p14 ARF deletion and methylation in genetic pathways to glioblastomas. Brain Pathology 2001; 11(2): 159-68.

[54] Peraud A, Kreth FW, Wiestler OD, Kleihues P, Reulen HJ. Prognostic Impact of TP53 Mutations and P53 Protein Overexpression in Supratentorial WHO Grade II Astrocytomas and Oligoastrocytomas. Clinical Cancer Research 2002; 8(5): 1117-24.

[55] Prognostic Impact of TP53 Mutation Status for Adult Patients with Supratentorial World Health Organization Grade II Astrocytoma or Oligoastrocytoma. Cancer 2004; 101(5):1028-35.

[56] Nasuha NA, Daud AH, Ghazali MM, Yusoff AA, Zainuddin N, Abdullah JM, Mutum SS, Biswal BM, Ariff AR, Sulong S, Isa MN. Molecular genetic analysis of anaplastic pleomorphic xanthoastrocytoma. Asian Journal of Surgery 2003; 26(2):120-5.

[57] Marton E, Feletti A, Orvieto E, Longatti P. Malignant progression in pleomorphic xanthoastrocytoma: personal experience and review of the literature. Journal of Neurological Sciences 2007; 252(2):144-53. Epub 2006 Dec 26.

[58] Paulus W, Lisle DK, Tonn JC, Wolf HK, Roggendorf W, Reeves SA, Louis DN. Molecular genetic alterations in pleomorphic xanthoastrocytoma. Acta Neuropathologica 1996; 91(3):293-7.

[59] Giannini C, Hebrink D, Scheithauer BW, Dei Tos AP, James CD. Analysis of TP53 mutation and expression in pleomorphic xanthoastrocytoma. Neurogenetics 2001; 3(3):159-62.

[60] Bettegowda C, Agrawal N, Jiao Y, Wang Y, Wood LD, Rodriguez FJ, Hruban RH, Gallia GL, Binder ZA, Riggins CJ, Salmasi V, Riggins GJ, Reitman ZJ, Rasheed A, Keir S, Shinjo S, Marie S, McLendon R, Jallo G, Vogelstein B, Bigner D, Yan H, Kinzler KW, Papadopoulos N. Exomic Sequencing of Four Rare Central Nervous System Tumor Types. Oncotarget 2013; 4(4):572-83.

[61] Ichimura K, Ohgaki H, Kleihues P, Collins VP. Molecular pathogenesis of astrocytic tumours. Journal of Neuro-oncology 2004; 70(2):137-60.

[62] Faria MH, Neves Filho EH, Alves MK, Burbano RM, de Moraes Filho MO, Rabenhorst SH. TP53 mutations in astrocytic gliomas: an association with histological grade, TP53 codon 72 polymorphism and p53 expression. APMIS 2012; 120(11):882-9.

[63] Ichimura K, Bolin MB, Goike HM, Schmidt EE, Moshref A, Collins VP. Deregulation of the p14ARF/MDM2/p53 pathway is a prerequisite for human astrocytic gliomas with G1-S transition control gene abnormalities. Cancer Research 2000; 60(2):417-24.

[64] Watanabe K, Sato K, Biernat W, Tachibana O, von Ammon K, Ogata N, Yonekawa Y, Kleihues P, Ohgaki H. Incidence and timing of p53 mutations during astrocytoma

progression in patients with multiple biopsies. Clinical Cancer Research 1997; 3(4): 523-30.

[65] Barnholtz-Sloan J, Sloan AE, Land S, Kupsky W, Monteiro AN. Somatic alterations in brain tumors. Oncology Reports 2008; 20(1):203-10.

[66] Zawlik I, Kita D, Vaccarella S, Mittelbronn M, Franceschi S, Ohgaki H. Common Polymorphisms in the MDM2 and TP53 Genes and the Relationship between TP53 Mutations and Patient Outcomes in Glioblastomas. Brain Pathology 2009; 19(2): 188-94.

[67] Ohgaki H, Dessen P, Jourde B, Horstmann S, Nishikawa T, Di Patre PL, Burkhard C, Schüler D, Probst-Hensch NM, Maiorka PC, Baeza N, Pisani P, Yonekawa Y, Yasargil MG, Lütolf UM, Kleihues P. Genetic pathways to glioblastoma: A population-based study. Cancer Research 2004; 64(19):6892-9.

[68] Meyer-Puttlitz B, Hayashi Y, Waha A, Rollbrocker B, Boström J, Wiestler OD, Louis DN, Reifenberger G, von Deimling A. Molecular genetic analysis of giant cell glioblastomas. The American Journal of Pathology 1997; 151(3):853-7.

[69] Peraud A, Watanabe K, Plate KH, Yonekawa Y, Kleihues P, Ohgaki H. p53 Mutations versus EGF receptor expression in giant cell glioblastomas. Journal of Neuropathology and Experimental Neurology 1997; 56(11):1236-41.

[70] Reis RM, Könü-Lebleblicioglu D, Lopes JM, Kleihues P, Ohgaki H. Genetic profile of the gliosarcoma. The American Journal of Pathology 2000; 156(2):425-32.

[71] Actor B, Cobbers JM, Büschges R, Wolter M, Knobbe CB, Lichter P, Reifenberger G, Weber RG. Comprehensive analysis of genomic alterations in gliosarcoma and its two tissue components. Genes, Chromosomes and Cancer 2002; 34(4):416-27.

[72] Biernat W, Kleihues P, Yonekawa Y, Ohgaki H. Amplification and overexpression of MDM2 in primary (de novo) glioblastomas. Journal of Neuropathology and Experimental Neurology 1997; 56(2):180-5.

[73] Smith JS, Tachibana I, Passe SM, Huntley BK, Borell TJ, Iturria N, O'Fallon JR, Schaefer PL, Scheithauer BW, James CD, Buckner JC, Jenkins RB. PTEN mutation, EGFR amplification, and outcome in patients with anaplastic astrocytoma and glioblastoma multiforme. Journal of the National Cancer Institute 2001; 93(16):1246-56.

[74] Simmons ML, Lamborn KR, Takahashi M, Chen P, Israel MA, Berger MS, Godfrey T, Nigro J, Prados M, Chang S, Barker FG 2nd, Aldape K. Analysis of complex relationships between age, p53, epidermal growth factor receptor, and survival in glioblastoma patients. Cancer Research 2001; 61(3):1122-8.

[75] Arshad H, Ahmad Z, Hasan SH. Gliomas: correlation of histologic grade, Ki67 and p53 expression with patient survival. Asian Pacific Journal of Cancer Prevention 2010; 11(6):1637-40.

[76] Schmidt MC, Antweiler S, Urban N, Mueller W, Kuklik A, Meyer-Puttlitz B, Wiestler OD, Louis DN, Fimmers R, von Deimling A. Impact of genotype and morphology on the prognosis of glioblastoma. Journal of Neuropathology and Experimental Neurology 2002; 61(4):321-8.

[77] El Hallani S, Ducray F, Idbaih A, Marie Y, Boisselier B, Colin C, Laigle-Donadey F, Rodéro M, Chinot O, Thillet J, Hoang-Xuan K, Delattre JY, Sanson M. Tp53 codon 72 polymorphism is associated with age at ons et of glioblastoma. Neurology 2009; 72(4):332-6.

[78] Murphy ME. Polymorphic variants in the p53 pathway. Cell Death and Differentiation 2006; 13(6):916-20.

[79] Rogler A, Rogenhofer M, Borchardt A, Lunz JC, Knoell A, Hofstaedter F, Tannapfel A, Wieland W, Hartmann A, Stoehr R. P53 codon 72 (Arg72Pro) polymorphism and prostate cancer risk: association between disease onset and proline genotype. Pathobiology. 2011;78(4):193-200.

[80] Blough MD, Beauchamp DC, Westgate MR, Kelly JJ, Cairncross JG. Effect of aberrant p53 function on temozolomide sensitivity of glioma cell lines and brain tumor initiating cells from glioblastoma. Journal of Neuro-oncology 2011; 102(1):1-7.

[81] Okamoto Y, Di Patre PL, Burkhard C, Horstmann S, Jourde B, Fahey M, Schüler D, Probst-Hensch NM, Yasargil MG, Yonekawa Y, Lütolf UM, Kleihues P, Ohgaki H. Population-based study on incidence, survival rates, and genetic alterations of low-grade diffuse astrocytomas and oligodendrogliomas. Acta Neuropathologica 2004; 108(1):49-56.

[82] Jeuken JW, von Deimling A, Wesseling P. Molecular pathogenesis of oligodendroglial tumors. Journal of Neuro-oncology 2004; 70(2):161-81.

[83] Kim YH, Nobusawa S, Mittelbronn M, Paulus W, Brokinkel B, Keyvani K, Sure U, Wrede K, Nakazato Y, Tanaka Y, Vital A, Mariani L, Stawski R, Watanabe T, De Girolami U, Kleihues P, Ohgaki H. Molecular Classification of Low-Grade Diffuse Gliomas. The American Journal of Pathology 2010; 177(6):2708-14.

[84] Mueller W, Hartmann C, Hoffmann A, Lanksch W, Kiwit J, Tonn J, Veelken J, Schramm J, Weller M, Wiestler OD, Louis DN, von Deimling A. Genetic signature of oligoastrocytomas correlates with tumor location and denotes distinct molecular subsets. The American Journal of Pathology 2002; 161(1):313-9.

[85] Reifenberger G, Louis DN. Oligodendroglioma: Toward Molecular Definitions in Diagnostic Neuro-Oncology. Journal of Neuropathology and Experimental Neurology 2003; 62(2):111-26.

[86] Watanabe T, Yokoo H, Yokoo M, Yonekawa Y, Kleihues P, Ohgaki H. Concurrent Inactivation of RB1 and TP53 Pathways in Anaplastic Oligodendrogliomas. Journal of Neuropathology and Experimental Neurology 2001; 60(12):1181-9.

[87] Ino Y, Betensky RA, Zlatescu MC, Sasaki H, Macdonald DR, Stemmer-Rachamimov AO, Ramsay DA, Cairncross JG, Louis DN. Molecular subtypes of anaplastic oligodendroglioma: Implications for patient management at diagnosis. Clinical Cancer Research 2001; 7(4):839-45.

[88] Gaspar N, Grill J, Geoerger B, Lellouch-Tubiana A, Michalowski MB, Vassal G. p53 Pathway dysfunction in primary childhood ependymomas. Pediatric Blood and Cancer 2006; 46(5):604-13.

[89] Biernat W, Zawrocki A. Molecular alterations in ependymomas. Folia Neuropathol 2007; 45(4):155-63.

[90] Fink KL, Rushing EJ, Schold SC Jr, Nisen PD. Infrequency of p53 gene mutations in ependymomas. Journal of Neuro-oncology 1996; 27(2):111-5.

[91] Shuangshoti S, Rushing EJ, Mena H, Olsen C, Sandberg GD. Supratentorial extraventricular ependymal neoplasms: A clinicopathologic study of 32 patients. Cancer 2005; 103(12):2598-605.

[92] Rushing EJ, Brown DF, Hladik CL, Risser RC, Mickey BE, White CL 3rd. Correlation of bcl-2, p53, and MIB-1 expression with ependymoma grade and subtype. Modern Pathology 1998; 11(5):464-70.

[93] Suzuki S, Oka H, Kawano N, Tanaka S, Utsuki S, Fujii K. Prognostic value of Ki-67 (MIB-1) and p53 in ependymomas. Brain Tumor Pathology 2001; 18(2):151-4.

[94] Sharma MC, Ghara N, Jain D, Sarkar C, Singh M, Mehta VS. A study of proliferative markers and tumor suppressor gene proteins in different grades of ependymomas. Neuropathology 2009; 29(2):148-55.

[95] Manasa LP, Uppin MS, Sundaram C. Correlation of p53 and KI 67 expression with grade and subtype of ependymoma. Indian Journal of Pathology and Microbiology 2012; 55(3):308-13.

[96] Zamecnik J, Snuderl M, Eckschlager T, Chanova M, Hladikova M, Tichy M, Kodet R. Pediatric intracranial ependymomas: prognostic relevance of histological, immunohistochemical, and flow cytometric factors. Modern Pathology 2003; 16(10):980-91.

[97] Kleihues P, Schäuble B, zur Hausen A, Estève J, Ohgaki H. Tumors associated with p53 germline mutations: a synopsis of 91 families. The American Journal of Pathology 1997; 150(1):1-13.

[98] Barel D, Avigad S, Mor C, Fogel M, Cohen IJ, Zaizov R. A novel germline mutation in the noncoding region of the p53 gene in a Li-Fraumeni family. Cancer Genetics and Cytogenetics 1998; 103(1):1-6.

[99] Tong WM, Ohgaki H, Huang H, Granier C, Kleihues P, Wang ZQ. Null mutation of DNA strand break-binding molecule poly(ADP-ribose) polymerase causes medulloblastomas in p53(–/–) mice. The American Journal of Pathology 2003; 162(1):343-52.

[100] Shakhova O, Leung C, van Montfort E, Berns A, Marino S. Lack of Rb and p53 delays cerebellar development and predisposes to large cell anaplastic medulloblastoma through amplification of N-Myc and Ptch2. Cancer Research 2006; 66(10):5190-200.

[101] Adesina AM, Nalbantoglu J, Cavenee WK. p53 gene mutation and mdm2 gene amplification are uncommon in medulloblastoma. Cancer Research 1994; 54(21):5649-51.

[102] Ferretti E, De Smaele E, Di Marcotullio L, Screpanti I, Gulino A. Hedgehog checkpoints in medulloblastoma: the chromosome 17p deletion paradigm. Trends in Molecular Medicine 2005; 11(12):537-45.

[103] Northcott PA, Korshunov A, Witt H, Hielscher T, Eberhart CG, Mack S, Bouffet E, Clifford SC, Hawkins CE, French P, Rutka JT, Pfister S, Taylor MD. Medulloblastoma comprises four distinct molecular variants. Journal of Clinical Oncology 2011; 29(11): 1408-14.

[104] Schwalbe EC, Lindsey JC, Straughton D, Hogg TL, Cole M, Megahed H, Ryan SL, Lusher ME, Taylor MD, Gilbertson RJ, Ellison DW, Bailey S, Clifford SC. Rapid diagnosis of medulloblastoma molecular subgroups. Clinical Cancer Research 2011; 17(7): 1883-94.

[105] Taylor MD, Northcott PA, Korshunov A, Remke M, Cho YJ, Clifford SC, Eberhart CG, Parsons DW, Rutkowski S, Gajjar A, Ellison DW, Lichter P, Gilbertson RJ, Pomeroy SL, Kool M, Pfister SM. Molecular subgroups of medulloblastoma: The current consensus. Acta Neuropathologica 2012; 123(4):465-72.

[106] Pfaff E, Remke M, Sturm D, Benner A, Witt H, Milde T, von Bueren AO, Wittmann A, Schöttler A, Jorch N, Graf N, Kulozik AE, Witt O, Scheurlen W, von Deimling A, Rutkowski S, Taylor MD, Tabori U, Lichter P, Korshunov A, Pfister SM. TP53 mutation is frequently associated with CTNNB1 mutation or MYCN amplification and is compatible with long-term survival in medulloblastoma. Journal Clinical of Oncology 2010; 28(35):5188-96.

[107] Lindsey JC, Hill RM, Megahed H, Lusher ME, Schwalbe EC, Cole M, Hogg TL, Gilbertson RJ, Ellison DW, Bailey S, Clifford SC. TP53 mutations in favorable-risk Wnt/wingless-subtype medulloblastomas. Journal of Clinical Oncology 2011; 29(12):e344-6.

[108] Gessi M, von Bueren AO, Rutkowski S, Pietsch T. p53 expression predicts dismal outcome for medulloblastoma patients with metastatic disease. Journal of Neuro-oncology 2012; 106(1):135-41.

[109] Pugh TJ, Weeraratne SD, Archer TC, Pomeranz Krummel DA, Auclair D, Bochicchio J, Carneiro MO, Carter SL, Cibulskis K, Erlich RL, Greulich H, Lawrence MS, Lennon NJ, McKenna A, Meldrim J, Ramos AH, Ross MG, Russ C, Shefler E, Sivachenko A, Sogoloff B, Stojanov P, Tamayo P, Mesirov JP, Amani V, Teider N, Sengupta S, Francois JP, Northcott PA, Taylor MD, Yu F, Crabtree GR, Kautzman AG, Gabriel SB, Getz G, Jäger N, Jones DT, Lichter P, Pfister SM, Roberts TM, Meyerson M, Pomeroy

SL, Cho YJ. Medulloblastoma exome sequencing uncovers subtype-specific somatic mutations. Nature 2012; 488(7409):106-10.

[110] Robinson G, Parker M, Kranenburg TA, Lu C, Chen X, Ding L, Phoenix TN, Hedlund E, Wei L, Zhu X, Chalhoub N, Baker SJ, Huether R, Kriwacki R, Curley N, Thiruvenkatam R, Wang J, Wu G, Rusch M, Hong X, Becksfort J, Gupta P, Ma J, Easton J, Vadodaria B, Onar-Thomas A, Lin T, Li S, Pounds S, Paugh S, Zhao D, Kawauchi D, Roussel MF, Finkelstein D, Ellison DW, Lau CC, Bouffet E, Hassall T, Gururangan S, Cohn R, Fulton RS, Fulton LL, Dooling DJ, Ochoa K, Gajjar A, Mardis ER, Wilson RK, Downing JR, Zhang J, Gilbertson RJ. Novel mutations target distinct subgroups of medulloblastoma. Nature. 2012 Aug 2;488(7409):43-8.

[111] Zhukova N, Ramaswamy V, Remke M, Pfaff E, Shih DJ, Martin DC, Castelo-Branco P, Baskin B, Ray PN, Bouffet E, von Bueren AO, Jones DT, Northcott PA, Kool M, Sturm D, Pugh TJ, Pomeroy SL, Cho YJ, Pietsch T, Gessi M, Rutkowski S, Bognar L, Klekner A, Cho BK, Kim SK, Wang KC, Eberhart CG, Fevre-Montange M, Fouladi M, French PJ, Kros M, Grajkowska WA, Gupta N, Weiss WA, Hauser P, Jabado N, Jouvet A, Jung S, Kumabe T, Lach B, Leonard JR, Rubin JB, Liau LM, Massimi L, Pollack IF, Shin Ra Y, Van Meir EG, Zitterbart K, Schüller U, Hill RM, Lindsey JC, Schwalbe EC, Bailey S, Ellison DW, Hawkins C, Malkin D, Clifford SC, Korshunov A, Pfister S, Taylor MD, Tabori U. Subgroup specific prognostic implications of TP53 mutation in medulloblastoma. Journal of Clinical Oncology 2013; 31(23):2927-35.

[112] Carvalho RM, Pinto GR, Yoshioka FK, Lima PD, Souza CR, Guimarães AC, Lamarão LM, Rey JA, Burbano RR. Prognostic value of the TP53 Arg72Pro single-nucleotide polymorphism and susceptibility to medulloblastoma in a cohort of Brazilian patients. Journal of Neuro-oncoly 2012; 110(1):49-57.

[113] Mendrysa SM, Ghassemifar S, Malek R. p53 in the CNS: Perspectives on Development, Stem Cells, and Cancer. Genes and Cancer 2011; 2(4):431-42.

[114] Ho YS, Hsieh LL, Chen JS, Chang CN, Lee ST, Chiu LL, Chin TY, Cheng SC. p53 gene mutation in cerebral primitive neuroectodermal tumor in Taiwan. Cancer Letters 1996; 104(1):103-13.

[115] Kraus JA, Felsberg J, Tonn JC, Reifenberger G, Pietsch T. Molecular genetic analysis of the TP53, PTEN, CDKN2A, EGFR, CDK4 and MDM2 tumour associated genes in supratentorial primitive neuroectodermal tumours and glioblastomas of childhood. Neuropathology and Applied Neurobiology 2002; 28(4):325-33.

[116] Postovsky S, Ben Arush MW, Elhasid R, Davidson S, Leshanski L, Vlodavsky E, Guilburd JN, Amikam D. A novel case of a CAT to AAT transversion in codon 179 of the p53 gene in a supratentorial primitive neuroectodermal tumor harbored by a young girl: case report and review of the literature. Oncology 2003; 65(1):46-51.

[117] Gessi M, Setty P, Bisceglia M, zur Muehlen A, Lauriola L, Waha A, Giangaspero F, Pietsch T. Supratentorial Primitive Neuroectodermal Tumors of the Central Nervous

System in Adults: Molecular and Histopathologic Analysis of 12 Cases. The American Journal of Surgical Pathology. 2011; 35(4):573-82.

[118] Eberhart CG, Chaudhry A, Daniel RW, Khaki L, Shah KV, Gravitt PE. Increased p53 immunopositivity in anaplastic medulloblastoma and supratentorial PNET is not caused by JC virus. BMC Cancer 2005; 17, 5:19.

[119] Woodburn RT, Azzarelli B, Montebello JF, Goss IE. Intense p53 staining is a valuable prognostic indicator for poor prognosis in medulloblastoma/central nervous system primitive neuroectodermal tumors. Journal of Neuro-oncology 2001; 52(1):57-62.

[120] Rosson GB, Hazen-Martin DJ, Biegel JA, Willingham MC, Garvin AJ, Oswald BW, Wainwright L, Brownlee NA, Wright CF. Establishment and molecular characterization of five cell lines derived from renal and extrarenal malignant rhabdoid tumors. Modern Pathology. 1998; 11(12):1228-37.

[121] Kinoshita Y, Shiratsuchi H, Tamiya S, Oshiro Y, Hachitanda Y, Oda Y, Suita S, Tsuneyoshi M. Mutations of the p53 gene in malignant rhabdoid tumors of soft tissue and the kidney: immunohistochemical and DNA direct sequencing analysis. Journal of Cancer Research and Clinical Oncology. 2001;127(6):351-8.

[122] Isakoff MS, Sansam CG, Tamayo P, Subramanian A, Evans JA, Fillmore CM, Wang X, Biegel JA, Pomeroy SL, Mesirov JP, Roberts CW. Inactivation of the Snf5 tumor suppressor stimulates cell cycle progression and cooperates with p53 loss in oncogenic transformation. Proceedings of National Academy of Science of USA 2005;102(49):17745-50.

[123] Kato H, Honma R, Sanda T, Fujiwara T, Ito E, Yanagisawa Y, Imai J, Okamoto T, Watanabe S. Knock down of hSNF5/Ini1 causes cell cycle arrest and apoptosis in a p53-dependent manner. Biochemical and Biophysical Research Communications 2007; 361(3):580-5.

[124] DelBove J, Kuwahara Y, Mora-Blanco EL, Godfrey V, Funkhouser WK, Fletcher CD, Van Dyke T, Roberts CW, Weissman BE. Inactivation of SNF5 cooperates with p53 loss to accelerate tumor formation in Snf5(+/–);p53(+/–) mice. Molecular Carcinogenesis 2009; 48(12):1139-48.

[125] Venneti S, Le P, Martinez D, Eaton KW, Shyam N, Jordan-Sciutto KL, Pawel B, Biegel JA, Judkins AR. p16 INK4A and p14 ARF Tumor Suppressor Pathways Are Deregulated in Malignant Rhabdoid Tumors. Journal of Neuropathology and Experimental Neurology 2011; 70(7):596-609.

[126] Varley JM, McGown G, Thorncroft M, James LA, Margison GP, Forster G, Evans DG, Harris M, Kelsey AM, Birch JM. Are there low-penetrance TP53 Alleles? Evidence from childhood adrenocortical tumors. American Journal of Human Genetics 1999; 65(4):995-1006.

[127] Gonzalez KD, Noltner KA, Buzin CH, Gu D, Wen-Fong CY, Nguyen VQ, Han JH, Lowstuter K, Longmate J, Sommer SS, Weitzel JN. Beyond Li Fraumeni syndrome:

Clinical characteristics of families with p53 germline mutations. Journal of Clinical Oncology 2009; 27(8):1250-6.

[128] Chompret A, Abel A, Stoppa-Lyonnet D, Brugiéres L, Pagés S, Feunteun J, Bonaïti-Pellié C. Sensitivity and predictive value of criteria for p53 germline mutation screening. Journal of Medical Genetics 2001; 38(1):43-7.

[129] Tinat J, Bougeard G, Baert-Desurmont S, Vasseur S, Martin C, Bouvignies E, Caron O, Bressac-de Paillerets B, Berthet P, Dugast C, Bonaïti-Pellié C, Stoppa-Lyonnet D, Frébourg T. 2009 Version of the Chompret criteria for Li Fraumeni syndrome. Journal of Clinical Oncology 2009 ; 27(26):e108-9.

[130] Wrede B, Hasselblatt M, Peters O, Thall PF, Kutluk T, Moghrabi A, Mahajan A, Rutkowski S, Diez B, Wang X, Pietsch T, Kortmann RD, Paulus W, Jeibmann A, Wolff JE. Atypical choroid plexus papilloma: clinical experience in the CPT-SIOP-2000 study. Journal of Neuro-oncology 2009; 95(3):383-92.

[131] Tabori U, Shlien A, Baskin B, Levitt S, Ray P, Alon N, Hawkins C, Bouffet E, Pienkowska M, Lafay-Cousin L, Gozali A, Zhukova N, Shane L, Gonzalez I, Finlay J, Malkin D. TP53 alterations determine clinical subgroups and survival of patients with choroid plexus tumors. Journal of Clinical Oncology 2010; 28(12):1995-2001.

[132] Krzyzankova M, Mertsch S, Koos B, Jeibmann A, Kruse A, Kordes U, Frühwald MC, Wolff JE, Paulus W, Hasselblatt M. Loss of TP53 expression in immortalized choroid plexus epithelialcells results in increased resistance to anticancer agents. Journal of Neuro-oncology. 2012; 109(3):449-55.

[133] Nagashima G, Aoyagi M, Yamamoto M, Yamamoto S, Wakimoto H, Ohno K, Yamamoto K, Hirakawa K. P53 overexpression and proliferative potential in malignant meningiomas. Acta Neurochirurgica (Wien). 1999;141(1):53-61.

[134] Joachim T, Ram Z, Rappaport ZH, Simon M, Schramm J, Wiestler OD, von Deimling A. Comparative analysis of the NF2, TP53, PTEN, KRAS, NRAS and HRAS genes in sporadic and radiation-induced human meningiomas. International Journal of Cancer 2001; 94(2):218-21.

[135] Verheijen FM, Sprong M, Kloosterman JM, Blaauw G, Thijssen JH, Blankenstein MA. TP53 mutations in human meningiomas. International Journal of Biological Markers. 2002; 17(1):42-8.

[136] Wang JL, Zhang ZJ, Hartman M, Smits A, Westermark B, Muhr C, Nistér M. Detection of TP53 gene mutation in human meningiomas: a study using immunohistochemistry, polymerase chain reaction/single-strand conformation polymorphism and DNA sequencing techniques on paraffin-embedded samples. International Journal of Cancer. 1995 Aug 22;64(4):223-8.

[137] Cho H, Ha SY, Park SH, Park K, Chae YS. Role of p53 gene mutation in tumor aggressiveness of intracranial meningiomas. Journal of Korean Medical Science. 1999; 14(2):199-205.

[138] Pavelin S, Bečić K, Forempoher G, Tomić S, Capkun V, Drmić-Hofman I, Mrklić I, Lušić I, Pogorelić Z. The Significance of Immunohistochemical Expression of Merlin, Ki-67, and p53 in Meningiomas. Applied Immunohistochemistry and Moecularl Morphology. 2013 Feb 28.

[139] Ohkoudo M, Sawa H, Hara M, Saruta K, Aiso T, Ohki R, Yamamoto H, Maemura E, Shiina Y, Fujii M, Saito I. Expression of p53, MDM2 protein and Ki-67 antigen in recurrent meningiomas. Journal of Neuro-oncology 1998; 38(1):41-9.

[140] Amatya VJ, Takeshima Y, Inai K. Methylation of p14(ARF) gene in meningiomas and its correlation to the p53 expression and mutation. Modern Pathology 2004; 17(6): 705-10.

[141] Al-Khalaf HH, Lach B, Allam A, AlKhani A, Alrokayan SA, Aboussekhra A. The p53/p21 DNA damage-signaling pathway is defective in most meningioma cells. Journal of Neuro-oncology 2007; 83(1):9-15.

[142] Kim H, Kwak NJ, Lee JY, Choi BH, Lim Y, Ko YJ, Kim YH, Huh PW, Lee KH, Rha HK, Wang YP. Merlin neutralizes the inhibitory effect of Mdm2 on p53. The Journal of Biological Chemistry. 2004; 279(9):7812-8.

[143] Das A, Tan WL, Smith DR. p53 point mutation is rare in meningiomas from Singaporean patients. Asian Journal of Surgery 2005; 28(1):7-10.

[144] Kamei Y, Watanabe M, Nakayama T, Kanamaru K, Waga S, Shiraishi T. Prognostic significance of p53 and p21WAF1/CIP1 immunoreactivity and tumor micronecrosis for recurrence of meningiomas. Journal of Neuro-oncology 2000; 46(3):205-13.

[145] Lanzafame S, Torrisi A, Barbagallo G, Emmanuele C, Alberio N, Albanese V. Correlation between histological grade, MIB-1, p53, and recurrence in 69 completely resected primary intracranial meningiomas with a 6 year mean follow-up. Pathology, Research and Practice 2000; 196(7):483-8.

[146] Hakin-Smith V, Battersby RD, Maltby EL, Timperley WR, Royds JA. Elevated p53 expression in benign meningiomas protects against recurrence and may be indicative of senescence. Neuropathology and Applied Neurobiology 2001; 27(1):40-9.

[147] Terzi A, Saglam EA, Barak A, Soylemezoglu F. The significance of immunohistochemical expression of Ki-67, p53, p21, and p16 in meningiomas tissue arrays. Pathology, Research and Practice ; 204(5):305-14.

[148] Nagarajan RP, Costello JF. Molecular Epigenetics and Genetics in Neuro-Oncology. Neurotherapeutics 2009; 6(3):436-46.

[149] Inbar-Feigenberg M, Choufani S, Butcher DT, Roifman M, Weksberg R. Basic concepts of epigenetics. Fertility and Sterility 2013; 99(3):607-15.

[150] Carén H, Pollard SM, Beck S. The good, the bad and the ugly: Epigenetic mechanisms in glioblastoma. Molecular Aspects of Medicine 2013; 34(4):849-62.

[151] Christensen BC, Smith AA, Zheng S, Koestler DC, Houseman EA, Marsit CJ, Wiemels JL, Nelson HH, Karagas MR, Wrensch MR, Kelsey KT, Wiencke JK. DNA methylation, isocitrate dehydrogenase mutation, and survival in glioma. Journal of the National Cancer Institute 2011; 103(2):143-53.

[152] Lima EM, Leal MF, Burbano RR, Khayat AS, Assumpção PP, Bello MJ, Rey JA, Smith MA, Casartelli C. Methylation status of ANAPC1, CDKN2A and TP53 promoter genes in individuals with gastric cancer. Brazilian Journal of Medical and Biological Research 2008; 41(6):539-43.

[153] Sidhu S, Martin E, Gicquel C, Melki J, Clark SJ, Campbell P, Magarey CJ, Schulte KM, Röher HD, Delbridge L, Robinson BG. Mutation and methylation analysis of TP53 in adrenal carcinogenesis. European Journal of Surgical Oncology 2005; 31(5):549-54.

[154] Tuck SP, Crawford L. Characterization of the human p53 gene promoter. Molecular and Cell Biology 1989; 9(5):2163-72.

[155] Schroeder M, Mass MJ. CpG methylation inactivates the transcriptional activity of the promoter of the human p53 tumor suppressor gene. Biochemistry and Biophysical Research Communication 1997; 235(2):403-6.

[156] Hurt EM, Thomas SB, Peng B, Farrar WL. Reversal of p53 epigenetic silencing in multiple myeloma permits apoptosis by a p53 activator. Cancer Biology and Therapy 2006; 5(9):1154-60.

[157] Gonzalez-Gomez P, Bello MJ, Lomas J, Arjona D, Alonso ME, Amiñoso C, Lopez-Marin I, Anselmo NP, Sarasa JL, Gutierrez M, Casartelli C, Rey JA. Aberrant methylation of multiple genes in neuroblastic tumours. relationship with MYCN amplification and allelic status at 1p. European Journal of Cancer 2003; 39(10): 1478-85.

[158] Alonso ME, Bello MJ, Gonzalez-Gomez P, Arjona D, Lomas J, de Campos JM, Isla A, Sarasa JL, Rey JA. Aberrant promoter methylation of multiple genes in oligodendrogliomas and ependymomas. Cancer Genetics and Cytogenetics 2003; 144(2):134-42.

[159] Amatya VJ, Naumann U, Weller M, Ohgaki H. TP53 promoter methylation in human gliomas. Acta Neuropathologica 2005; 110(2):178-84.

[160] Almeida LO, Custódio AC, Pinto GR, Santos MJ, Almeida JR, Clara CA, Rey JA, Casartelli C. Polymorphisms and DNA methylation of gene TP53 associated with extra-axial brain tumors. Genetics and Molecular Research 2009; 8(1):8-18.

[161] Weber MA, Giesel FL, Stieltjes B. MRI for identification of progression in brain tumors: from morphology to function. Expert Review of Neurotherapeutics 2008; 8(10): 1507-25.

[162] Barajas RF Jr, Cha S. Imaging diagnosis of brain metastasis. Progress in Neurological Surgery 2012; 25:55-73.

[163] Filipowicz W, Bhattacharyya SN, Sonenberg N. Mechanisms of post-transcriptional regulation by microRNAs: are the answers in sight? Nature Reviews Genetics 2008; 9(2):102-14.

[164] McDermott R, Gabikian P, Sarvaiya P, Ulasov I, Lesniak MS. MicroRNAs in brain metastases: big things come in small packages. Journal of Molecular Medicine 2013; 91(1):5-13.

[165] Blower PE, Chung JH, Verducci JS, Lin S, Park JK, Dai Z, Liu CG, Schmittgen TD, Reinhold WC, Croce CM, Weinstein JN, Sadee W. MicroRNAs modulate the chemosensitivity of tumor cells. Molecular Cancer Therapeutics 2008; 7(1):1-9.

[166] Calin GA, Croce CM. MicroRNA signatures in human cancers. Nature Reviews Cancer 2006; 6(11):857-66.

[167] Cummins JM, Velculescu VE. Implications of micro-RNA profiling for câncer diagnosis. Oncogene 2006; 25(46):6220-7.

[168] Kumar MS, Lu J, Mercer KL, Golub TR, Jacks T. Impaired microRNA processing enhances cellular transformation and tumorigenesis. Nature Genetics 2007; 39(5):673-7.

[169] Calin GA, Liu CG, Ferracin M, Hyslop T, Spizzo R, Sevignani C, Fabbri M, Cimmino A, Lee EJ, Wojcik SE, Shimizu M, Tili E, Rossi S, Taccioli C, Pichiorri F, Liu X, Zupo S, Herlea V, Gramantieri L, Lanza G, Alder H, Rassenti L, Volinia S, Schmittgen TD, Kipps TJ, Negrini M, Croce CM. Ultraconserved regions encoding ncRNAs are altered in human leukemias and carcinomas. Cancer Cell 2007; 12(3):215-29.

[170] Schmittgen TD, Lee EJ, Jiang J, Sarkar A, Yang L, Elton TS, Chen C. Real-time PCR quantification of precursor and mature microRNA. Methods 2008; 44(1):31-8.

[171] Liu CG, Spizzo R, Calin GA, Croce CM. Expression profiling of microRNA using oligo DNA arrays. Methods 2008; 44(1):22-30.

[172] Wienholds E, Kloosterman WP, Miska E, Alvarez-Saavedra E, Berezikov E, de Bruijn E, Horvitz HR, Kauppinen S, Plasterk RH. MicroRNA expression in zebrafish embryonic development. Science. 2005 Jul 8;309(5732):310-1.

[173] Cummins JM, He Y, Leary RJ, Pagliarini R, Diaz LA Jr, Sjoblom T, Barad O, Bentwich Z, Szafranska AE, Labourier E, Raymond CK, Roberts BS, Juhl H, Kinzler KW, Vogelstein B, Velculescu VE. The colorectal microRNAome. Proceedings of National Academy of Science of USA 2006; 103(10):3687-92.

[174] He L, He X, Lowe SW, Hannon GJ. microRNAs join the p53 network-another piece in the tumour-suppression puzzle. Nature Reviews Cancer. 2007 Nov;7(11):819-22.

[175] Park SY, Lee JH, Ha M, Nam JW, Kim VN. miR-29 miRNAs activate p53 by targeting p85 alpha and CDC42. Nature Structural and Molecular Biology 2009; 16(1):23-9.

[176] Zhang Y, Gao JS, Tang X, Tucker LD, Quesenberry P, Rigoutsos I, Ramratnam B. MicroRNA 125ª and its regulation of the p53 tumor suppressor gene. FEBS Letters 2009; 583(22):3725-30.

[177] He L, He X, Lim LP, de Stanchina E, Xuan Z, Liang Y, Xue W, Zender L, Magnus J, Ridzon D, Jackson AL, Linsley PS, Chen C, Lowe SW, Cleary MA, Hannon GJ. A microRNA component of the p53 tumour suppressor network. Nature 2007; 447(7148): 1130-4.

[178] Luan S, Sun L, Huang F. MicroRNA-34a: A Novel Tumor Suppressor in p53-mutant Glioma Cell Line U251. Archives of Medical Research 2010; 41(2):67-74.

[179] Lee YS, Dutta A. MicroRNAs in Cancer. Annual Review Pathology 2009; 4:199-227.

[180] Bommer GT, Gerin I, Feng Y, Kaczorowski AJ, Kuick R, Love RE, Zhai Y, Giordano TJ, Qin ZS, Moore BB, MacDougald OA, Cho KR, Fearon ER. p53-mediated activation of miRNA34 candidate tumor-suppressor genes. Current Biology 2007; 17(15): 1298-307.

[181] Chang TC, Wentzel EA, Kent OA, Ramachandran K, Mullendore M, Lee KH, Feldmann G, Yamakuchi M, Ferlito M, Lowenstein CJ, Arking DE, Beer MA, Maitra A, Mendell JT. Transactivation of miR-34a by p53 broadly influences gene expression and promotes apoptosis. Molecular Cell 2007; 26(5):745-52.

[182] Raver-Shapira N, Marciano E, Meiri E, Spector Y, Rosenfeld N, Moskovits N, Bentwich Z, Oren M. Transcriptional activation of miR-34a contributes to p53-mediated apoptosis. Molecular Cell ; 26(5):731-43.

[183] Welch C, Chen Y, Stallings RL. MicroRNA-34a functions as a potential tumor suppressor by inducing apoptosis in neuroblastoma cells. Oncogene 2007; 26(34):5017-22.

[184] Corney DC, Flesken-Nikitin A, Godwin AK, Wang W, Nikitin AY. MicroRNA-34b and microRNA-34c are targets of p53 and cooperate in control of cell proliferation and adhesion-independent growth. Cancer Research 2007; 67(18):8433-8.

[185] Le MT, Teh C, Shyh-Chang N, Xie H, Zhou B, Korzh V, Lodish HF, Lim B. MicroRNA-125b is a novel negative regulator of p53. Genes and Development 2009; 23(7): 862-76.

[186] Hu W, Chan CS, Wu R, Zhang C, Sun Y, Song JS, Tang LH, Levine AJ, Feng Z. Negative regulation of tumor suppressor p53 by microRNA miR-504. Molecular Cell 2010; 38(5):689-99.

[187] Hermeking H. p53 Enters the MicroRNA World. Cancer Cell 2007; 12(5):414-8.

[188] Weeraratne SD, Amani V, Neiss A, Teider N, Scott DK, Pomeroy SL, Cho YJ. miR-34a confers chemosensitivity through modulation of MAGE-A and p53 in medulloblastoma. Neuro-Oncology 2011; 13(2):165-75.

[189] Suh SS, Yoo JY, Nuovo GJ, Jeon YJ, Kim S, Lee TJ, Kim T, Bakàcs A, Alder H, Kaur B, Aqeilan RI, Pichiorri F, Croce CM. MicroRNAs/TP53 feedback circuitry in glioblastoma multiforme. Proceedings of National Academy of Science of USA 2012; 109(14): 5316-21.

[190] Heywood RM, Marcus HJ, Ryan DJ, Piccirillo SG, Al-Mayhani TM, Watts C. A review of the role of stem cells in the development and treatment of glioma. Acta Neurochirurgica 2012; 154(6):951-69.

[191] Gangemi R, Paleari L, Orengo AM, Cesario A, Chessa L, Ferrini S, Russo P. Cancer Stem Cells: A New Paradigm for Understanding Tumor Growth and Progression and Drug Resistance. Current Medical Chemistry 2009;16(14):1688-703.

[192] Sugihara E, Saya H. Complexity of cancer stem cells. International Journal of Cancer 2013; 132(6):1249-59.

[193] Bonnet D, Dick JE. Human acute myeloid leukemia is organized as a hierarchy that originates from a primitive hematopoietic cell. Nature Medicine 1997; 3(7):730-7.

[194] Hope KJ, Jin L, Dick JE. Acute myeloid leukemia originates from a hierarchy of leukemic stem cell classes that differ in self-renewal capacity. Nature Immunology 2004; 5(7):738-43.

[195] Lee C, Dunn SE, Yip S. Stem Cells in Brain Tumour Development and Therapy-Two-Sides of the Same Coin. The Canadian Journal of Neurological Science 2012; 39(2): 145-56.

[196] Wang K, Wu X, Wang J, Huang J. Cancer stem cell theory: therapeutic implications for nanomedicine. International Journal of Nanomedicine 2013; 8:899-908.

[197] Stiles CD, Rowitch DH. Glioma Stem Cells: A Midterm Exam. Neuron 2008; 58(6): 832-46.

[198] Ji J, Black KL, Yu JS. Glioma stem cell research for the development of immunotherapy.

[199] Cicalese A, Bonizzi G, Pasi CE, Faretta M, Ronzoni S, Giulini B, Brisken C, Minucci S, Di Fiore PP, Pelicci PG. The tumor suppressor p53 regulates polarity of self-renewing divisions in mammary stem cells. Cell 2009; 138(6):1083-95.

[200] Liu Y, Elf SE, Asai T, Miyata Y, Liu Y, Sashida G, Huang G, Di Giandomenico S, Koff A, Nimer SD. The p53 tumor suppressor protein is a critical regulator of hematopoietic stem cell behavior. Cell Cycle 2009; 8(19):3120-4.

[201] Lin T, Chao C, Saito S, Mazur SJ, Murphy ME, Appella E, Xu Y. p53 induces di ff erentiation of mouse embryonic stem cells by suppressing Nanog expression. Nature Cell Biology 2005; 7(2):165-71.

[202] Meletis K, Wirta V, Hede SM, Nistér M, Lundeberg J, Frisén J. p53 suppresses the self-renewal of adult neural stem cells. Development 2006; 133(2):363-9.

[203] Armesilla-Diaz A, Bragado P, Del Valle I, Cuevas E, Lazaro I, Martin C, Cigudosa JC, Silva A. p53 REGULATES THE SELF-RENEWAL AND DIFFERENTIATION OF NEURAL PRECURSORS. Neuroscience 2009; 158(4):1378-89.

[204] Medrano S, Scrable H. Maintaining appearances-the role of p53 in adult neurogenesis. Biochemical and Biophysical Research Communications 2005; 331(3):828-33.

[205] Medrano S, Burns-Cusato M, Atienza MB, Rahimi D, Scrable H. Regenerative capacity of neural precursors in the adult mammalian brain is under the control of p53. Neurobiology of Aging 2009; 30(3):483-97.

[206] Billon N, Terrinoni A, Jolicoeur C, McCarthy A, Richardson WD, Melino G, Raff M. Roles for p53 and p73 during oligodendrocyte development. Development 2004; 131(6):1211-20.

[207] Wosik K, Antel J, Kuhlmann T, Brück W, Massie B, Nalbantoglu J. Oligodendrocyte injury in multiple sclerosis: a role for p53. Journal of Neurochemistry 2003; 85(3): 635-44.

[208] Vescovi AL, Galli R, Reynolds BA. Brain tumour stem cells. Nature Reviews Cancer 2006; 6(6):425-36.

[209] Shackleton M. Normal stem cells and cancer stem cells: similar and different. Seminars in Cancer Biology 2010; 20(2):85-92.

[210] Holland EC, Hively WP, DePinho RA, Varmus HE. A constitutively active epidermal growth factor receptor cooperates with disruption of G1 cell-cycle arrest pathways to induce glioma-like lesions in mice. Genes and Development 1998; 12(23):3675-85.

[211] Holland EC, Celestino J, Dai C, Schaefer L, Sawaya RE, Fuller GN. Combined activation of Ras and Akt in neural progenitors induces glioblastoma formation in mice. Nature Genetics 2000; 25(1):55-7.

[212] Bachoo RM, Maher EA, Ligon KL, Sharpless NE, Chan SS, You MJ, Tang Y, DeFrances J, Stover E, Weissleder R, Rowitch DH, Louis DN, DePinho RA. Epidermal growth factor receptor and Ink4a/Arf: convergent mechanisms governing terminal differentiation and transformation along the neural stem cell to astrocyte axis. Cancer Cell 2002; 1(3):269-77.

[213] Muller PA, Vousden KH, Norman JC. p53 and its mutants in tumor cell migration and invasion. The Journal of Cell Biology 2011; 192(2):209-18.

[214] Burness ML, Sipkins DA. The stem cell niche in health and malignancy. Seminars in Cancer Biology 2010; 20(2):107-15.

[215] Lane DP, Cheok CF, Lain S. p53-based cancer therapy. Cold Spring Harbor Perspectives in Biology 2010; 2(9):a001222.

[216] Murphy AM, Rabkin SD. Current status of gene therapy for brain tumors. Translational Research 2013; 161(4):339-54.

[217] Stupp R, Hegi ME, van den Bent MJ, Mason WP, Weller M, Mirimanoff RO, Cairncross JG. Changing paradigms–an update on the multidisciplinary management of malignant glioma. The Oncologist 2006; 11(2):165-80.

[218] Wen PY, Kesari S. Malignant gliomas in adults. The New England Journal of Medicine 2008 ; 359(5):492-507.

[219] Stupp R, Mason WP, van den Bent MJ, Weller M, Fisher B, Taphoorn MJ, Belanger K, Brandes AA, Marosi C, Bogdahn U, Curschmann J, Janzer RC, Ludwin SK, Gorlia T, Allgeier A, Lacombe D, Cairncross JG, Eisenhauer E, Mirimanoff RO. Radiotherapy plus concomitant and adjuvant temozolomide for glioblastoma. The New England Journal of Medicine 2005; 352(10):987-96.

[220] Stupp R, Hegi ME, Mason WP, van den Bent MJ, Taphoorn MJ, Janzer RC, Ludwin SK, Allgeier A, Fisher B, Belanger K, Hau P, Brandes AA, Gijtenbeek J, Marosi C, Vecht CJ, Mokhtari K, Wesseling P, Villa S, Eisenhauer E, Gorlia T, Weller M, Lacombe D, Cairncross JG, Mirimanoff RO. Effects of radiotherapy with concomitant and adjuvant temozolomide versus radiotherapy alone on survival in glioblastoma in a randomised phase III study: 5-year analysis of the EORTC-NCIC trial. The Lancet Oncology 2009; 10(5):459-66.

[221] Lefranc F, Brotchi J, Kiss R. Possible future issues in the treatment of glioblastomas: special emphasis on cell migration and the resistance of migrating glioblastoma cells to apoptosis. Journal of Clinical Oncology 2005; 23(10):2411-22.

[222] Amberger-Murphy V. Hypoxia helps glioma to fight therapy. Current Cancer Drug Targets 2009; 9(3):381-90.

[223] Chinot OL, Barrié M, Fuentes S, Eudes N, Lancelot S, Metellus P, Muracciole X, Braguer D, Ouafik L, Martin PM, Dufour H, Figarella-Branger D. Correlation between O6-methylguanine-DNA methyltransferase and survival in inoperable newly diagnosed glioblastoma patients treated with neoadjuvant temozolomide. Journal of Clinical Oncology 2007; 25(12):1470-5.

[224] Sathornsumetee S, Rich JN. Designer therapies for glioblastoma multiforme. Annals of th New York Academy of Science 2008; 1142:108-32.

[225] Kastan MB. Wild-Type p53: Tumors Can't Stand It. Cell 2007; 128(5):837-4.

[226] Vassilev LT, Vu BT, Graves B, Carvajal D, Podlaski F, Filipovic Z, Kong N, Kammlott U, Lukacs C, Klein C, Fotouhi N, Liu EA. In vivo activation of the p53 pathway by small-molecule antagonists of MDM2. Science 2004; 303(5659):844-8.

[227] Künkele A, De Preter K, Heukamp L, Thor T, Pajtler KW, Hartmann W, Mittelbronn M, Grotzer MA, Deubzer HE, Speleman F, Schramm A, Eggert A, Schulte JH. Pharmacological activation of the p53 pathway by nutlin-3 exerts anti-tumoral effects in medulloblastomas. Neuro-Oncology 2012; 14(7):859-69.

[228] Shen J, Vakifahmetoglu H, Stridh H, Zhivotovsky B, Wiman KG. PRIMA-1MET induces mitochondrial apoptosis through activation of caspase-2. Oncogene 2008; 27(51):6571-80.

[229] Wang T, Lee K, Rehman A, Daoud SS. PRIMA-1 induces apoptosis by inhibiting JNK signaling but promoting the activation of Bax. Biochemical and Biophysical Research Communications. 2007; 352(1):203-12.

[230] Mercer WE, Shields MT, Amin M, Sauve GJ, Appella E, Romano JW, Ullrich SJ. Negative growth regulation in a glioblastoma tumor cell line that conditionally expresses human wild-type p53. Proceedings of National Academy of Science of USA 1990; 87(16):6166-70.

[231] Köck H, Harris MP, Anderson SC, Machemer T, Hancock W, Sutjipto S, Wills KN, Gregory RJ, Shepard HM, Westphal M, Maneval DC. Adenovirus-mediated p53 gene transfer suppresses growth of human glioblastoma cells in vitro and in vivo. International Journal of Cancer 1996; 67(6):808-15.

[232] Gomez-Manzano C, Fueyo J, Kyritsis AP, McDonnell TJ, Steck PA, Levin VA, Yung WK. Characterization of p53 and p21 functional interactions in glioma cells en route to apoptosis. Journal of the National Cancer Institute 1997; 89(14):1036-44.

[233] Lang FF, Bruner JM, Fuller GN, Aldape K, Prados MD, Chang S, Berger MS, McDermott MW, Kunwar SM, Junck LR, Chandler W, Zwiebel JA, Kaplan RS, Yung WK. Phase I trial of adenovirus-mediated p53 gene therapy for recurrent glioma: biological and clinical results. Journal of Clinical Oncology 2003; 21(13):2508-18.

[234] Candolfi M, Yagiz K, Foulad D, Alzadeh GE, Tesarfreund M, Muhammad AK, Puntel M, Kroeger KM, Liu C, Lee S, Curtin JF, King GD, Lerner J, Sato K, Mineharu Y, Xiong W, Lowenstein PR, Castro MG. Release of HMGB1 in response to proapoptotic glioma killing strategies: efficacy and neurotoxicity. Clinical Cancer Research 2009; 15(13):4401-14.

[235] Sur S, Pagliarini R, Bunz F, Rago C, Diaz LA Jr, Kinzler KW, Vogelstein B, Papadopoulos N. A panel of isogenic human cancer cells suggests a therapeutic approach for cancers with inactivated p53. Proceedings of National Academy of Science of USA 2009; 106(10):3964-9.

[236] Shchors K, Persson AI, Rostker F, Tihan T, Lyubynska N, Li N, Swigart LB, Berger MS, Hanahan D, Weiss WA, Evan GI. Using a preclinical mouse model of high-grade

astrocytoma to optimize p53 restoration therapy. Proceedings of National Academy of Science of USA 2013; 110(16):E1480-9.

[237] Vasconcelos, DS, da Silva FP, Quintana LG, Anselmo NP, Othman MA, Liehr T, de Oliveira EH. Numerical aberrations of chromosome 17 and TP53 in brain metastases derived from breast cancer. Genetics and Molecular Research. 2013; 12(3):2594-600.

Section 4

Angiogenesis and Immune Therapy – New Therapeutical Approaches

Chapter 7

Anti-Angiogenesis, Gene Therapy, and Immunotherapy in Malignant Gliomas

Paula Province, Alexis Bashinski Shaefer,
Benjamin McCullough and
Hassan M Fathallah-Shaykh

Additional information is available at the end of the chapter

http://dx.doi.org/10.5772/58320

1. Introduction

Malignant gliomas remain associated with poor prognosis and the cause of significant morbidity. In 2010, there was excitement that recent spectacular advancements in our basic understanding of their molecular pathogenesis, angiogenesis and new gene transfer technologies will turn the tide in our favor. The negative results of several costly phase III clinical trials are sobering; unfortunately, they take us back to the drawing board in terms of how we can improve our methods and why brain cancer has this incredible ability to resist therapy. This chapter is organized as follows. We start by an overview of the classification and significance of malignant gliomas. We proceed to reviewing the molecular pathogenesis of angiogenesis and the development of new treatment modalities against anti-angiogenesis targets, some of which were tested in Phase III clinical trials. Before considering immunotherapy strategies and targets for malignant gliomas, we review basic concepts in immunology and discuss the unique immunological features of the central nervous system (CNS). Finally, we discuss gene therapy vectors, strategies, and clinical trials in malignant gliomas. We conclude by an analysis of our current limitations, possible tumor mechanisms for resisting treatments, and what we can do to improve the outcome.

INTECH
open science | open minds

© 2014 The Author(s). Licensee InTech. This chapter is distributed under the terms of the Creative Commons Attribution License (http://creativecommons.org/licenses/by/3.0), which permits unrestricted use, distribution, and reproduction in any medium, provided the original work is properly cited.

2. Overview and significance

2.1. Classification of gliomas

CNS neoplasms are diverse and demonstrate a great deal of variability in terms of clinical presentation, aggressiveness, and response to therapy, with distinctions in histology and cellular and molecular composition being primarily responsible for these variations (Brat and Mapstone 2003; Omuro and DeAngelis 2013). Gliomas are the most frequent primary brain tumors in adults and, of this group, anaplastic astrocytomas and glioblastoma (GBM) are the two highest-grade astrocytic neoplasms (Brat and Mapstone 2003; Ricard, Idbaih et al. 2012). The World Health Organization (WHO) system classifies astrocytomas into four grades. These histological grades are defined by increasing degrees of undifferentiation, anaplasia, and aggressiveness (Louis, Ohgaki et al. 2007; Omuro and DeAngelis 2013). Grade I and II tumors, the lower grade tumors, are well-differentiated with limited cell density. The characteristic features of grade III astrocytomas (anaplastic) are increased vessel and cell density, cellular atypias, and high mitotic activity. Grade IV astrocytoma (GBM) is characterized by vascular proliferation or necrosis (Westphal and Lamszus 2011; Omuro and DeAngelis 2013). Glioblastoma and other malignant gliomas are highly infiltrative tumors. Of note, there is also a WHO grading system for oligodendrogliomas and oligoastrocytomas, but they will not be discussed in this chapter (Omuro and DeAngelis 2013).

2.2. Significance of malignant gliomas

The annual incidence of malignant glioma is 5.26 per 100 thousand and this group accounts for approximately 80% of the total number of new cases of malignant primary brain tumors diagnosed in the United States each year (Omuro and DeAngelis 2013). The overall incidence of gliomas is highest among Caucasians, as compared to other ethnic groups, and is higher among males as compared to females (7.2 versus 5.0 per 100,000 persons-years) (Peak and Levin 2010). Malignant gliomas can occur in any age group; however, the incidence increases in the fifth decade of life and peaks at about 65 years of age (Brat and Mapstone 2003). GBM is the most aggressive glioma. Stupp and colleagues reported that 27.2 and 9.8 percent of GBM patients treated by concomitant and adjuvant Temozolamide and radiotherapy remained alive at 2 years and 5 years, respectively (Stupp, Mason et al. 2005; Stupp, Hegi et al. 2009). For patients diagnosed with anaplastic astrocytoma, the median survival time is higher at approximately 2 to 5 years (Wen and Kesari 2008).

3. Angiogenesis

3.1. History

The theory that tumor growth is dependent on angiogenesis and that anti-angiogenic therapy may be a potential cancer treatment was first proposed by Dr. Folkman in the 1970s (Folkman 1972). Since that time, understanding the mechanism of action of angiogenesis and developing targeted therapies have been a high priority.

3.2. Summary of angiogenesis

Angiogenesis is the process by which the vascular system is formed through growth of new capillaries from pre-existing vessels (Plate, Scholz et al. 2012). Angiogenesis plays a critical role in key physiologic and formative processes such as embryogenesis, regeneration, and wound healing. Angiogenesis is also involved in various pathologic processes including age-related macular degeneration, rheumatoid arthritis, and tumor growth and development (Wang, Fei et al. 2004).

The process of angiogenesis can be briefly summarized as follows. First, there is vasodilation, in response to nitric oxide, and increased permeability of the existing vessels. This is followed by degradation of the existing vessel's basement membrane. Next, endothelial precursor cells migrate to the area and begin to proliferate and mature into capillaries via a balance of both growth and inhibition. The final steps involve recruitment of vascular smooth muscle cells and pericytes that form a new network of mature vessels (Shinkaruk, Bayle et al. 2003).

3.3. Molecular signals of angiogenesis

Although there are numerous factors and signals that contribute to angiogenesis, the chemical signal that seems to play the most critical role in the process is Vascular Endothelial Growth Factor (VEGF). VEGF is a pro-angiogenic growth factor, which is secreted by many cells, including mesenchymal, stromal, and especially tumor cells. VEGF induces the migration of the endothelial precursor cells to sites of angiogenesis and is responsible for their proliferation and differentiation. The VEGF gene is located on chromosome 6p12 and the gene family is composed of five members, namely VEGF-A, VEGF-B, VEGF-C, VEGF-D, and placental-derived growth factor (PlGF). Of these, VEGF-A, B, and PIGF are involved in the development of the vascular system and VEGF-C and D are involved in the development of the lymphatic system (Ahluwalia and Gladson 2010). VEGF primarily signals through its receptor VEGFR2 which is a tyrosine kinase receptor that is expressed by many cells, including endothelial cells, endothelial cell precursors, and tumor cells (Jain, di Tomaso et al. 2007). Other chemical signals that play an important role in angiogenesis are fibroblast growth factor, hepatocyte growth factor (HGF), tumor necrosis factor-alpha (TNF-α), transforming growth factor-beta (TGF-β), angiopoietins, and platelet derived growth factor (PDGF). Their various roles include involvement in extracellular matrix degradation, endothelial proliferation and migration, and neo-vessel stabilization and maturation (Martin and Jiang 2010; Ucuzian, Gassman et al. 2010).

3.4. Angiogenesis in tumors

Seven different cellular mechanisms appear to contribute to tumor angiogenesis: (1) classical sprouting angiogenesis, (2) vascular co-option, (3) myeloid cell-driven angiogenesis, (4) vessel intussusception, (5) vasculogenic mimicry, (6) bone marrow derived vasculogenesis, and (7) cancer stem-like cell derived vasculogenesis (Carmeliet and Jain 2011; Plate, Scholz et al. 2012). Of the above-listed mechanisms, the first three seem to have a clear role in glioma vascularization, as supported by pre-clinical tumor models (Plate, Scholz et al. 2012).

1. *Classical sprouting angiogenesis*. This is believed to be the primary modulator of neovascularization of the brain during development and in pathological conditions (Plate, Breier

et al. 1994; Risau 1997; Kurz, Korn et al. 2001; Plate, Scholz et al. 2012). In this model, a vascular sprout is led by tip cells toward an angiogenic stimulus that is produced by tumor cells. This sprout then elongates via dividing stalk cells. The newly formed vessel undergoes remodeling to create a vascular lumen that allows blood flow (Plate, Scholz et al. 2012). There is evidence to support that both tip and stalk cell phenotypes co-exist in the glioblastoma vasculature (Plate, Breier et al. 1994; Broholm and Laursen 2004; Dieterich, Mellberg et al. 2012; Plate, Scholz et al. 2012)

2. *Vascular co-option*. This is the process by which tumor cells infiltrate into normal tissue and adopt pre-existing vasculature (Holash, Wiegand et al. 1999; Plate, Scholz et al. 2012). This pathway seems to be enhanced through activity of pro-angiogenic molecules, like VEGF and Angiopoeitin-2 (Holash, Wiegand et al. 1999).

3. *Myeloid cell-driven angiogenesis*. Tumor-associated macrophages contribute to angiogenesis by secreting pro-angiogenic factors such as fibroblast growth factor 2 (FGF2), VEGF, and matrix metalloproteinases (MMPs) (Plate, Scholz et al. 2012). Tumor-associated macrophages may also assist two vascular sprouts to form a direct connection through a process referred to as anastomosis (Plate, Scholz et al. 2012).

The role of the remaining four mechanisms in glioma angiogenesis is not yet fully understood. Briefly, *vessel intussusception* is the process by which a new vessel is formed by internal division of the pre-existing capillary plexus without sprouting through a series of steps that include vascular invagination, intra-luminar pillar formation and remodeling, and splitting (Djonov, Schmid et al. 2000; Plate, Scholz et al. 2012). *Vasculogenic mimicry* refers to the process by which cancer cells form *de novo* vasculature as a result of their high plasticity (Plate, Scholz et al. 2012; Seftor, Hess et al. 2012). *Bone marrow-derived vasculogenesis* refers to the process by which circulating endothelial precursor cells are recruited to the tumor and are incorporated into the vessel wall (Plate, Scholz et al. 2012; Huang, Peng et al. 2013). *Cancer stem-like derived vasculogenesis* is the process by which tumor-derived cells trans-differentiate into endothelial cells (Ricci-Vitiani, Pallini et al. 2010; Plate, Scholz et al. 2012). It is not the goal of this chapter to study these mechanisms in detail, but instead to provide an overview of angiogenesis in glioma and discuss key molecules involved and possible therapeutic options that target them.

4. Targets for anti-angiogenics

4.1. VEGF receptor blockers

4.1.1. Bevacizumab

Bevacizumab (Avastin) is a recombinant humanized monoclonal antibody that targets VEGF. It was the first anti-angiogenesis agent to be approved by the United States Food and Drug Administration (FDA) in 2004. Bevacizumab was initially approved for use in metastatic colorectal cancer, but its clinical use has been extended to other cancer types (Van Meter and Kim 2010). Bevacizumab has six VEGF binding residues that neutralize the ability of VEGF to bind to its target receptors on endothelial cells. This neutralization has been shown to have efficacy not only in *in vitro* studies, but also in *in vivo* ones.

Recently, two phase III clinical trials investigating Bevacizumab as a first-line treatment for newly diagnosed GBM tumors were completed. Unfortunately, both trials were consistent in showing no statistically-significant prolongation of overall survival time (OS) but there was a slight improvement in progression-free survival time (PFS). The two trials had a similar design, namely double-blinded prospective trials where newly diagnosed GBM patients were randomized to either standard of care with Bevacizumab or with placebo; the standard of care consisted of radiation therapy with adjuvant and concomitant Temozolomide. A total of 637 and 921 adult participants were randomized in the Radiation Therapy Oncology Group (RTOG) and AVAglio trials, respectively. The median OS was 16.1 vs. 15.7 months, in the RTOG trial ($p = 0.11$). The median PFS was longer in patients who received Bevacizumab, 7.3 vs. 10.7 months ($p = 0.004$) and 6.2 vs. 10.6 months ($p<0.0001$) in the RTOG and Avaglio trials, respectively. In addition, the results also showed a higher incidence of adverse reactions in the Bevacizumab arm, including neutropenia, hypertension, and deep vein thromboembolism and pulmonary emboli (Gilbert, Dignam et al. 2013). The AVAglio trial noted delayed time to definitive deterioration in terms of health-related quality of life ($p<0.0001$) and Karnofsky Performance Scale, and increased time to corticosteroid initiation (HR 0.71, 95% CI 0.57-0.88; median 12.3 vs. 3.7 months) (Henriksson, Bottomley et al. 2013). These results are discouraging and do not justify the use of Bevacizumab in a GBM patient who has had a reasonable surgical resection.

The data support the idea that Bevacizumab may be reserved until the time of recurrence as several prospective phase II clinical trials have shown prolongation of the 6-month PFS rates ranging from 25 to 42.6 percent and median OS times from 6.5 to 9.2 months. However, a significant limitation of these trials is that the comparison was made to historical controls (Friedman, Prados et al. 2009; Kreisl, Kim et al. 2009; Raizer, Grimm et al. 2010).

4.1.2. VEGF-trap

VEGF-Trap (drug name Aflibercept) is a recombinant fusion protein that acts as a decoy receptor for VEGF, thereby blocking its interaction with its normal receptors and interrupting the VEGF signaling pathway (Holash, Davis et al. 2002). VEGF-Trap was developed by incorporating domains of both VEGF receptor 1 and VEGF receptor 2 fused to the constant region of human immunoglobulin G1. VEGF Trap has a high affinity for all isoforms of VEGF-A, as well as for PlGF, another pro-angiogenic agent that primarily acts on VEGF receptor 1 (Holash, Davis et al. 2002; Gomez-Manzano, Holash et al. 2008; de Groot, Lamborn et al. 2011). Preclinical studies demonstrated efficacy of VEGF-trap in glioma animal models (Haapa-Paananen, Chen et al. 2013). de Groot et al. conducted a Phase II study of Aflibercept in recurrent malignant glioma; unfortunately, their results revealed that Aflibercept had minimal activity as a single-agent against recurrent GBM (de Groot, Lamborn et al. 2011).

4.1.3. Sunitinib

Sunitinib is a small-molecule inhibitor of VEGF receptors 1 and 2, PDGFR alpha and beta, stem-cell factor receptor (SCFR), fms-like tyrosine kinase 3 (FLT-3), colony-stimulating factor-1 receptor (CSF-1R), and the *RET* oncogene tyrosine kinase (*RET*) (Chow and Eckhardt 2007; Kreisl, Smith et al. 2013). It has FDA approval for use in metastatic renal-cell carcinoma, gastorintestical stromal tumors refractory to imatinib mesylate, and advanced pancreatic neuroendocrine neoplasms (Kreisl, Smith et al. 2013). Recently, a phase II clinical trial was completed investigating the role of continuous daily Sunitinib in recurrent GBM in both Bevacizumab exposed and Bevacizumab naïve patients (Kreisl, Smith et al. 2013). Unfortunately, the results did not demonstrate an improvement in PFS in either population. Recent evidence by Costa et al suggests that silencing of micro-RNA 21 (miR-21), a small, non-coding RNA that regulates gene expression, may enhance the anti-tumoral effect of Sunitinib (Costa, Cardoso et al. 2013).

4.1.4. Nintedanib

Nintedanib (BIBF 1120) is a small, orally available triple angio-kinase inhibitor that targets VEGF receptors 1-3, FGFRs 1-3, and PDGFR alpha and beta. It is still in phase III development, but preclinical models demonstrated effective growth inhibition of both endothelial and perivascular cells when the above listed pathways were simultaneously interrupted (Hilberg, Roth et al. 2008; Muhic, Poulsen et al. 2013). Phase I/II clinical trial results have demonstrated tumor stabilization rates of 46-76%, when tested in various tumor types (Mross, Stefanic et al. 2010; Okamoto, Kaneda et al. 2010; Richeldi, Costabel et al. 2011; Muhic, Poulsen et al. 2013) Muhic et al. conducted an uncontrolled phase II trial assessing the efficacy of single-agent Nintedanib in patients with recurrent GBM who had previously failed 1-2 lines of therapy; unfortunately, this study was stopped prematurely secondary to futility (Muhic, Poulsen et al. 2013).

4.1.5. Vandetanib

Vandetanib is a multi-targeted tyrosine kinase inhibitor of VEGF receptor 2, epidermal growth factor receptor (EGFR) 2, and the rearranged-during-transfection oncogene that results in the simultaneous blocking of several pathways, including angiogenesis (Kreisl, McNeill et al. 2012). Preclinical rat and mice glioma xenografts have shown anti-tumor effects of Vandetanib (Sandstrom, Johansson et al. 2004; Rich, Sathornsumetee et al. 2005; Kreisl, McNeill et al. 2012). Kreisl et al. conducted a phase I/II trial of Vandetanib in patients with recurrent malignant glioma and found that it did not have activity as a single agent in this population (Kreisl, McNeill et al. 2012).

4.2. Integrins

Integrins are cell surface receptors that play key roles in mediating the migration of endothelial cells. They are receptors for many different extracellular matrix (ECM) ligands and they play an important role in angiogenesis via the processes of integrin-mediated adhesion, migration, proliferation, survival, and differentiation of cells that form the vasculature (Hynes, Bader et al. 1999; Tchaicha, Mobley et al. 2010). The αv integrin subfamily has five members- $\alpha v\beta 1$, $\alpha v\beta 3$, $\alpha v\beta 5$, $\alpha v\beta 6$, and $\alpha v\beta 8$- and the $\alpha v\beta 8$ member, in particular, has been shown in mouse models to be a central regulator of angiogenesis in the developing brain (McCarty, Monahan-Earley et al. 2002; Zhu, Motejlek et al. 2002; Tchaicha, Reyes et al. 2011).

Cilengitide, a selective inhibitor of $\alpha v\beta 3$ and $\alpha v\beta 5$ integrins, demonstrated preclinical activity against angiogenesis in GBMs and it is also being investigated clinically (MacDonald, Taga et al. 2001; Onishi, Kurozumi et al. 2013). A phase II study of Cilengitide conducted by Reardon et al. was associated with a median survival of 9.9 months and a PFS rate of 15% in recurrent glioma patients. Unfortunately, the CENTRIC phase III trial revealed that Cilengitide failed to prolong PFS or OS in patients with newly diagnosed GBM and a methylated MGMT promoter (Onishi, Kurozumi et al. 2013).

4.3. Notch signaling

4.3.1. Ligands

Notch signaling in host endothelial cells is important for angiogenesis. Recent evidence has shown that delta-like ligand 4 (DLL4), a member of the Notch ligand family, is expressed in tumor cells and can activate Notch signaling in host endothelial cells and can therefore affect the vascular function of tumors. In fact, DLL4 expression appears to be regulated by VEGF and the tumor's hypoxic microenvironment (Patel, Li et al. 2005; Li, Gong et al. 2012). Increased levels of VEGF lead to an up-regulation of DLL4 expression which results in endothelial cells expressing Notch receptors to down-regulate VEGF-induced vessel sprouting and branching and ultimately resulting in productive and efficient angiogenesis (Li, Gong et al. 2012). Furthermore, it has also been demonstrated that blockade of DLL4 can result in non-productive angiogenesis by causing tumor growth inhibition and a decrease in tissue perfusion (Scehnet, Jiang et al. 2007; Li, Gong et al. 2012). Li et al. recently conducted a study to investigate the role of DLL4 in malignant gliomas, specifically in terms of vascular quantity and quality and showed that DLL4 expression was significantly up-regulated in malignant human gliomas as compared to normal brain tissue. Additionally, they also demonstrated that DLL4-positive malignant glioma tissues have increased proliferation of vascular endothelial cells and pericyte recruitment, as compared to DLL4-negative malignant glioma tissue, and that DLL4-positive tissues had a higher vessel maturation index (VMI). These results provide evidence that DLL4 inhibition may alter glioma vessel maturity and, in turn, may improve the effects of anti-angiogenic agents (Li, Gong et al. 2012).

4.3.2. Gamma secretase

Gamma secretase is a pre-senilin dependent protease that acts as a regulator of angiogenesis through a series of complex steps that are beyond the scope of this chapter. However, part of its role in angiogenesis is related to Notch signaling (Jain, di Tomaso et al. 2007; Boulton, Cai et al. 2008). RO4929097 is a potent and selective gamma secretase inhibitor of Notch signaling that is being investigated as an anti-tumor agent. Phase I studies have demonstrated safety and phase II studies are underway to assess its role in recurrent GBM when given alone and in combination with Bevacizumab (Tolcher, Messersmith et al. 2012).

4.4. Transforming growth factor beta (TGF-β)

TGF-β is a multifunctional protein that is involved in the regulation of proliferation, differentiation, and survival of many cells, including glioma cells and endothelial cells (Bertolino, Deckers et al. 2005). TGF-β1 and TGF-β2, members of the TGF-β family, stimulate expression of VEGF, the plasminogen activator inhibitor, and some metalloproteinases that are involved in vascular remodeling, angiogenesis, and degradation of the extracellular matrix. Animal models demonstrate that inhibitors of TGF-β signaling reduce viability and invasion of gliomas (Kaminska, Kocyk et al. 2013). Fresolimumab, a human monoclonal antibody that inactivates all forms of TGF-β, is being investigated as a potential therapeutic for glioma (Trachtman, Fervenza et al. 2011).

4.5. Topoisomerase I inhibitors

Topoisomerase I is critical for efficient DNA replication and cell division. Topoisomerase I activity is increased in malignant gliomas and inhibitors of topoisomerase I activity, such as Camptothecin, Irinotecan, and the indolocarbazoles, have been tested as potential glioma therapies (Pommier 2006; Feun and Savaraj 2008; Vredenburgh, Desjardins et al. 2009; Lampropoulou, Manioudaki et al. 2011). Recently, Lampropoulou et al. have shown that inhibition of topoisomerase I activity by the pyrrolo[2,3-α]carbazole derivatives may be linked to a decrease in the number of viable glioma and endothelial cells *in vitro* and may also be related to inhibition of angiogenesis *in vivo* (Lampropoulou, Manioudaki et al. 2011).

4.6. Oncoproteins

B-cell specific Moloney murine leukemia virus integration site 1 (Bmi-1) is an oncoprotein that plays a role in the development and progression of cancers including breast, lung, prostate, and interestingly, brain (Jagani, Wiederschain et al. 2010). Bmi-1 is a member of the Polycomb gene family of proteins that function as epigenetic silencers of genes that control self-renewal, differentiation, and proliferation; dysregulation of Bmi-1 has been associated with cancer cell proliferation, invasion, and repression of apoptosis or senescence (Jiang, Song et al. 2013). In particular, Bmi-1 promotes growth and survival of glioma tumor cells (Li, Gong et al. 2010; Jiang, Song et al. 2013); furthermore, Bmi-1 promotes angiogenesis of gliomas by activating the NF-κB signaling pathway *in vitro* as well as *in vivo* (Jiang, Song et al. 2013). Thus, targeting Bmi-1 is a promising aim in gliomas.

4.7. Other potential therapeutics in development

4.7.1. Carboxyamidotriazole orotate (CTO)

CTO is a triazole orotate formulation of carboxyamidotriazole (CAI), which is an inhibitor of receptor-operated calcium channel-mediated calcium influx. CTO has anti-proliferative, anti-invasive, as well as anti-angiogenic properties in several human cancer cell lines including glioblastoma (Ge, Rempel et al. 2000; Fiorio Pla, Grange et al. 2008; Karmali, Maxuitenko et al. 2011). In initial clinical development, CAI was shown to have poor bioavailability, limited efficacy, and high toxicity. CTO, however, appears to have much better bioavailability and less toxicity (Grover, Kelly et al. 2007; Karmali, Maxuitenko et al. 2011).

4.7.2. TRC105

TRC105 is a novel, first-in-class antibody against endoglin (CD 105), an endothelial cell receptor that is essential to angiogenesis and acts primarily through its effects on TGF-β and BMP-9 signaling. A phase I trial conducted by Rosen et al. demonstrated that this drug is well-tolerated at clinically relevant doses and multiple phase II trials are ongoing to evaluate its potential role in other malignancies, including malignant glioma (Rosen, Hurwitz et al. 2012).

4.7.3. Thalidomide and lenalidomide

Thalidomide and its analogue Lenalidomide have both been shown to have anti-angiogenic and anti-tumor effects in preclinical models (D'Amato, Loughnan et al. 1994; Short, Traish et al. 2001). The anti-angiogenic effects are thought to be related to a hepatic metabolite that inhibits endothelial growth, although the exact mechanism is unclear (Short, Traish et al. 2001). Additionally, an early clinical trial conducted by Baumann et al. showed that the combination of Thalidomide with Temozolomide appeared to be more effective than Thalidomide alone in the treatment of GBM (Baumann, Bjeljac et al. 2004). Additional studies are underway to examine the role of Thalidomide in combination with other anti-glioma agents.

4.7.4. Tandutinib

Tandutinib (MLN0518) is an active inhibitor of type III receptor kinases with activity against PDGF receptors alpha and beta, FLT3, and c-KIT. Its anti-angiogenic effects appear to be mediated by interruption of PDGF/PDGFR. It is currently being investigated in combination therapy with other agents against malignant glioma (Boult, Terkelsen et al. 2013).

5. Immunotherapy for malignant gliomas

Our immune system can be viewed as an intricate balance of opposing functions that lead to either immunity or tolerance. Perturbations that disrupt this stable equilibrium could lead to autoimmune disease or tolerance to malignant cells. In general, the immune system has the ability to recognize and to react to foreign antigens, which leads to their removal as well as to the destruction of cells that express them. Before attempting immunotherapy for cancer, one needs to understand the crucial balancing acts of the immune response that eventually lead to a desired outcome; in addition, the central nervous system has unique features that require special considerations.

In this section, our goals are to introduce the readers to the basics of peripheral immunology focusing on how foreign antigens activate the immune response leading to immunity vs. tolerance. Nevertheless, a detailed discussion of immunity is not within our scope; in some disciplines, we will just be scratching the surface. We will detail antigen processing and presentation, T cell priming, with attention to the synapse between T cells and the antigen-presenting cell (APC) and clonal expansion. Because of our interest in brain tumors, we will compare the systemic immune response to that of the CNS, discussing the historical thoughts of the immune privileges of the CNS and more recent evidence of processing of CNS antigens via the glymphatic pathway. The stage will be set for a discussion of immunotherapy for brain tumors, including priming in the periphery, priming in the CNS, and passive transfer of immunity. The last section lists the clinical trials that employ immunotherapy for brain tumors and their proposed modes of action.

5.1. Peripheral immunology

As part of the adaptive immune system, antigens enter the body through epithelium and are immediately met in the infected tissue by APCs, most commonly dendritic cells (DCs), which then process the antigens into protein fragments (Hugues 2010; Joffre, Segura et al. 2012; Abbas, Lichtman et al. 2014). DCs are a type of APC that can induce priming of naïve CD4+ and CD8+ T cells into helper and cytotoxic T cells through a series of steps that include antigen processing, antigen presentation, and interactions with co-stimulatory molecules, in addition to the secretion of various cytokines (Hivroz, Chemin et al. 2012). If not processed locally by an APC, the antigens drain into lymph nodes via lymphatic vessels where an APC will be waiting (Abbas, Lichtman et al. 2014). These antigens are processed internally through degradation in the cytosol, processing in the endoplasmic reticulum, and transportation to the cell surface by the Golgi apparatus (Joffre, Segura et al. 2012). APCs then travel to the lymph nodes, where naïve T cells can recognize displayed protein fragments of antigens (Abbas, Lichtman et al. 2014). DCs serve as the most specialized of the APCs and assist in differentiating naïve T cells into both effector and memory cells. Once activated, effector cells then travel via the blood stream to the site of infection where they can recognize antigens being presented by other types of cells and initiate cytotoxic responses (Abbas, Lichtman et al. 2014).

All nucleated cells in the body display a major histocompatibility complex (MHC) I molecule for presenting processed pathogens or infected cells to T lymphocytes once detected (Joffre, Segura et al. 2012). Only CD8+ T cells bear receptors for MHC I; CD4+ T cells bear receptors for MHC II, typically expressed by dendritic cells, macrophages, and B cells (Abbas, Lichtman et al. 2014). Nucleated cells produce peptide antigens from viruses living in the cell, phagocytosed and endocytosed organisms, and proteins derived from mutated self-genes (Joffre, Segura et al. 2012; Abbas, Lichtman et al. 2014). Traditionally, exogenous antigens are presented via MHC II-bearing cells and endogenous antigens by MHC I cells, but cross-presentation permits MHC I cells to present exogenous antigens (Jarry, Jeannin et al. 2013). Additionally, DCs can ingest virally-infected host cells and present the processed antigens via MHC I to CD8+ naïve T cells through cross-priming (Abbas, Lichtman et al. 2014). Similarly, infected DCs can prime CD8+ T cells via MHC I by directly presenting the processed antigen

(Joffre, Segura et al. 2012). This cross-priming process has been implicated in immune responses not only to infection, but also to cancer and autoimmune disease (Jarry, Jeannin et al. 2013)

5.1.2. T cell priming and activation

T cell priming by DCs induces activation, cytokine secretion, and clonal proliferation (Mempel, Henrickson et al. 2004). For T-cell activation, both the MHC-bound antigen and the MHC itself must be recognized by the T-cell receptor (TCR) and the co-receptor, respectively (Abbas, Lichtman et al. 2014). This process of priming naïve T cells into effector and helper cells occurs in lymphoid organs (Joffre, Segura et al. 2012). DCs prime the T cells during three stages: 1. Contact for exchange of information between the T cell and the dendrite in the lymphocyte pool, 2. The formation of a stable bond followed by secretion of interleukin-2 and interferon-γ, and 3. Rapid movement and clonal expansion (Mempel, Henrickson et al. 2004).

The synapse between the T cell and the APC requires the interaction of not only the TCR and MHC, but also adhesion molecules and co-receptors to receive signals from the APC (see section 5.1.3 below). Early on during this process various cytokines are released. Certain cytokines lead to clonal expansion of antigen-specific lymphocytes, some of which become differentiated into effector T cells that can remove infected cells. Others differentiate into memory T cells that serve to remain inactive until re-exposed to the same antigen (Abbas, Lichtman et al. 2014). During future encounters, DC-bearing antigens will migrate to the paracortical region in the lymph node to search for a T cell that recognizes its antigen, ultimately activating clonal expansion (Bousso, 2003).

5.1.2.1. T lymphocyte — Antigen presenting cell contact

To begin the process of priming T cells, the DC must physically contact the naïve T cell. This process tends to occur in lymphoid tissue, specifically in the draining lymph nodes, spleen, and Peyer's patches, after infiltration of antigen-APC complexes from peripheral tissue through lymph vessels (Mempel, Henrickson et al. 2004; Hugues 2010). Mempel et al. showed that naïve T cells re-circulate continually between the blood and lymph nodes searching for antigen. In the absence of antigen, the T cells move randomly in the three dimensions in a stop-and-go manner leading to approximately 500-5000 T cells contacting one DC per hour (Mempel, Henrickson et al. 2004; Miller, Hejazi et al. 2004; Hugues 2010). In the absence of antigen, DCs enter the lymph node via the sub-capsular cortex and travel to the paracortex where T cells are localized. Then, the dendrites on DCs scan the T cells which results in transient interactions of up to a few minutes (Hugues 2010). In the presence of antigen, the data supports a three-phase model. First, within a few hours of lymph node entry, contact between naïve T cell-DC with peptide increases in duration, now lasting up to five minutes. Within ten hours of antigen entry into the lymph node, mobility slows dramatically as T cells and DCs form more stable bonds, which will persist from two to twenty four hours. This step also promotes the up-regulation of activation markers. After thirty hours, the bonds separate and this is followed by increased mobility of T cells, corresponding with T cell proliferation (Miller, Wei et al. 2002; Mempel, Henrickson et al. 2004; Hugues 2010).

5.1.2.2. Naïve T lymphocyte — Antigen presenting cell synapse

Naïve T cells are constantly searching for presented antigen on the MHC-antigen complex of mature DCs, from which the T cell and its receptor will require co-stimulation (Mempel, Henrickson et al. 2004). T cell activation relies on the successful synapse of the T cell receptor (TCR) with the peptide-MHC complex on the APC. Additionally, several signaling complexes must connect between the TCR and the adaptor protein linker for activation of T cells and subsequent filamentous actin (F-actin)-dependent TCR cluster formation (Dustin and Depoil 2011). The role of co-stimulatory and co-inhibitory proteins is to modulate the TCR signal to increase or decrease activation of the T cell or to direct the response of that cell down a particular differentiation pathway (Dustin and Depoil 2011).

Antigen recognition and adhesion involves simultaneous recognition of many molecules. In the receptor layer, antigen recognition occurs by the TCR to the peptide with its co-receptor CD4 or CD8 binding MHC II or MHC I, respectively. This is the first step in the signal cascade. For signal transduction and co-stimulation, several transmembrane signaling molecules, including CD3 and ζ chain, form part of the TCR complex and bind the MHC/antigen complex. Additionally, CD28 (and CTLA-4) on the T cell binds B7-1 (CD80)/B7-2 (CD86) on the APC (Dustin and Depoil 2011). The B7 proteins are created by APC in response to an antigen to ensure that T cells are not activated by self-antigens. This key bond is essential for signaling and thus activation of naïve T cells. Concurrently, the CD40 Ligand on the T cell and CD40 on the APC unite and promote increased production of B7 and secretion of cytokines in the APC in order to further encourage T cell activation (Abbas, Lichtman et al. 2014). For adhesion, the T-cell integrin LFA-1 (Leukocyte function-associated antigen 1) binds ICAM-1 (Intercellular adhesion molecule) on the APC (Dustin and Depoil 2011; Abbas, Lichtman et al. 2014).

The co-stimulatory signals play a key role in determining immunity or tolerance. Due to the required co-receptors and signal transduction, many mechanisms are set in place to prevent T cells from activating against self-protein. Through early central tolerance mechanisms designed to prevent autoimmune disease, immature T cells that react to self-proteins undergo apoptosis early in development (Luptrawan, Liu et al. 2008). This activation-induced cell death is assisted through the interaction of Fas, which is expressed everywhere and in high concentration in the thymus, with Fas Ligand on T lymphocytes and NK cells (Maher, Toomey et al. 2002); a similar process results in clonally expanded T cells after they are no longer needed. Similarly, if a T cell encounters an antigen on an APC without the appropriate co-stimulation, it is susceptible to developing tolerance to that antigen such that on future encounters it will ignore it, even if given the appropriate co-stimulation (Luptrawan, Liu et al. 2008; Abbas, Lichtman et al. 2014). On cross-presentation by dendritic cells with MHC I and CD8+ T cells, clonal deletion, functional inactivation (anergy) or programming into a suppressive (regulatory) T cell phenotype can result (Joffre, Segura et al. 2012).

5.1.2.3. Clonal expansion

To amplify activation, T cells and APCs secrete various cytokines. Initially, T cells secrete interleukin-2 (IL-2), which facilitates the binding of IL-2 by augmenting the presence of IL-2 receptors. IL-2, by acting on the T cell that secreted it, supports the production of T cells specific to the antigen. IL-2 is also needed to maintain regulatory T cells (Abbas, Lichtman et al. 2014).

Clonal expansion transpires in 1-2 days, leading to the creation of antigen-specific CD4+ and CD8+ cells. CD8+ cells develop into effector cells that ultimately migrate to the site of infection to interact with the specific antigen to which they were primed. CD4+ cells further develop into T helper I (Th1) and T helper 2 (Th2) lymphocytes. Antigen-exposed macrophages and DCs release IL-12 and natural killer cells secrete interferon-γ, thereby promoting the differentiation of Th 1 cells (Abbas, Lichtman et al. 2014). Th1 cells secrete IL-2, interferon-γ, and lymphotoxin-a which leads to type 1 immunity with enhanced macrophage activation and phagocytosis (Spellberg and Edwards 2001). Interferon-γ also increases the expression of MHC I and II molecules to amplify antigen presentation (Spellberg and Edwards 2001). Th2 cells, stimulated by IL-4, also release IL-4, IL-5, IL-9, IL-10, and IL-13 promoting production of antibodies and type 2 immunity, which minimizes phagocytosis and decreases inflammation (Spellberg and Edwards 2001). In times of overwhelming systemic response or immunosuppression, a type 2 response can supersede the appropriate type 1 response (Spellberg and Edwards 2001).

All the aforementioned steps have to be executed flawlessly to achieve immunity against a tumor or a tumor antigen. The body is set up to have low affinity to self-antigens, as would be expressed on tumor cells (Luptrawan, Liu et al. 2008). Along those lines, dendritic cells, which have been discovered in tumors, play a large role in presentation of tumor antigens; however, that does not necessarily predict the nature of the immune response. In particular, any flaw in dendritic cells, from cross presentation to IL-12 production, will lead to tolerance and impaired CD8+ T cell response to tumors (Joffre, Segura et al. 2012).

5.2. Central nervous system immunology

The CNS was once thought to be immunologically-privileged because of its unique immunological features, including 1) lack of immunological surveillance due to low expression of MHC molecules, 2) lack of distinct lymphatic drainage, and 3) protection by the blood brain barrier (BBB), which limits the movement of naïve T cells into the CNS (Chavarria and Cardenas 2013). Nonetheless, the CNS has more recently been discovered to have a finely tuned immune surveillance managed by APC, believed to be microglia, DC, perivascular macrophages and meningeal dendritic cells (Fathallah-Shaykh, Gao et al. 1998; Yang, Han et al. 2010; D'Agostino, Gottfried-Blackmore et al. 2012; Ousman and Kubes 2012; Romo-Gonzalez, Chavarria et al. 2012; Chavarria and Cardenas 2013). Furthermore, more recent evidence, as can be found in gliomas and multiple sclerosis, suggests that the CNS microglia coordinate with peripheral T cells and APC (Yang, Han et al. 2010). Such evidence describes more active inspection of the BBB in specific regions of the brain most notably the meninges, ventricles, circumventricular organs, and choroid plexus (D'Agostino, Gottfried-Blackmore et al. 2012).

5.2.1. Centrally-acting peripheral immune cells

In addition to resident microglia, the primary immune cell in the CNS, peripheral immune cells including peripherally activated T lymphocytes, macrophages, and DC circulate in small numbers within the CNS. They are predominantly in specialized CNS compartments located outside the parenchyma with ability to gain access to the parenchyma through various mechanisms that include the choroid plexus, perivascular or Virchow-Robin spaces, meningeal vessel branch points into the subarachnoid space, and through post-capillary venules (Ousman and Kubes 2012). As in the periphery, these cells are capable of mounting an activated immune response if they encounter an antigen (Ousman and Kubes 2012; Jarry, Jeannin et al. 2013). Additionally, perivascular macrophages sample CSF and can phagocytose suspected antigens (Ousman and Kubes 2012). There is also separate evidence of drainage of CNS antigens to deep cervical lymph nodes, based on intracranial injection of labeled antigen (D'Agostino, Gottfried-Blackmore et al. 2012; Ousman and Kubes 2012). Despite controversy over poor immune surveillance due to low expression of MHC II, it is thought that pre-activated T cells can release IFN-γ and TNF-α to simulate MHC II molecule expression (Romo-Gonzalez, Chavarria et al. 2012). Also of debate is the function of central antigen presentation by central DCs. It is known that the integrity of the BBB is compromised during times of infection, trauma, aging, and autoimmunity due to weakening of the vascular endothelium as a result of cytokine release by astrocytes and microglia (D'Agostino, Gottfried-Blackmore et al. 2012; Romo-Gonzalez, Chavarria et al. 2012).

5.2.2. Microglia

Microglia play a large role in both innate and adaptive immune responses, in addition to regulatory roles in the CNS (Yang, Han et al. 2010). They comprise 5-12% of all CNS cells and are uniformly distributed throughout the CNS parenchyma (D'Agostino, Gottfried-Blackmore et al. 2012). Similar to the peripheral immune APCs, microglia express MHC I and II molecules and CD 80/86 and CD40 co-stimulatory molecules that once activated, proliferate and phagocytose in response to both CD4+ and CD8+ T cells (Fathallah-Shaykh, Gao et al. 1998; Yang, Han et al. 2010; Ousman and Kubes 2012). In the latent state, microglia survey the microenvironment via pinocytosis. Once they sense infection, neuronal injury, or neurodegenerative disease, they up-regulate the expression of MHC and co-stimulatory molecules and release cytokines including IL-1, IL-6, and TNF-alpha as well as neurotrophic and cytotoxic factors, and chemokines for lymphocyte recruitment (Yang, Han et al. 2010; Jarry, Jeannin et al. 2013). These pro-inflammatory cytokines then make the BBB more soluble for entry of peripheral immune cells and potentially naïve T lymphocytes (Yang, Han et al. 2010). Microglia's phagocytic and cytotoxic features are also up-regulated with the triggering of an immune response (Yang, Han et al. 2010). As in the peripheral immune response, microglia CD80/CD86 and CD40 bind the T cell's CD28 and CD40L, respectively (Yang, Han et al. 2010). IFN-γ release sustains this response and promotes phagocytosis and direct tumor-cell cytotoxicity (Fathallah-Shaykh, Gao et al. 1998; Yang, Han et al. 2010; D'Agostino, Gottfried-Blackmore et al. 2012).

Similar to peripheral tolerance, if there is insufficient co-stimulatory response, the interaction of Fas ligand (FASL) on microglia and Fas receptor on the T cell leads to activation-induced T cell apoptosis. Microglia also express FAS molecules themselves, which induce apoptosis upon binding FASL (Yang, Han et al. 2010). Nitric oxide released by microglia in response to activation can also potentiate effector cell death (Yang, Han et al. 2010). Furthermore, microglia display B7-H1 molecules which also support immunosuppression by stimulating T cell apoptosis (Yang, Han et al. 2010). Additionally, glycoprotein CD200 down regulates activated microglia (via CD200 ligand on microglia) and perivascular macrophages in the CNS, acting as an anti-inflammatory and serving to keep microglia in a quiescent state (Ousman and Kubes 2012; Chavarria and Cardenas 2013).

5.2.3. *The glymphatic pathway*

The CNS lacks lymphoid tissue. For appropriate immune surveillance, both antigens and APC must be able to travel to lymphoid tissue, ideally via lymphatic channels, for T cell priming (Romo-Gonzalez, Chavarria et al. 2012). For small and hydrophobic molecules as well as transporter substrates, exit through the BBB is easy. Other substances are cleared from CSF through arachnoid granulations or peripheral lymphatics on cranial nerves. Clearance of large particles and matter deep within the parenchyma is more difficult and is ascribed to a high rate of flow of interstitial fluid (Iliff and Nedergaard 2013). This flow of fluid transports antigens from the brain parenchyma for presentation in cervical lymph nodes (Romo-Gonzalez, Chavarria et al. 2012). Through what has been termed the glio-vascular or glymphatic pathway, interstitial solutes are cleared from the brain to the peripheral lymphatic system via perivascular water channels from the para-arterial CSF influx pathway through the interstitium and along the para-venous clearance route (Iliff and Nedergaard 2013). Once filtered from the CNS, antigens are captured by APCs in the cervical lymph nodes and activate lymphocytes that then migrate to the CNS in search for remaining antigens (Romo-Gonzalez, Chavarria et al. 2012). As noted above, several hypotheses for lymph-like drainage of antigens exist including efferent flow via CSF and interstitial fluid past the optic, trigeminal, and acoustic nerves to the cervical lymph nodes, reabsorption through arachnoid villi into the venous sinuses, and through perivascular APC including macrophages and DC (Romo-Gonzalez, Chavarria et al. 2012).

A more recent study by Jarry et al. showed that adult microglia can cross-present antigen to naïve CD8+ T cells for priming if there is appropriate microglial activation (Jarry, Jeannin et al. 2013). Their study involved injecting naïve T cells into the brain, as the natural presence of naïve T cells in the brain is limited, with restriction of entry to activated T cells instead. Their study suggests that if naïve T lymphocytes are given the ability for entry into the brain, typically during stressful inflammatory illnesses, coupled with the appropriate microglial response, cross-priming of naïve T cells is possible (Jarry, Jeannin et al. 2013).

5.2.4. *Glioma-associated microglia*

Glioma-associated microglia/macrophages cannot mount a successful anti-tumor T cell response (Yang, Han et al. 2010). Microglia, along with some T lymphocytes, infiltrate gliomas in a pattern that was initially thought to be an immune response against tumor cells but has been more recently realized to actually encourage tumor growth by promoting immunosuppression (Yang, Han et al. 2010). Pathological examination typically reveals a large numbers of microglia dispersed within the tumor and not just in necrotic tissue (Yang, Han et al. 2010). The data of Okada et al. suggest that the glioma-infiltrating cells may compose up to 30% of the glioma tumor, correlating in volume with degree of malignancy (Okada, Kohanbash et al. 2009). The lack of phagocytosis by the microglia is thought be related to decreased expression of MHC II and co-stimulatory molecules CD80/86 and CD40, thus prohibiting appropriate T cell activation (Okada, Kohanbash et al. 2009; Yang, Han et al. 2010). Glioma cells appear to attract microglia by secreting chemoattractants and growth factors including Macrophage Chemoattractive Protein-1 (MCP-1), which binds to the microglial MCP-1 receptor, as well as colony stimulating factor-1, Granulocyte-CSF, and hepatocyte growth factor/scatter factor (Yang, Han et al. 2010). Microglial secretion of epidermal growth factor (EGF), VEGF and MCP-1 promote tumor propagation and angiogenesis (Okada, Kohanbash et al. 2009; Yang, Han et al. 2010). Additionally, the release by microglia of MMPs assists in tumor dispersal (Yang, Han et al. 2010). Interestingly, tumors depleted of microglia actually become less invasive (Okada, Kohanbash et al. 2009).

In addition to altering the response of microglial cells, gliomas take an active role in down-regulating the immune response. Recent data has shown that reduced phagocytic activity by glioma-associated microglia stems from defective antigen presentation for T cell activation due to decreased MHC II expression as well as suppression of pro-inflammatory cytokine (TNF-α) release, especially in high-grade gliomas (Yang, Han et al. 2010). Instead, glioma cells favor TGF- β, IL-10, and PGE2 secretion, which inhibits both cytotoxic function of T cells and IFN-γ-induced MHC II expression in microglial cells (Luptrawan, Liu et al. 2008; Okada, Kohanbash et al. 2009; Yang, Han et al. 2010). PGE2 specifically inhibits T cell activation, suppresses natural killers cell activity, and favors a Th2 response by increasing cytokines Il-4, Il-10, and Il-6 while suppressing the Th1 cytokines Il-2, IFN-gamma, and TNF-α (Luptrawan, Liu et al. 2008). Additionally, glioma cells do not express adequate co-stimulatory molecules required for appropriate T cell activation, potentiating anergy through tolerance (Luptrawan, Liu et al. 2008). A homologue to the B7 family (B71/2 (CD80/86)), B7-H1 expression on the surface of glioma cells inhibits CD4+ and CD8+ T cell activation. IFN- γ not only enhances antigen processing but also promotes increased B7-H1 expression, ultimately reducing T lymphocyte effectiveness in the presence of gliomas (Okada, Kohanbash et al. 2009). Additionally, some gliomas display Fas-L leading to apoptosis of Fas-labeled T cells contacting the tumor cells (Okada, Kohanbash et al. 2009).

6. Immunotherapy strategies and targets

Immunotherapy for malignant gliomas is based on various strategies aimed at the induction of anti-tumor immunity. Nevertheless, though curing a mouse from a brain tumor using immunotherapy is rather easy, this goal has proven to be more challenging in humans especially when coupled with the globally impaired immune response and increased tumor tolerance in patients with GBM (Luptrawan, Liu et al. 2008). Because of the aforementioned data, the goal of immunotherapy for gliomas should be not only to activate the cytotoxic T cell response, but also to counteract the active immunological depressive effects by the tumor itself. We will not list an exhaustive search of all immunotherapeutic strategies but will instead discuss an outline of the approaches than can be used. A thorough discussion can be found in Okada et al. (Okada, Kohanbash et al. 2009). Here, we will emphasize the different categories and discuss limitations of immunotherapy.

6.1. Priming in the periphery

Initiating an immune response against tumors is typically difficult due to poor antigen presentation and the active immunosuppressive effects by tumor cells (Luptrawan, Liu et al. 2008). Peripheral vaccination has been performed using purified antigen and irradiated genetically modified tumor cells. Through vaccination with a tumor antigen, one hopes to induce an immune response peripherally, which translates to CNS immunity as activated T cells cross the BBB. This goal may be achieved by processing the antigen via APCs at the subcutaneous injection site, migration to lymph nodes, and priming naïve T cells. Nevertheless, choosing an appropriate antigen is crucial so as to avoid an autoimmune response causing encephalitis (Okada, Kohanbash et al. 2009).

Peptide-based vaccines (see Table 1) for glioma epitopes are synthetically derived for specific antigens and run less risk of autoimmune encephalitis. This process has the potential to be individually tailored based on assessment of the patient's peripheral blood for positive response to the various antigens (Okada, Kohanbash et al. 2009). Many antigen epitopes exist and will be briefly covered. Il-13Rα2 appears as a membrane protein in more than 80% of gliomas but not in normal brain tissue, making it a target for immunotherapy (Debinski, Gibo et al. 1999). The tyrosine kinase receptor EphA2, which is involved in cell-cell contact in normal cells, contributes to malignant nature of tumor cells (Kinch, Moore et al. 2003). T-cell epitopes of Survivin, an apoptosis inhibitor protein present in several human cancers, have shown promise via vaccination for patients with pancreatic cancer and melanoma (Otto, Andersen et al. 2005; Wobser, Keikavoussi et al. 2006). These proteins are found in 100% of astrocytomas but not in normal brain tissue (Uematsu, Ohsawa et al. 2005; Okada, Kohanbash et al. 2009). Wilm's Tumor 1 gene, a transcription factor oncogene, is also present in many tumor types, including the majority of GBM but not in normal glial cells (Sugiyama 2002). The transcriptional cofactor family SOX, Sry-Related High-Mobility Group Box, is present in normal tissue development and is upregulated in various tumors, including gliomas. Vaccinations with SOX have been shown to be therapeutic in mice with gliomas (Ueda, Kinoshita et al. 2008; Okada, Kohanbash et al. 2009). HER-2/neu, in the EGFR family, promotes tumor growth by inhibiting apoptosis and stimulating migration, adhesion, and angiogenesis in many tumor-types, most notably breast, ovarian, colorectal, pancreatic, renal-cell, and GBM (Meric-Bernstam and Hung 2006; Okada, Kohanbash et al. 2009). Additional epitopes have been identified involving EGFR variant III, found in 30-50% of GBMs, Squamous Cell Carcinoma Antigen Recognized by T Cells 1 (SART-1), a gene-coding tumor antigen in many cancer types, including glioma but not in normal tissue, and Cytomegalovirus, which infects a large number of gliomas and may contribute to glioma pathogenesis (Cobbs, Harkins et al. 2002; Saikali, Avril et al. 2007; Okada, Kohanbash et al. 2009).

In addition to using purified antigen as above, whole glioma cells may be used for vaccination (See Table 2). In this process, tumor cells, either autologous or allogeneic, are grown *in vitro*, irradiated, and injected back into the patient (Wikstrand and Bigner 1980; Zhang, Eguchi et al. 2007). The benefit of whole cell vaccinations is the availability of multiple associated antigens and, specifically, the ones expressed by the individual patient's glioma (Okada, Kohanbash et al. 2009).

As a means of bypassing local antigen presentation at the site of the tumor, DC vaccination has also been a source for many clinical trials with various techniques of uniting the DC with the antigen (See Table 3). Some have used DCs pulsed with autologous glioma cell peptides and have shown promise when the DC vaccines were given both into the tumor and subcutaneously (Yamanaka, Homma et al. 2005; Okada, Kohanbash et al. 2009; D'Agostino, Gottfried-Blackmore et al. 2012). Through loading autologous DCs, one can use either tumor lysates, apoptotic tumor cells or tumor-based cDNA (D'Agostino, Gottfried-Blackmore et al. 2012). DC-glioma cell fusion, to create a multinucleated cell such that the DC can present tumor antigen, has also shown potential (D'Agostino, Gottfried-Blackmore et al. 2012). The results of DC vaccinations are encouraging; in one study, repeat surgical resection showed infiltration into the tumor of appropriate CD8+ T cells (Luptrawan, Liu et al. 2008). Furthermore, DC vaccination was well tolerated by 12 GBM patients; the median OS was 23.4 months as compared to 18.3 months in controls. In addition to best method of preparing the vaccine, several questions remain unanswered including the best DC subtypes to use, ideal conditions and co-stimulation, prime route of administration, and the correct vaccination dosing and frequency (Okada, Kohanbash et al. 2009). Additional obstacles include the initial immune state of the host prior to vaccination; for example, patients with increased tumor burden have elevated levels of TGF- β and Il-10, which inhibit entry into a cytotoxic response (Luptrawan, Liu et al. 2008).

6.2. Priming in the brain

Fathallah-Shaykh et al. showed that priming in the brain elicits an anti-tumor response leading to destruction of the brain tumor as well as to anti-tumor systemic immunity in animals (Fathallah-Shaykh, Gao et al. 1998). The basic mechanisms for eliciting such an immune response in the CNS are detailed above. One possible method consists of injecting DCs directly into the tumor; the goal is to enhance local antigen processing followed by glymphatic drainage and priming in cervical lymph nodes (Luptrawan, Liu et al. 2008). Early preliminary results in humans are encouraging. In a study of 10 patients with glioma, half received subcutaneous vaccination of pulsed DC with autologous tumor lysate and the other half received both subcutaneous vaccine and intra-tumoral injection of immature autologous DC. On follow-up imaging, the patients who received both therapies showed diminution of contrast-enhancing tumor (Yamanaka, Yajima et al. 2003; Luptrawan, Liu et al. 2008). A phase I/II trial including 24 patients with Grade III or IV glioma at first recurrence evaluated the safety and benefits of DC immunotherapy given either via subcutaneous injection near a cervical lymph node or both subcutaneously and intra-tumorally via an Ommaya reservoir. The study revealed that patients with both intratumoral and intradermal administrations had a longer survival times than patients with intradermal administration only (Yamanaka, Homma et al. 2005; Luptrawan, Liu et al. 2008). Another method, which has shown promise in animal models was used by Choi et al and involves the injection of chimeric antigen receptors-transduced T cells targeting EGFR variant III into mice gliomas. The results show a dose-dependent increase in survival, while at the same time sparing cytotoxicity to normal brain tissue (Choi, Suryadevara et al. 2013).

6.3. Passive transfer of immunity

In passive immunotherapy, the patient is given *effector* cells or molecules. Such therapies include monoclonal antibodies, radio-nucleotides that are conjugated to monoclonal antibodies, coupled toxins, and T cells.

6.3.1. Transfer of monoclonal antibodies

The use of monoclonal antibodies (see Table 4) for CNS targets necessitates overcoming important barriers (Okada, Kohanbash et al. 2009); for instance, the size of monoclonal antibodies, around 150kDa, impairs their diffusion into the CNS. However, evidence suggests that the BBB both in normal patients and those with malignancy tolerates the entry of monoclonal antibodies (Chen and Mitchell 2012). Additionally, antibodies bound to the tumor boundary layer create a concentration gradient that makes it difficult for additional antibodies to permeate against a concentration gradient, essentially not being able to reach the core of the tumor. This option may be more valid for use in conjunction with surgical resection and convection enhanced delivery (CED) where the agent of choice is given at high pressure and in bulk through an intracranial catheter into the brain tumor and parenchyma (Okada, Kohanbash et al. 2009). As opposed to using diffusion, this method uses bulk flow and has been implemented in several clinical trials. While bypassing the BBB and limiting systemic toxicities, a limitation of this method is that it can be slow and thus difficult to deliver high volumes of molecules (Bobo, Laske et al. 1994; Ferguson and Lesniak 2007; Okada, Kohanbash et al. 2009).

Several targets for monoclonal antibodies have been investigated in clinical trials. Epidermal growth factor receptor (EGFR) antibodies target the EGFR on glioma cells, over-expressed on 40-50% of tumors (Rivera, Vega-Villegas et al. 2008; Okada, Kohanbash et al. 2009). EGFR is a transmembrane receptor responsible for initiating gene transcription and thus increased tumor growth and spread(Baselga 2001). A variant of EGFR, EGFR variant III, is often found in GBM (Batra, Castelino-Prabhu et al. 1995). The monoclonal antibody Cetuximab inhibits this EGFR pathway, including glioma cells expression variant EGFR (Fukai, Nishio et al. 2008). Nimotuzumab works similarly (Ramos, Figueredo et al. 2006).

Radio-immunotherapy (RIT) via radionucleotides conjugated to monoclonal antibodies is another technique for targeting specific tumor antigens (see Table 5). This technique delivers localized, cytotoxic radiation to tumor cells resulting in cell death. This method is used concurrently with surgical resection into the surgical cavity. Specifically, antitenascin has been most studied for RIT due to high prevalence of the glycoprotein tenascin on the surface of high-grade gliomas, including 90% of GBMs (Zalutsky 2004). Duke University has developed the specific antibody 81C6, which has shown promise when given into the tumor cavity concurrently with resection (Zalutsky, Moseley et al. 1989; Okada, Kohanbash et al. 2009). Several other clinical trials have used similar approaches with RIT and glycoprotein tenascin. Other targets include the DNA/Histone H1 complex, the extra domain B of fibronectin, and the alpha chain of the IL-2 receptor (Okada, Kohanbash et al. 2009).

6.3.2. Transfer of ligands (cytokines)

Via coupled targeted toxins, cytokines fused with toxins can be delivered to tumor cells (see Table 6). Specifically, IL-4R and IL-13Rα2 expression is increased in high-grade gliomas making them ideal targets for chimeric fused proteins. For these chimeras, pseudomonas exotoxin is fused to IL-4 and IL-13, creating IL4-PE and IL13-PE, respectively (Debinski, Obiri et al. 1995; Joshi, Leland et al. 2001). These proteins are then delivered via CED (Okada, Kohanbash et al. 2009). By combining toxins with cytokines, one can target tumor receptors and induce cytotoxicity. Additional chimeras have been made using diphtheria toxin, which bonds to transferring, and TGFα, which binds to Pseudomonas exotoxin.

6.3.3. Transfer of cells

For the adoptive transfer of tumor-reactive autologous cytotoxic T lymphocytes (see Table 7), various techniques are used to create an antigen-specific receptor on a CD8+ T cell that can prompt T cell activation (Okada, Kohanbash et al. 2009). This process has previously been used in conjunction with IL-2 infusion for the treatment of melanoma. Antigen-specific cytotoxic T cells from peripheral blood or from tumor nodules are isolated from the patient. The T cells will then undergo clonal expansion *in vitro* with specificity for tumor antigen, possibly with the aid of IL-2. These cells are then returned to the patient where they would in theory perform cytotoxic responses upon recognition of tumor-associated antigen in the brain parenchyma (Okada, Kohanbash et al. 2009). In terms of usage in gliomas, the first steps would be creating a library of highly avid cytotoxic T cell clones from which to build highly selective TCR gene pairs to create transgenic cytotoxic T cells. Adoptive therapy is not limited to CD8+ T cells and has been also tried using NK cells and CD4+ T cells, both of which can be similarly removed, expanded, and injected back into the patient. Blancher et al treated 13 GBM by recombinant IL-2, with and without lymphokine activated killer cells, given directly via a catheter into the tumor resection bed. Unfortunately, the treatment had no effects on tumor progression. The adverse reactions included cerebral edema, confusion, and fever (Blancher, Roubinet et al. 1993).

Some obstacles with the adoptive process include creating T cells with TCR of appropriate avidity (Okada, Kohanbash et al. 2009). Further difficulties arise with T cell reproduction; many of these specialized T cell populations are thought to be terminally differentiated and thus unable to propagate long-term existence (Wherry, Teichgraber et al. 2003). Additionally, these transgenic T cells must also overcome the immunosuppressive features of GBM and, in fact, do so better than natural T cells due to the ability to manipulate them and strengthen them with specific chemokines and integrin receptors (Okada, Kohanbash et al. 2009).

6.4. Limitations of immunotherapy

The limitations of immunotherapy for malignant gliomas include: 1) physical obstacles of drug administration due to the BBB, 2) direct and indirect down-regulation of the immune response by gliomas, 3) the high mutation rate of the tumor, which will select for tumor cells that do not express the target of the immune response. In fact, cancer genomes are unstable as evidenced by microsatellite instability of the tumor cells, which aides in tumor evolution and progression (van de Kelft and Verlooy 1994; Yip, Miao et al. 2009; Milinkovic, Bankovic et al. 2012). Additional limitations include difficulty in monitoring the tumor response to treatment because inducing an inflammatory response may create MRI changes that mimic tumor growth. Immunotherapy is also complicated by the common use of steroids, which suppress the immune system.

In our opinion, the most significant limitation of immunotherapy is the limited understanding of the dynamics of the interactions of cytotoxic T lymphocytes with the tumor microenvironment. Clinical trials using immunotherapy have failed to show a clinically significant therapeutic response despite demonstrating the presence of circulating tumor-specific CTL (Lasalvia-Prisco, Garcia-Giralt et al. 2008; Leffers, Lambeck et al. 2009). The key obstacle that we need to overcome is not the induction of a systemic anti-tumor immune response, but making that immune response effective within the tumor microenvironment

7. Immunotherapy clinical trials for brain tumors

- A Pilot Study of Glioma Associated Antigen Vaccines in Conjunction With Poly-ICLC in Pediatric Gliomas
- A Study of Rindopepimut/GM-CSF in Patients With Relapsed EGFRvIII-Positive Glioblastoma
- Biological Therapy Following Surgery and Radiation Therapy in Treating Patients With Primary or Recurrent Astrocytoma or Oligodendroglioma
- Effects of Vaccinations With HLA-A2-Restricted Glioma Antigen-Peptides in Combination With Poly-ICLC for Adults With High-Risk WHO Grade II Astrocytomas and Oligo-Astrocytomas
- GP96 Heat Shock Protein-Peptide Complex Vaccine in Treating Patients With Recurrent or Progressive Glioma
- HLA-A2-Restricted Glioma Antigen-Peptides Vaccinations With Poly-ICLC for Recurrent WHO Grade II Gliomas
- HSPPC-96 Vaccine With Temozolomide in Patients With Newly Diagnosed GBM
- Immunotherapy for Recurrent Ependymomas in Children Treatment for Recurrent Ependymomas Using HLA-A2 Restricted Tumor Antigen Peptides in Combination With Imiquimod
- Peptide Vaccine for Glioblastoma Against Cytomegalovirus Antigens
- Peptide-based Glioma Vaccine IMA950 in Patients With Glioblastoma
- Phase I Study of Safety and Immunogenicity of ADU-623
- Phase I/II Trial of IMA950 Multi-peptide Vaccine Plus Poly-ICLC in Glioblastoma
- Phase II Study of Rindopepimut (CDX-110) in Patients With Glioblastoma Multiforme

- Phase III Study of Rindopepimut/GM-CSF in Patients With Newly Diagnosed Glioblastoma (uses EGFR)
- Poliovirus Vaccine for Recurrent Glioblastoma Multiforme (GBM)
- Vaccine Therapy and Sargramostim in Treating Patients With Malignant Glioma
- Vaccine Therapy and Sargramostim in Treating Patients With Sarcoma or Brain Tumor
- Vaccine Therapy in Treating Patients With Newly Diagnosed Glioblastoma Multiforme
- Vaccine Therapy, Temozolomide, and Radiation Therapy in Treating Patients With Newly Diagnosed Glioblastoma Multiforme

Table 1. Tumor Antigen Vaccine

www.clinicaltrials.gov

The above table lists several current clinical trials using tumor-derived antigens for developing peripheral vaccination against CNS tumors. See section 4.1 above.

- Chemotherapy and Vaccine Therapy Followed by Bone Marrow or Peripheral Stem Cell Transplantation and Interleukin-2 in Treating Patients With Recurrent or Refractory Brain Cancer
- Derivation of Tumor Specific Hybridomas
- Imiquimod/Brain Tumor Initiating Cell (BTIC) Vaccine in Brain Stem Glioma
- Phase I/II Study To Test The Safety and Efficacy of TVI-Brain-1 As A Treatment For Recurrent Grade IV Glioma
- Pilot Immunotherapy Trial for Recurrent Malignant Gliomas
- Study to Evaluate the Effects of Imiquimod and Tumor Lysate Vaccine Immunotherapy in Adults With High Risk or Recurrent/Post-Chemotherapy WHO Grade II Gliomas
- Study To Test the Safety and Efficacy of TVI-Brain-1 As A Treatment for Recurrent Grade IV Glioma
- Vaccination With Lethally Irradiated Glioma Cells Mixed With GM-K562 Cells in Patients Undergoing Craniotomy For Recurrent Tumor

Table 2. Tumor Lysate or Cell Vaccine

The above table lists several current clinical trials using whole tumor cells to develop peripheral vaccines against multiple antigens found on CNS tumors. See section 4.1 above.

- A Study of ICT-107 Immunotherapy in Glioblastoma Multiforme (GBM)
- Biological Therapy in Treating Patients With Glioblastoma Multiforme
- Daclizumab in Treating Patients With Newly Diagnosed Glioblastoma Multiforme Undergoing Targeted Immunotherapy and Temozolomide-Caused Lymphopenia
- Dendritic Cell Cancer Vaccine for High-grade Glioma
- Dendritic Cell Vaccine For Malignant Glioma and Glioblastoma Multiforme in Adult and Pediatric Subjects

http://dx.doi.org/10.5772/58320

- Dendritic Cell Vaccine for Patients With Brain Tumors
- Dendritic Cell Vaccine Therapy With In Situ Maturation in Pediatric Brain Tumors
- Dendritic Cell Vaccine With Imiquimod for Patients With Malignant Glioma
- Efficacy & Safety of Autologous Dendritic Cell Vaccination in Glioblastoma Multiforme After Complete Surgical Resection
- Immunotherapy for Patients With Brain Stem Glioma and Glioblastoma
- Phase II Feasibility Study of Dendritic Cell Vaccination for Newly Diagnosed Glioblastoma Multiforme
- Proteome-based Personalized Immunotherapy of Glioblastoma
- Safe Study of Dendritic Cell (DC) Based Therapy Targeting Tumor Stem Cells in Glioblastoma
- Study of a Drug [DCVax®-L] to Treat Newly Diagnosed GBM Brain Cancer
- Study of DC Vaccination Against Glioblastoma
- Surgical Resection With Gliadel Wafer Followed by Dendritic Cells Vaccination for Malignant Glioma Patients
- Tumor Lysate Pulsed Dendritic Cell Immunotherapy for Patients With Brain Tumors
- Vaccination With Dendritic Cells Loaded With Brain Tumor Stem Cells for Progressive Malignant Brain Tumor
- Vaccination-Dendritic Cells With Peptides for Recurrent Malignant Gliomas
- Vaccine for Patients With Newly Diagnosed or Recurrent Low-Grade Glioma
- Vaccine Immunotherapy for Recurrent Medulloblastoma and Primitive Neuroectodermal Tumor
- Vaccine Therapy and Temozolomide in Treating Patients With Newly Diagnosed Glioblastoma
- Vaccine Therapy in Treating Patients Undergoing Surgery for Recurrent Glioblastoma Multiforme
- Vaccine Therapy in Treating Patients With Malignant Glioma
- Vaccine Therapy in Treating Patients With Newly Diagnosed Glioblastoma Multiforme
- Vaccine Therapy in Treating Young Patients Who Are Undergoing Surgery for Malignant Glioma
- Vaccine Therapy With or Without Sirolimus in Treating Patients With NY-ESO-1 Expressing Solid Tumors

Table 3. Dendritic Cell Vaccine

The above table lists several current clinical trials using dendritic cells combined with tumor antigen as a method of delivering peripheral vaccination against CNS tumors. See section 4.1 above.

- A Phase 2 Evaluation of TRC105 in Combination with Bevacizumab for the Treatment of Recurrent or Progressive Glioblastoma That Has Progressed on Bevacizumab
- Chemotherapy, Radiation Therapy, and Vaccine Therapy With Basiliximab in Treating Patients With Glioblastoma Multiforme That Has Been Removed by Surgery
- Use of Racotumomab in Patients With Pediatric Tumors Expressing N-glycolylated Gangliosides (anti-idiotype antibody)

• Vaccine Therapy With Bevacizumab Versus Bevacizumab Alone in Treating Patients With Recurrent Glioblastoma Multiforme That Can Be Removed by Surgery

Table 4. Vaccine with monoclonal antibody

The above table lists several current clinical trials using passive immunotherapy by means of delivering monoclonal antibodies directed at tumor cells. See section 4.3.1 above.

• Convection-Enhanced Delivery of 124I-8H9 for Patients With Non-Progressive Diffuse Pontine Gliomas Previously Treated With External Beam Radiation Therapy

• Intrathecal Radioimmunotherapy, Radiation Therapy, and Chemotherapy After Surgery in Treating Patients with Medullolblastoma

• Radiolabeled Monoclonal Antibody Therapy in Treating Patients with Primary or Metastatic Brain Tumors

• Radiosurgery Plus Bevacizumab in Glioblastoma

Table 5. Radioimmunotherapy with monoclonal antibody

The above table lists current clinical trials using cytotoxic radiation coupled to monoclonal antibodies to kill tumor cells. See section 4.3.1 above.

• IL-4 (38-37)-PE38KDEL Immunotoxin in Treating Patients With Recurrent Malignant Astrocytoma

• Imaging Study of the Distribution of IL13-PE38QQR Infused Before and After Surgery in Adult Patients With Recurrent Malignant Glioma

• NBI-3001 Followed by Surgery in Treating Patients with Recurrent Glioblastoma Multiforme

• TP-38 Toxin in Treating Young Patients with Recurrent or Progressive Supratentorial High-Grade Glioma

Table 6. Transfer of Ligands

The above table lists current clinical trials using molecules fused with toxins as a means of killing tumor cells.

• A Phase I Study to Investigate Tolerability and Efficacy of ALECSAT Administered to Glioblastoma Multiforme Patients

• Autologous Natural Killer T Cells Infusion for the Treatment of Cancer

• Cellular Adoptive Immunotherapy in Treating Patients With Glioblastoma Multiforme

• Cellular Adoptive Immunotherapy Using Genetically Modified T-Lymphocytes in Treating Patients With Recurrent or Refractory High-Grade Malignant Glioma

• Cellular Immunotherapy Study for Brain Cancer

• CMV-specific Cytotoxic T Lymphocytes Expressing CAR Targeting HER2 in Patients with GBM (HERT-GBM)

• Evaluation of Recovery From Drug-Induced Lymphopenia Using Cytomegalovirus-specific T-cell Adoptive Transfer
• Phase I Study of Cellular Immunotherapy for Recurrent/Refractory Malignant Glioma Using Intratumoral Infusions of GRm13Z40-2, An Allogeneic CD8+ Cytolitic T-Cell Line Genetically Modified to Express the IL 13-Zetakine and HyTK and to be Resistant to Glucocorticoids, in Combination With Interleukin-2
• Safety and Effectiveness Study of Autologous Natural Killer and Natural Killer T Cells on Cancer
• White Blood Cells With Anti-EGFR-III for Malignant Gliomas

Table 7. Adoptive Immunotherapy

The above table lists several current clinical trials using adoptive immunotherapy as a way of applying passive immunotherapy to return autologous tumor-antigen-specific T cells back to the patient as a means of targeting CNS tumors. See section 4.3.3 above.

8. Gene therapy

Gene therapy as it relates to malignant gliomas is based on tumor-specific introduction of genetic material for the purpose of treatment. It involves direct injection of a gene transfer vector or vector producing cells (VPC) into the tumor itself or into the cavity left after resection. Although preclinical studies have been quite promising, unfortunately therapeutic response to gene therapy clinical trials remains low (Tobias, Ahmed et al. 2013). Three classes of genetic therapy treatment have taken center stage over the last several decades: prodrug/suicide genes, oncolytic viruses, and gene immunotherapy. Although each is its own distinct entity, they all facilitate delivery of genetic material through the use of one or more vectors as described below.

8.1. Vectors

8.1.1. Retroviral vectors

Retroviruses and retroviral vector producing cells (RVPCs) may be used to deliver specific genes to glioma cells; they are perhaps the most widely-studied class of vectors for treatment of GBM. This class of virus is advantageous in that its transduction is limited to rapidly dividing cells, meaning that normal brain cells remain unaltered. However, the transduction rate is low secondary to rapid inactivation of free retroviral vectors by complement as well as a lack of movement of virus to sites distant to the injection. It should be noted that transduction of circulating cells by vectors may occur, thus putting the patient at risk of cancer initiation via insertional mutagenesis (Barzon, Zanusso et al. 2006).

8.1.2. Adenoviral vectors

Adenoviruses belong to a family of 90-100 nm non-enveloped viruses made up of a nucleo-capsid and double-stranded linear DNA. They account for roughly one tenth of all upper respiratory tract infections in children, infecting the host via introduction of their genome into the nucleus of the host organism's cells where the viral DNA remains free. This is in opposition to the retroviral mechanism involving incorporation of genetic material into the host cell's genomic structure.

Adenovirus enters the host cell by way of 2 distinct sets of interactions. Firstly, the knob domain of the virus's fiber protein binds to the cell receptor (either CD46 or coxsackievirus adenovirus receptor). This is followed by the interaction of a specialized motif in the penton base protein with an integrin molecule, which prompts internalization of the virus via an endosome. Thereafter the capsid components dissociate and the virion is released into the cytoplasm. Viral DNA enters the nucleus via the nuclear pore, later associating with histones. Following nuclear invasion, the viral genome is reproduced along with the host cell's DNA. However, the progeny of the original host cell will not carry the newly-introduced viral DNA. This necessitates numerous rounds of viral introduction in the treatment of cancer (Doloff and Waxman 2013).

8.1.3. Reoviral vectors

The genome of Reoviridae is segmented, double-stranded RNA, and the virus has the ability to make use of a non-functional protein kinase R (PKR) pathway in glioma cells to allow for viral replication. This is advantageous as the virus does not require genetic engineering. Other advantages include small size (70-80nm) and an absence of known consequent encephalitis in humans (Clarke, Debiasi et al. 2005).

8.1.4. Nonviral vectors

There are several nonviral vectors either currently in use or being considered for use in gene therapy such as synthetic vectors, nanoparticles, and stem cells/progenitor cells. From this group, perhaps the most studied is the liposome (included in the category of nanoparticles). Cationic Liposomes are easy to produce, have relatively low immunogenicity and toxicity, and typically exhibit long-term stability (Tobias, Ahmed et al. 2013).

8.2. Gene therapy strategies

8.2.1. Prodrug activating genes/suicide genes

Prodrug/suicide genes represent an ingenious wing of gene therapy. The basis of this antitumor modality is introduction of genes, either into the host genome or the intranuclear milieu, which imparts susceptibility to a subsequent therapeutic agent. The vectors themselves are genetically modified to produce an enzyme which converts a prodrug, given systemically, into toxic metabolites which act specifically on the malignancy.

Perhaps the earliest/most-studied example of prodrug/suicide gene utility when addressing gliomas is that of Herpes Simplex Type 1 Thymidine Kinase (HSV-tk). After incorporation of this gene into tumor cells (often residual cells status-post resection) and the endothelium of their vasculature, the host is treated with an antiviral such as gancyclovir (GCV). HSV-TK phosphorylates the prodrug of GCV into its active compound, whose mechanism of action involves DNA cross-linking, which leads to cell death. Following treatment with GCV, there may also be an observed "bystander effect" which involves the killing of non-transduced adjacent cells or even distant cells via immune response (T Cells, NK Cells) and toxic metabolites received via gap junctions (Ram, Culver et al. 1997; Floeth, Shand et al. 2001; Matuskova, Hlubinova et al. 2010). In a xenograft glioma model, a significant therapeutic effect was found when only approximately 10% of tumor cells were transduced with HSV-tk (Chen, Chang et al. 1995; Sandmair, Loimas et al. 2000). Introduction of HSV-tk/GCV may also increase response to standard measures such as radio- and chemotherapy (Rainov, Fels et al. 2001; Chiocca, Broaddus et al. 2004). This method has also been hypothesized to stimulate an immune response and provide an anti-angiogenic effect (Culver, Ram et al. 1992; Ayala, Satoh et al. 2006; Chiocca, Aguilar et al. 2011). Although there have been numerous enzyme-prodrug clinical trials ranging from Phase I to Phase III, endpoints such as median survival have not been overly impressive (Iwami, Natsume et al. 2010; Kroeger, Muhammad et al. 2010).

8.2.2. Retrovirally-mediated therapy

Intratumor injection of RVPCs has shown a high percentage of tumor regression in some studies (Ram, Culver et al. 1997; Pulkkanen and Yla-Herttuala 2005). Rainov et al. conducted a Phase III, multicenter, open-label, randomized trial of newly diagnosed GBM comparing standard therapy vs. standard therapy with adjuvant gene therapy of the tumor bed by HSV-tk. Although this mode of treatment was shown to be safe, there was no significant difference in 12-month survival rates or progression-free median survival (Rainov 2000). A recent Phase I head-to-head trial of intra-operative HSV-tk introduction via retrovirus vs. adenovirus showed promising results for adenoviral vectors in a small number of patients (Sandmair, Loimas et al. 2000).

8.2.3. Adenovirally-mediated therapy

It should also be noted that unlike retroviral vectors, adenovirus can transduce both dividing and non-dividing cells. The majority of adenoviruses used for this purpose are E1-deleted adenoviral vectors, which may be injected at a higher titer than RVPCs; however high doses may indeed lead to serious side effects, including confusion, seizures, fever, leukocytosis, and hyponatremia that appear to be secondary to immune response to the vector (Trask, Trask et al. 2000). This same immune response lowers the yield of viral delivery but also aids in tumor reduction (Trask, Trask et al. 2000; Lang, Bruner et al. 2003). Notably, the adenoviral vector may be found transiently in blood but has not been found as a replication-competent entity.

Preliminary clinical data suggest that adenoviral mediated gene transfer of suicide genes (AdvHSV-tk) may have clinical utility (Germano, Fable et al. 2003; Immonen, Vapalahti et al. 2004). A Phase IIB randomized controlled trial of patients with malignant gliomas reported a significant increase in OS from 37.7 weeks in the control arm (n=19) to 62.4 weeks in the adenoviral treated arm (AdvHSV-tk, n=17) (Immonen, Vapalahti et al. 2004). A recent Phase 1B trial showed treatment with adenovirus-HSV-tk followed by Valacyclovir, when paired with resection, chemotherapy and radiotherapy, was safe and without dose-limiting toxicity (Chiocca, Aguilar et al. 2011).

Despite the aforementioned promising results from a small number of patients, the Phase III international open-label, randomized ASPECT clinical trial, which studied the intra-operative administration of adenoviral-HSV-tk followed by GCV (n=124) as compared to resection and standard of care alone (n=126), was not positive. Unfortunately, the data revealed no difference between the groups in terms of OS; furthermore, more patients in the experimental group had one or more treatment-related adverse events than those in the control group (88 [71%] vs 51 [43%]) (Westphal, Yla-Herttuala et al. 2013).

8.2.4. Nanopartical/Neural stem cell-mediated therapy

Synthetic vectors, including nanoparticles have been applied to deliver DNA plasmids, RNA and siRNA (Jin and Ye 2007; Germano and Binello 2009; Jin, Bae et al. 2011). Liposomes are perhaps the most-researched of all nanoparticles (Tobias, Ahmed et al. 2013). Given through convection-enhanced delivery via stereotactically-placed catheters a liposome-DNA complex has been used to deliver HSV-tk in a small number of patients. The treatment was well-tolerated without major side effects (Jacobs, Voges et al. 2001; Voges, Reszka et al. 2003).

Pleuripotent neural stem cells procured from the subgranular zone of the hippocampus and the areas surrounding the lateral ventricles have the ability to migrate to areas of parenchymal damage (Luskin 1993). Neural stem cell clones may migrate to areas of tumor infiltration and thus were examined as vehicles for delivery of suicide genes, cytokines, or tumor necrosis factor-related apoptosis-inducing ligand (TRAIL); there is evidence of potential efficacy in animal models but no clinical utility data yet (Aboody, Brown et al. 2000; Marsh, Goldfarb et al. 2013).

8.2.5. Tumor suppressor gene replacement

A well-documented characteristic of GBM is its inherent inactivation of the p53 tumor suppressor gene. Animal trials have shown that re-introduction of the wild-type p53 gene is pro-apoptotic leading to increased sensitivity to current modalities of treatment such as chemo- and radiotherapy. A Phase 1 trial of adenoviral gene transfer of intra-tumoral wild-type p53 in recurrent malignant glioma proved to be safe, but the transfected cells were not found in a radius large enough to be therapeutically effective (Lang, Bruner et al. 2003).

8.3. Oncolytic gene therapy

The realm of oncolytic virus therapy involves the use of replication-competent viruses with the ability to selectively replicate and kill cancer cells, with or without gene transfer. This is in opposition to prodrug/suicide gene therapy which makes use of replication-incompetent modalities. In order to combat the inefficiency of suicide gene therapy, oncolytic treatment employs tumor-specific, conditionally replicating viral vectors (Tobias, Ahmed et al. 2013). The mechanism of action involves viral replication which eventually leads to lysis of the host tumor cell and subsequent release of additional copies of competent virus which may lead to further tumor reduction. This method is tumor-specific as it makes use of either attenuated viruses containing inactivated genes which replicate in tumor cells only, or viruses with replication-essential genes in tumor-specific promoters (Chiocca 2002). This method employs herpes simplex virus (HSV), Adenovirus, Reovirus, Poliovirus, Newcastle Disease Virus (NDV), and Measles virus.

8.3.1. Oncolytic HSV-1

Herpes Simplex is an enveloped, doubled-stranded DNA virus which exhibits inherent action upon the human nervous system; it can replicate in both active and quiescent cells. Consequently, safety was an original concern with this viral vector. Approximately 8 different HSV-1 genes have been altered or deleted to promote tumor specificity and lower collateral CNS damage (Tobias, Ahmed et al. 2013). There are two strains of replication-competent HSV-1 which have been significantly studied: G207 and HSV1716. G207 is the more widely-examined of the two and possesses a mechanism of action involving alteration of the gene which produces ribonucleotide reductase. In a recent phase 1B clinical trial, patients received injections of this virus both before and after tumor resection. Although viral replication was observed, treatment efficacy was sparse (Markert, Liechty et al. 2009). Additional studies have likewise shown adequate safety but minimal efficacy (Todo, Martuza et al. 2001).

G207 overcomes host defenses mediated by protein kinase R (PKR), which normally shuts down translation in infected cells through phosphorylation of eIF-2 alpha (Barzon, Zanusso et al. 2006). In a Phase I study by Markert et al., conditionally replicating G207 virus (given by stereotactic intratumor injection) was not found to lead to the development of herpes encephalitis (Markert, Medlock et al. 2000). Additionally, replication-competent HSV1716 administration in a Phase 1 dose-escalation study by Rampling et al. did not lead to encephalitis. Furthermore, no viral shedding was noted and no viral genome was found in tumor biopsies performed months after treatment (Rampling, Cruickshank et al. 2000).

8.3.2. Oncolytic adenoviruses

Adenoviruses carrying mutations in E1A or E1B can also act on GBM via oncolysis. Their mechanism of action involves tumor-specific binding and inactivation of apoptotic proteins like pRB family and p53. Of note, adenovirus is inherently non-neurotropic, which may lend itself to superior safety versus HSV. One adenovirus, *ONYX-015,* has been found to preferentially replicate in p53 deficient cells secondary to its deletion for p53-inactivating protein E1B-55K. In one clinical trial it was injected into the surgical cavity after resection and found to have no serious adverse effects; however; almost all patients involved in the trial had progression of their GBM (Chiocca, Abbed et al. 2004). It should also be noted that Geoerger et al found human xenografts to be responsive to ONYX-015 without correlation to their p53 status (Geoerger, Grill et al. 2003).

8.3.3. Oncolytic NDV

NDV is an avian paramyxovirus, which does not harm humans except for rare pulmonary infection in poultry farmers; certain strains harm neoplastic cells via a currently unknown mechanism (Reichard, Lorence et al. 1992). Interestingly, NDV also has pleiotropic immune-modulatory properties (Schirrmacher, Haas et al. 1999). It should be noted that treatment with NDV necessitates starting at a low dose as there have been examples of treatment-related death with *NDV PV701 and solid cancers* (Pecora, Rizvi et al. 2002). *MTH-68/H*, a live attenuated oncolytic viral strain of NDV, has shown promising results is a small number of GBM patients (Csatary, Gosztonyi et al. 2004).

8.3.2. Oncolytic reoviruses

Reovirus is a double-stranded RNA-containing virus that replicates in GBM cells because of a hyperactive ras signaling; it distinctively does not replicate in normal brain cells. A phase I clinical trial of intrattumoral administration of genetically unmodified virus was well tolerated by patients with recurrent malignant gliomas (Forsyth, Roldan et al. 2008). Further studies involving reovirus are currently underway.

8.4. Gene immunotherapy

Treatment of gliomas with immune therapy is based on harnessing of the patient's T-Cell mediated response to tumor cells. Typically, gene-immune therapy falls into the category of priming in the brain by the transfer of cytokine genes, like IL-2, IL-4, IL-12, and interferons gamma and beta (Freeman, Abboud et al. 1993; Borden, Lindner et al. 2000; Candolfi, Xiong et al. 2010; Denbo, Williams et al. 2011; Ryu, Park et al. 2011; Markert, Cody et al. 2012). A phase I clinical trial of the injection of cationic liposomes carrying the human IFN-Beta gene into the postsurgical cavity showed low toxicity (Wakabayashi, Natsume et al. 2008). A phase 1 trial of adenovirus-mediated gene transfer of INF-Beta was also well tolerated (Chiocca, Smith et al. 2008). Furthermore, a small pilot study of liposomal-mediated IFN-Beta gene transfer into the postsurgical cavity showed promising results (Yoshida, Mizuno et al. 2004).

Another important strategy combines cytokine gene transfer (human IL-2) paired with HSV-TK/GCV treatment (Palu, Cavaggioni et al. 1999; Colombo, Barzon et al. 2005). The results are promising in a small number of patients (Colombo, Barzon et al. 2005); in particular, biopsy following treatment showed tumor necrosis at site of administration as well as significant immune response in the form of activated cytotoxic T cells, macrophages and T-Helper/inducer lymphocytes (Barzon, Zanusso et al. 2006).

9. Conclusion

The aforementioned negative results of several key phase III clinical trials in GBM demonstrate that current proof of efficacy in preclinical models is a necessary but not sufficient condition

http://dx.doi.org/10.5772/58320

for clinical utility. The consistency in obtaining negative results in GBM is remarkable. How can we improve and what do we do to turn the tide in our favor?

It is becoming evident that the phenotypes of GBM are not created by few solitary molecules but rather by dynamic networks with positive and negative loops that react and respond to a therapeutic intervention. The good news is that these networks are finite dimensional. Furthermore, because of the instability of cancer genomes, random mutations are introduced in the population of rapidly dividing glioma cells; hence, a particular therapy could merely delay growth by selecting a resistant subpopulation. We suggest that we should elevate the threshold by mandating stringent criteria before proceeding to very costly phase III clinical trials, as follows.

1. Phase II clinical trials must include a control arm with appropriate stratification instead of historical controls.

2. Preclinical models must include proof of feasibility in at least 8-10 different cell lines/ animal models.

3. We ought to invest in developing a better understanding of the structure of the oncogenic molecular networks in GBM and demand laboratory data depicting the reactions of these networks to a new therapeutic strategy.

4. We need to develop mathematical models, results, and simulations of these molecular networks and acquire the ability to test therapeutic strategies in silico.

We believe that investing in the aforementioned endeavors will increase the likelihood that a chosen therapy will have proven clinical utility against GBM. Maintaining the status quo, by forging ahead with large phase III clinical trials costing about $50-100 million each, is not attractive.

Author details

Paula Province, Alexis Bashinski Shaefer, Benjamin McCullough and Hassan M Fathallah-Shaykh

The University of Alabama at Birmingham, Birmingham, Alabama, USA

References

[1] Abbas, A. K, Lichtman, A. H, et al. (2014). Basic immunology : functions and disorders of the immune system. Philadelphia, W.B. Saunders Co.

[2] Aboody, K. S, Brown, A, et al. (2000). Neural stem cells display extensive tropism for pathology in adult brain: evidence from intracranial gliomas." Proc Natl Acad Sci U S A , 97(23), 12846-12851.

[3] Ahluwalia, M. S, & Gladson, C. L. (2010). Progress on antiangiogenic therapy for patients with malignant glioma." J Oncol 2010: 689018.

[4] Ayala, G, Satoh, T, et al. (2006). Biological response determinants in HSV-tk + ganciclovir gene therapy for prostate cancer." Mol Ther , 13(4), 716-728.

[5] Barzon, L, Zanusso, M, et al. (2006). Clinical trials of gene therapy, virotherapy, and immunotherapy for malignant gliomas." Cancer Gene Ther , 13(6), 539-554.

[6] Baselga, J. (2001). The EGFR as a target for anticancer therapy--focus on cetuximab." Eur J Cancer 37 Suppl 4: S, 16-22.

[7] Batra, S. K, Castelino-prabhu, S, et al. (1995). Epidermal growth factor ligand-independent, unregulated, cell-transforming potential of a naturally occurring human mutant EGFRvIII gene." Cell Growth Differ , 6(10), 1251-1259.

[8] Baumann, F, Bjeljac, M, et al. (2004). Combined thalidomide and temozolomide treatment in patients with glioblastoma multiforme." J Neurooncol 67(1-2): 191-200.

[9] Bertolino, P, Deckers, M, et al. (2005). Transforming growth factor-beta signal transduction in angiogenesis and vascular disorders." Chest 128(6 Suppl): 585S-590S.

[10] Blancher, A, Roubinet, F, et al. (1993). Local immunotherapy of recurrent glioblastoma multiforme by intracerebral perfusion of interleukin-2 and LAK cells." Eur Cytokine Netw , 4(5), 331-341.

[11] Bobo, R. H, Laske, D. W, et al. (1994). Convection-enhanced delivery of macromolecules in the brain." Proc Natl Acad Sci U S A , 91(6), 2076-2080.

[12] Borden, E. C, Lindner, D, et al. (2000). Second-generation interferons for cancer: clinical targets." Semin Cancer Biol , 10(2), 125-144.

[13] Boult, J. K, Terkelsen, J, et al. (2013). A multi-parametric imaging investigation of the response of C6 glioma xenografts to MLN0518 (tandutinib) treatment." PLoS One 8(4): e63024.

[14] Boulton, M. E, Cai, J, et al. (2008). gamma-Secretase: a multifaceted regulator of angiogenesis." J Cell Mol Med , 12(3), 781-795.

[15] Brat, D. J, & Mapstone, T. B. (2003). Malignant glioma physiology: cellular response to hypoxia and its role in tumor progression." Ann Intern Med , 138(8), 659-668.

[16] Broholm, H, & Laursen, H. (2004). Vascular endothelial growth factor (VEGF) receptor neuropilin-1's distribution in astrocytic tumors." APMIS 112(4-5): 257-263.

[17] Candolfi, M, Xiong, W, et al. (2010). Gene therapy-mediated delivery of targeted cytotoxins for glioma therapeutics." Proc Natl Acad Sci U S A , 107(46), 20021-20026.

[18] Carmeliet, P, & Jain, R. K. (2011). Molecular mechanisms and clinical applications of angiogenesis." Nature , 473(7347), 298-307.

[19] Chavarria, A, & Cardenas, G. (2013). Neuronal influence behind the central nervous system regulation of the immune cells." Front Integr Neurosci 7: 64.

[20] Chen, C. Y, Chang, Y. N, et al. (1995). Effect of herpes simplex virus thymidine kinase expression levels on ganciclovir-mediated cytotoxicity and the "bystander effect"." Hum Gene Ther , 6(11), 1467-1476.

[21] Chen, K. S, & Mitchell, D. A. (2012). Monoclonal antibody therapy for malignant glioma." Adv Exp Med Biol , 746, 121-141.

[22] Chiocca, E. A. (2002). Oncolytic viruses." Nat Rev Cancer , 2(12), 938-950.

[23] Chiocca, E. A, Abbed, K. M, et al. (2004). A phase I open-label, dose-escalation, multi-institutional trial of injection with an E1B-Attenuated adenovirus, ONYX-015, into the peritumoral region of recurrent malignant gliomas, in the adjuvant setting." Mol Ther , 10(5), 958-966.

[24] Chiocca, E. A, Aguilar, L. K, et al. (2011). Phase IB study of gene-mediated cytotoxic immunotherapy adjuvant to up-front surgery and intensive timing radiation for malignant glioma." J Clin Oncol , 29(27), 3611-3619.

[25] Chiocca, E. A, Broaddus, W. C, et al. (2004). Neurosurgical delivery of chemotherapeutics, targeted toxins, genetic and viral therapies in neuro-oncology." J Neurooncol 69(1-3): 101-117.

[26] Chiocca, E. A, Smith, K. M, et al. (2008). A phase I trial of Ad.hIFN-beta gene therapy for glioma." Mol Ther , 16(3), 618-626.

[27] Choi, B. D, Suryadevara, C. M, et al. (2013). Intracerebral delivery of a third generation EGFRvIII-specific chimeric antigen receptor is efficacious against human glioma." J Clin Neurosci.

[28] Chow, L. Q, & Eckhardt, S. G. (2007). Sunitinib: from rational design to clinical efficacy." J Clin Oncol , 25(7), 884-896.

[29] Clarke, P, Debiasi, R. L, et al. (2005). Mechanisms of reovirus-induced cell death and tissue injury: role of apoptosis and virus-induced perturbation of host-cell signaling and transcription factor activation." Viral Immunol , 18(1), 89-115.

[30] Cobbs, C. S, Harkins, L, et al. (2002). Human cytomegalovirus infection and expression in human malignant glioma." Cancer Res , 62(12), 3347-3350.

[31] Colombo, F, Barzon, L, et al. (2005). Combined HSV-TK/IL-2 gene therapy in patients with recurrent glioblastoma multiforme: biological and clinical results." Cancer Gene Ther , 12(10), 835-848.

[32] Costa, P. M, Cardoso, A. L, et al. (2013). MicroRNA-21 silencing enhances the cytotoxic effect of the antiangiogenic drug sunitinib in glioblastoma." Hum Mol Genet , 22(5), 904-918.

[33] Csatary, L. K, Gosztonyi, G, et al. (2004). MTH-68/H oncolytic viral treatment in human high-grade gliomas." J Neurooncol 67(1-2): 83-93.

[34] Culver, K. W, Ram, Z, et al. (1992). In vivo gene transfer with retroviral vector-producer cells for treatment of experimental brain tumors." Science , 256(5063), 1550-1552.

[35] Agostino, D, Gottfried-blackmore, P. M. , A, et al. (2012). Brain dendritic cells: biology and pathology." Acta Neuropathol , 124(5), 599-614.

[36] Amato, D, Loughnan, R. J. , M. S, et al. (1994). Thalidomide is an inhibitor of angiogenesis." Proc Natl Acad Sci U S A , 91(9), 4082-4085.

[37] De Groot, J. F, Lamborn, K. R, et al. (2011). Phase II study of aflibercept in recurrent malignant glioma: a North American Brain Tumor Consortium study." J Clin Oncol , 29(19), 2689-2695.

[38] Debinski, W, Gibo, D. M, et al. (1999). Receptor for interleukin 13 is a marker and therapeutic target for human high-grade gliomas." Clin Cancer Res , 5(5), 985-990.

[39] Debinski, W, Obiri, N. I, et al. (1995). Human glioma cells overexpress receptors for interleukin 13 and are extremely sensitive to a novel chimeric protein composed of interleukin 13 and pseudomonas exotoxin." Clin Cancer Res , 1(11), 1253-1258.

[40] Denbo, J. W, Williams, R. F, et al. (2011). Continuous local delivery of interferon-beta stabilizes tumor vasculature in an orthotopic glioblastoma xenograft resection model." Surgery , 150(3), 497-504.

[41] Dieterich, L. C, Mellberg, S, et al. (2012). Transcriptional profiling of human glioblastoma vessels indicates a key role of VEGF-A and TGFbeta2 in vascular abnormalization." J Pathol , 228(3), 378-390.

[42] Djonov, V, Schmid, M, et al. (2000). Intussusceptive angiogenesis: its role in embryonic vascular network formation." Circ Res , 86(3), 286-292.

[43] Doloff, J. C, & Waxman, D. J. (2013). Adenoviral Vectors for Prodrug Activation-based Gene Therapy for Cancer." Anticancer Agents Med Chem.

[44] Dustin, M. L, & Depoil, D. (2011). New insights into the T cell synapse from single molecule techniques." Nat Rev Immunol , 11(10), 672-684.

[45] Fathallah-shaykh, H. M, Gao, W, et al. (1998). Priming in the brain, an immunologically privileged organ, elicits anti-tumor immunity." Int J Cancer , 75(2), 266-276.

[46] Ferguson, S, & Lesniak, M. S. (2007). Convection enhanced drug delivery of novel therapeutic agents to malignant brain tumors." Curr Drug Deliv , 4(2), 169-180.

[47] Feun, L, & Savaraj, N. (2008). Topoisomerase I inhibitors for the treatment of brain tumors." Expert Rev Anticancer Ther , 8(5), 707-716.

[48] Fiorio PlaA., C. Grange, et al. ((2008). Arachidonic acid-induced Ca2+ entry is involved in early steps of tumor angiogenesis." Mol Cancer Res , 6(4), 535-545.

[49] Floeth, F. W, Shand, N, et al. (2001). Local inflammation and devascularization--in vivo mechanisms of the "bystander effect" in VPC-mediated HSV-Tk/GCV gene therapy for human malignant glioma." Cancer Gene Ther , 8(11), 843-851.

[50] Folkman, J. (1972). Anti-angiogenesis: new concept for therapy of solid tumors." Ann Surg , 175(3), 409-416.

[51] Forsyth, P, Roldan, G, et al. (2008). A phase I trial of intratumoral administration of reovirus in patients with histologically confirmed recurrent malignant gliomas." Mol Ther , 16(3), 627-632.

[52] Freeman, S. M, Abboud, C. N, et al. (1993). The "bystander effect": tumor regression when a fraction of the tumor mass is genetically modified." Cancer Res , 53(21), 5274-5283.

[53] Friedman, H. S, Prados, M. D, et al. (2009). Bevacizumab alone and in combination with irinotecan in recurrent glioblastoma." J Clin Oncol , 27(28), 4733-4740.

[54] Fukai, J, Nishio, K, et al. (2008). Antitumor activity of cetuximab against malignant glioma cells overexpressing EGFR deletion mutant variant III." Cancer Sci , 99(10), 2062-2069.

[55] Ge, S, Rempel, S. A, et al. (2000). Carboxyamido-triazole induces apoptosis in bovine aortic endothelial and human glioma cells." Clin Cancer Res , 6(4), 1248-1254.

[56] Geoerger, B, Grill, J, et al. (2003). Potentiation of radiation therapy by the oncolytic adenovirus dl1520 (ONYX-015) in human malignant glioma xenografts." Br J Cancer , 89(3), 577-584.

[57] Germano, I. M, & Binello, E. (2009). Gene therapy as an adjuvant treatment for malignant gliomas: from bench to bedside." J Neurooncol , 93(1), 79-87.

[58] Germano, I. M, Fable, J, et al. (2003). Adenovirus/herpes simplex-thymidine kinase/ganciclovir complex: preliminary results of a phase I trial in patients with recurrent malignant gliomas." J Neurooncol , 65(3), 279-289.

[59] Gilbert, M. R, Dignam, J, et al. (2013). RTOG 0825: Phase III double-blind placebo-controlled trial evaluating bevacizumab (Bev) in patients (Pts) with newly diagnosed glioblastoma (GBM)." ASCO Meeting Abstracts 31(18_suppl): 1.

[60] Gomez-manzano, C, Holash, J, et al. (2008). VEGF Trap induces antiglioma effect at different stages of disease." Neuro Oncol , 10(6), 940-945.

[61] Grover, G, Kelly, J, et al. (2007). Comparative pharmacokinetic profile of carboxyamidotriazole and carboxyamidotriazole-orotate." Cancer Therapy , 5, 437-442.

[62] Haapa-paananen, S, Chen, P, et al. (2013). Functional profiling of precursor MicroRNAs identifies MicroRNAs essential for glioma proliferation." PLoS One 8(4): e60930.

[63] Henriksson, R, Bottomley, A, et al. (2013). Progression-free survival (PFS) and health-related quality of life (HRQoL) in AVAglio, a phase III study of bevacizumab (Bv), temozolomide (T), and radiotherapy (RT) in newly diagnosed glioblastoma (GBM)." ASCO Meeting Abstracts 31(15_suppl): 2005.

[64] Hilberg, F, Roth, G. J, et al. (2008). BIBF 1120: triple angiokinase inhibitor with sustained receptor blockade and good antitumor efficacy." Cancer Res , 68(12), 4774-4782.

[65] Hivroz, C, Chemin, K, et al. (2012). Crosstalk between T lymphocytes and dendritic cells." Crit Rev Immunol , 32(2), 139-155.

[66] Holash, J, Davis, S, et al. (2002). VEGF-Trap: a VEGF blocker with potent antitumor effects." Proc Natl Acad Sci U S A , 99(17), 11393-11398.

[67] Holash, J, Wiegand, S. J, et al. (1999). New model of tumor angiogenesis: dynamic balance between vessel regression and growth mediated by angiopoietins and VEGF." Oncogene , 18(38), 5356-5362.

[68] Huang, S, Peng, L, et al. (2013). Hypoxia of PC-3 prostate cancer cells enhances migration and vasculogenesis in vitro of bone marrow-derived endothelial progenitor cells by secretion of cytokines." Oncol Rep , 29(6), 2369-2377.

[69] Hugues, S. (2010). Dynamics of dendritic cell-T cell interactions: a role in T cell outcome." Semin Immunopathol , 32(3), 227-238.

[70] Hynes, R. O, Bader, B. L, et al. (1999). Integrins in vascular development." Braz J Med Biol Res , 32(5), 501-510.

[71] Iliff, J. J, & Nedergaard, M. (2013). Is there a cerebral lymphatic system?" Stroke 44(6 Suppl 1): S, 93-95.

[72] Immonen, A, Vapalahti, M, et al. (2004). AdvHSV-tk gene therapy with intravenous ganciclovir improves survival in human malignant glioma: a randomised, controlled study." Mol Ther , 10(5), 967-972.

[73] Iwami, K, Natsume, A, et al. (2010). Gene therapy for high-grade glioma." Neurol Med Chir (Tokyo) , 50(9), 727-736.

[74] Jacobs, A, Voges, J, et al. (2001). Positron-emission tomography of vector-mediated gene expression in gene therapy for gliomas." Lancet , 358(9283), 727-729.

[75] Jagani, Z, Wiederschain, D, et al. (2010). The Polycomb group protein Bmi-1 is essential for the growth of multiple myeloma cells." Cancer Res , 70(13), 5528-5538.

[76] Jain, R. K, & Di, E. Tomaso, et al. ((2007). Angiogenesis in brain tumours." Nat Rev Neurosci , 8(8), 610-622.

[77] Jarry, U, Jeannin, P, et al. (2013). Efficiently stimulated adult microglia cross-prime naive CD8+ T cells injected in the brain." Eur J Immunol , 43(5), 1173-1184.

[78] Jiang, L, Song, L, et al. (2013). Bmi-1 promotes glioma angiogenesis by activating NF-kappaB signaling." PLoS One 8(1): e55527.

[79] Jin, J, Bae, K. H, et al. (2011). In vivo specific delivery of c-Met siRNA to glioblastoma using cationic solid lipid nanoparticles." Bioconjug Chem , 22(12), 2568-2572.

[80] Jin, S, & Ye, K. (2007). Nanoparticle-mediated drug delivery and gene therapy." Biotechnol Prog , 23(1), 32-41.

[81] Joffre, O. P, Segura, E, et al. (2012). Cross-presentation by dendritic cells." Nat Rev Immunol , 12(8), 557-569.

[82] Joshi, B. H, Leland, P, et al. (2001). In situ expression of interleukin-4 (IL-4) receptors in human brain tumors and cytotoxicity of a recombinant IL-4 cytotoxin in primary glioblastoma cell cultures." Cancer Res , 61(22), 8058-8061.

[83] Kaminska, B, Kocyk, M, et al. (2013). TGF beta signaling and its role in glioma pathogenesis." Adv Exp Med Biol , 986, 171-187.

[84] Karmali, R, Maxuitenko, Y, et al. (2011). Carboxyamidotriazole Orotate and Cytotoxic Chemotherapy have a Synergistic Effect on Tumor Inhibition in Glioblastoma and Colon Xenograft Mouse Models." Cancer Therapy , 8, 71-80.

[85] Kinch, M. S, Moore, M. B, et al. (2003). Predictive value of the EphA2 receptor tyrosine kinase in lung cancer recurrence and survival." Clin Cancer Res , 9(2), 613-618.

[86] Kreisl, T. N, Kim, L, et al. (2009). Phase II trial of single-agent bevacizumab followed by bevacizumab plus irinotecan at tumor progression in recurrent glioblastoma." J Clin Oncol , 27(5), 740-745.

[87] Kreisl, T. N, Mcneill, K. A, et al. (2012). A phase I/II trial of vandetanib for patients with recurrent malignant glioma." Neuro Oncol , 14(12), 1519-1526.

[88] Kreisl, T. N, Smith, P, et al. (2013). Continuous daily sunitinib for recurrent glioblastoma." J Neurooncol , 111(1), 41-48.

[89] Kroeger, K. M, Muhammad, A. K, et al. (2010). Gene therapy and virotherapy: novel therapeutic approaches for brain tumors." Discov Med , 10(53), 293-304.

[90] Kurz, H, Korn, J, et al. (2001). Embryonic central nervous system angiogenesis does not involve blood-borne endothelial progenitors." J Comp Neurol , 436(3), 263-274.

[91] Lampropoulou, E, Manioudaki, M, et al. (2011). Pyrrolo[2,3-alpha]carbazole derivatives as topoisomerase I inhibitors that affect viability of glioma and endothelial cells in vitro and angiogenesis in vivo." Biomed Pharmacother , 65(3), 142-150.

[92] Lang, F. F, Bruner, J. M, et al. (2003). Phase I trial of adenovirus-mediated gene therapy for recurrent glioma: biological and clinical results." J Clin Oncol 21(13): 2508-2518., 53.

[93] Lasalvia-prisco, E, Garcia-giralt, E, et al. (2008). Randomized phase II clinical trial of chemo-immunotherapy in advanced nonsmall cell lung cancer." Biologics , 2(3), 555-561.

[94] Leffers, N, Lambeck, A. J, et al. (2009). Immunization with a synthetic long peptide vaccine induces P53-specific immune responses in ovarian cancer patients, a phase II trial." Int J Cancer 125(9): 2104-2113., 53.

[95] Li, J, Gong, L. Y, et al. (2010). Oncoprotein Bmi-1 renders apoptotic resistance to glioma cells through activation of the IKK-nuclear factor-kappaB Pathway." Am J Pathol , 176(2), 699-709.

[96] Li, Z. Q, Gong, L. L, et al. (2012). Delta-like ligand 4 correlates with endothelial proliferation and vessel maturation in human malignant glioma." Onkologie , 35(12), 763-768.

[97] Louis, D. N, Ohgaki, H, et al. (2007). The 2007 WHO classification of tumours of the central nervous system." Acta Neuropathol , 114(2), 97-109.

[98] Luptrawan, A, Liu, G, et al. (2008). Dendritic cell immunotherapy for malignant gliomas." Rev Recent Clin Trials , 3(1), 10-21.

[99] Luskin, M. B. (1993). Restricted proliferation and migration of postnatally generated neurons derived from the forebrain subventricular zone." Neuron , 11(1), 173-189.

[100] MacDonaldT. J., T. Taga, et al. ((2001). Preferential susceptibility of brain tumors to the antiangiogenic effects of an alpha(v) integrin antagonist." Neurosurgery , 48(1), 151-157.

[101] Maher, S, Toomey, D, et al. (2002). Activation-induced cell death: the controversial role of Fas and Fas ligand in immune privilege and tumour counterattack." Immunol Cell Biol , 80(2), 131-137.

[102] Markert, J. M, Cody, J. J, et al. (2012). Preclinical evaluation of a genetically engineered herpes simplex virus expressing interleukin-12." J Virol , 86(9), 5304-5313.

[103] Markert, J. M, Liechty, P. G, et al. (2009). Phase Ib trial of mutant herpes simplex virus G207 inoculated pre-and post-tumor resection for recurrent GBM." Mol Ther , 17(1), 199-207.

[104] Markert, J. M, Medlock, M. D, et al. (2000). Conditionally replicating herpes simplex virus mutant, G207 for the treatment of malignant glioma: results of a phase I trial." Gene Ther , 7(10), 867-874.

[105] Marsh, J. C, Goldfarb, J, et al. (2013). Current status of immunotherapy and gene therapy for high-grade gliomas." Cancer Control , 20(1), 43-48.

[106] Martin, T. A, & Jiang, W. G. (2010). Hepatocyte growth factor and its receptor signalling complex as targets in cancer therapy." Anticancer Agents Med Chem , 10(1), 2-6.

[107] Matuskova, M, Hlubinova, K, et al. (2010). HSV-tk expressing mesenchymal stem cells exert bystander effect on human glioblastoma cells." Cancer Lett , 290(1), 58-67.

[108] Mccarty, J. H, Monahan-earley, R. A, et al. (2002). Defective associations between blood vessels and brain parenchyma lead to cerebral hemorrhage in mice lacking alphav integrins." Mol Cell Biol , 22(21), 7667-7677.

[109] Mempel, T. R, Henrickson, S. E, et al. (2004). T-cell priming by dendritic cells in lymph nodes occurs in three distinct phases." Nature , 427(6970), 154-159.

[110] Meric-bernstam, F, & Hung, M. C. (2006). Advances in targeting human epidermal growth factor receptor-2 signaling for cancer therapy." Clin Cancer Res , 12(21), 6326-6330.

[111] Milinkovic, V, Bankovic, J, et al. (2012). Genomic instability and alterations in patients with malignant glioma." Exp Mol Pathol 93(2): 200-206., 53.

[112] Miller, M. J, Hejazi, A. S, et al. (2004). T cell repertoire scanning is promoted by dynamic dendritic cell behavior and random T cell motility in the lymph node." Proc Natl Acad Sci U S A , 101(4), 998-1003.

[113] Miller, M. J, Wei, S. H, et al. (2002). Two-photon imaging of lymphocyte motility and antigen response in intact lymph node." Science , 296(5574), 1869-1873.

[114] Mross, K, Stefanic, M, et al. (2010). Phase I study of the angiogenesis inhibitor BIBF 1120 in patients with advanced solid tumors." Clin Cancer Res , 16(1), 311-319.

[115] Muhic, A, Poulsen, H. S, et al. (2013). Phase II open-label study of nintedanib in patients with recurrent glioblastoma multiforme." J Neurooncol , 111(2), 205-212.

[116] Okada, H, Kohanbash, G, et al. (2009). Immunotherapeutic approaches for glioma." Crit Rev Immunol , 29(1), 1-42.

[117] Okamoto, I, Kaneda, H, et al. (2010). Phase I safety, pharmacokinetic, and biomarker study of BIBF 1120, an oral triple tyrosine kinase inhibitor in patients with advanced solid tumors." Mol Cancer Ther , 9(10), 2825-2833.

[118] Omuro, A, & Deangelis, L. M. (2013). Glioblastoma and other malignant gliomas: a clinical review." JAMA , 310(17), 1842-1850.

[119] Onishi, M, Kurozumi, K, et al. (2013). Mechanisms of Tumor Development and Anti-angiogenic Therapy in Glioblastoma Multiforme." Neurol Med Chir (Tokyo) , 53(11), 755-763.

[120] Otto, K, Andersen, M. H, et al. (2005). Lack of toxicity of therapy-induced T cell responses against the universal tumour antigen survivin." Vaccine , 23(7), 884-889.

[121] Ousman, S. S, & Kubes, P. (2012). Immune surveillance in the central nervous system." Nat Neurosci , 15(8), 1096-1101.

[122] Palu, G, Cavaggioni, A, et al. (1999). Gene therapy of glioblastoma multiforme via combined expression of suicide and cytokine genes: a pilot study in humans." Gene Ther , 6(3), 330-337.

[123] Patel, N. S, Li, J. L, et al. (2005). Up-regulation of delta-like 4 ligand in human tumor vasculature and the role of basal expression in endothelial cell function." Cancer Res , 65(19), 8690-8697.

[124] Peak, S. J, & Levin, V. A. (2010). Role of bevacizumab therapy in the management of glioblastoma." Cancer Manag Res , 2, 97-104.

[125] Pecora, A. L, Rizvi, N, et al. (2002). Phase I trial of intravenous administration of PV701, an oncolytic virus, in patients with advanced solid cancers." J Clin Oncol , 20(9), 2251-2266.

[126] Plate, K. H, Breier, G, et al. (1994). Molecular mechanisms of developmental and tumor angiogenesis." Brain Pathol , 4(3), 207-218.

[127] Plate, K. H, Breier, G, et al. (1994). Vascular endothelial growth factor and glioma angiogenesis: coordinate induction of VEGF receptors, distribution of VEGF protein and possible in vivo regulatory mechanisms." Int J Cancer , 59(4), 520-529.

[128] Plate, K. H, Scholz, A, et al. (2012). Tumor angiogenesis and anti-angiogenic therapy in malignant gliomas revisited." Acta Neuropathol , 124(6), 763-775.

[129] Pommier, Y. (2006). Topoisomerase I inhibitors: camptothecins and beyond." Nat Rev Cancer , 6(10), 789-802.

[130] Pulkkanen, K. J, & Yla-herttuala, S. (2005). Gene therapy for malignant glioma: current clinical status." Mol Ther , 12(4), 585-598.

[131] Rainov, N. G. (2000). A phase III clinical evaluation of herpes simplex virus type 1 thymidine kinase and ganciclovir gene therapy as an adjuvant to surgical resection and radiation in adults with previously untreated glioblastoma multiforme." Hum Gene Ther , 11(17), 2389-2401.

[132] Rainov, N. G, Fels, C, et al. (2001). Temozolomide enhances herpes simplex virus thymidine kinase/ganciclovir therapy of malignant glioma." Cancer Gene Ther , 8(9), 662-668.

[133] Raizer, J. J, Grimm, S, et al. (2010). A phase 2 trial of single-agent bevacizumab given in an every-3-week schedule for patients with recurrent high-grade gliomas." Cancer , 116(22), 5297-5305.

[134] Ram, Z, Culver, K. W, et al. (1997). Therapy of malignant brain tumors by intratumoral implantation of retroviral vector-producing cells." Nat Med , 3(12), 1354-1361.

[135] Ramos, T. C, Figueredo, J, et al. (2006). Treatment of high-grade glioma patients with the humanized anti-epidermal growth factor receptor (EGFR) antibody h-R3: report from a phase I/II trial." Cancer Biol Ther , 5(4), 375-379.

[136] Rampling, R, Cruickshank, G, et al. (2000). Toxicity evaluation of replication-competent herpes simplex virus (ICP 34.5 null mutant 1716) in patients with recurrent malignant glioma." Gene Ther , 7(10), 859-866.

[137] Reichard, K. W, Lorence, R. M, et al. (1992). Newcastle disease virus selectively kills human tumor cells." J Surg Res , 52(5), 448-453.

[138] Ricard, D, Idbaih, A, et al. (2012). Primary brain tumours in adults." Lancet , 379(9830), 1984-1996.

[139] Ricci-vitiani, L, Pallini, R, et al. (2010). Tumour vascularization via endothelial differentiation of glioblastoma stem-like cells." Nature , 468(7325), 824-828.

[140] Rich, J. N, Sathornsumetee, S, et al. (2005). ZD6474, a novel tyrosine kinase inhibitor of vascular endothelial growth factor receptor and epidermal growth factor receptor, inhibits tumor growth of multiple nervous system tumors." Clin Cancer Res , 11(22), 8145-8157.

[141] Richeldi, L, Costabel, U, et al. (2011). Efficacy of a tyrosine kinase inhibitor in idiopathic pulmonary fibrosis." N Engl J Med , 365(12), 1079-1087.

[142] Risau, W. (1997). Mechanisms of angiogenesis." Nature , 386(6626), 671-674.

[143] Rivera, F, Vega-villegas, M. E, et al. (2008). Current situation of Panitumumab, Matuzumab, Nimotuzumab and Zalutumumab." Acta Oncol , 47(1), 9-19.

[144] Romo-gonzalez, T, Chavarria, A, et al. (2012). Central nervous system: a modified immune surveillance circuit?" Brain Behav Immun , 26(6), 823-829.

[145] Rosen, L. S, Hurwitz, H. I, et al. (2012). A Phase I First-in-Human Study of TRC105 (Anti-Endoglin Antibody) in Patients with Advanced Cancer." Clinical Cancer Research , 18(17), 4820-4829.

[146] Ryu, C. H, Park, S. H, et al. (2011). Gene therapy of intracranial glioma using interleukin 12-secreting human umbilical cord blood-derived mesenchymal stem cells." Hum Gene Ther , 22(6), 733-743.

[147] Saikali, S, Avril, T, et al. (2007). Expression of nine tumour antigens in a series of human glioblastoma multiforme: interest of EGFRvIII, IL-13Ralpha2, gp100 and TRP-2 for immunotherapy." J Neurooncol , 81(2), 139-148.

[148] Sandmair, A. M, Loimas, S, et al. (2000). Thymidine kinase gene therapy for human malignant glioma, using replication-deficient retroviruses or adenoviruses." Hum Gene Ther , 11(16), 2197-2205.

[149] Sandstrom, M, Johansson, M, et al. (2004). The tyrosine kinase inhibitor ZD6474 inhibits tumour growth in an intracerebral rat glioma model." Br J Cancer , 91(6), 1174-1180.

[150] Scehnet, J. S, Jiang, W, et al. (2007). Inhibition of Dll4-mediated signaling induces proliferation of immature vessels and results in poor tissue perfusion." Blood , 109(11), 4753-4760.

[151] Schirrmacher, V, Haas, C, et al. (1999). Human tumor cell modification by virus infection: an efficient and safe way to produce cancer vaccine with pleiotropic immune stimulatory properties when using Newcastle disease virus." Gene Ther , 6(1), 63-73.

[152] Seftor, R. E, Hess, A. R, et al. (2012). Tumor cell vasculogenic mimicry: from controversy to therapeutic promise." Am J Pathol , 181(4), 1115-1125.

[153] Shinkaruk, S, Bayle, M, et al. (2003). Vascular endothelial cell growth factor (VEGF), an emerging target for cancer chemotherapy." Curr Med Chem Anticancer Agents , 3(2), 95-117.

[154] Short, S. C, Traish, D, et al. (2001). Thalidomide as an anti-angiogenic agent in relapsed gliomas." J Neurooncol , 51(1), 41-45.

[155] Spellberg, B, & Edwards, J. E. Jr. ((2001). Type 1/Type 2 immunity in infectious diseases." Clin Infect Dis , 32(1), 76-102.

[156] Stupp, R, Hegi, M. E, et al. (2009). Effects of radiotherapy with concomitant and adjuvant temozolomide versus radiotherapy alone on survival in glioblastoma in a randomised phase III study: 5-year analysis of the EORTC-NCIC trial." Lancet Oncol , 10(5), 459-466.

[157] Stupp, R, Mason, W. P, et al. (2005). Radiotherapy plus concomitant and adjuvant temozolomide for glioblastoma." N Engl J Med , 352(10), 987-996.

[158] Sugiyama, H. (2002). Cancer immunotherapy targeting WT1 protein." Int J Hematol , 76(2), 127-132.

[159] Tchaicha, J. H, Mobley, A. K, et al. (2010). A mosaic mouse model of astrocytoma identifies alphavbeta8 integrin as a negative regulator of tumor angiogenesis." Oncogene , 29(31), 4460-4472.

[160] Tchaicha, J. H, Reyes, S. B, et al. (2011). Glioblastoma angiogenesis and tumor cell invasiveness are differentially regulated by beta8 integrin." Cancer Res , 71(20), 6371-6381.

[161] Tobias, A, Ahmed, A, et al. (2013). The art of gene therapy for glioma: a review of the challenging road to the bedside." J Neurol Neurosurg Psychiatry , 84(2), 213-222.

[162] Todo, T, Martuza, R. L, et al. (2001). Oncolytic herpes simplex virus vector with enhanced MHC class I presentation and tumor cell killing." Proc Natl Acad Sci U S A , 98(11), 6396-6401.

[163] Tolcher, A. W, Messersmith, W. A, et al. (2012). Phase I study of RO4929097, a gamma secretase inhibitor of Notch signaling, in patients with refractory metastatic or locally advanced solid tumors." J Clin Oncol , 30(19), 2348-2353.

[164] Trachtman, H, Fervenza, F. C, et al. (2011). A phase 1, single-dose study of fresolimumab, an anti-TGF-beta antibody, in treatment-resistant primary focal segmental glomerulosclerosis." Kidney Int , 79(11), 1236-1243.

[165] Trask, T. W, Trask, R. P, et al. (2000). Phase I study of adenoviral delivery of the HSV-tk gene and ganciclovir administration in patients with current malignant brain tumors." Mol Ther , 1(2), 195-203.

[166] Ucuzian, A. A, Gassman, A. A, et al. (2010). Molecular mediators of angiogenesis." J Burn Care Res , 31(1), 158-175.

[167] Ueda, R, Kinoshita, E, et al. (2008). Induction of protective and therapeutic antitumor immunity by a DNA vaccine with a glioma antigen, SOX6." Int J Cancer , 122(10), 2274-2279.

[168] Uematsu, M, Ohsawa, I, et al. (2005). Prognostic significance of the immunohistochemical index of survivin in glioma: a comparative study with the MIB-1 index." J Neurooncol , 72(3), 231-238.

[169] van de KelftE. and J. Verlooy ((1994). Instability of short tandem repeats (microsatellites) in human gliomas." J Neurosurg Sci , 38(4), 203-208.

[170] Van Meter, M. E, & Kim, E. S. (2010). Bevacizumab: current updates in treatment." Curr Opin Oncol , 22(6), 586-591.

[171] Voges, J, Reszka, R, et al. (2003). Imaging-guided convection-enhanced delivery and gene therapy of glioblastoma." Ann Neurol , 54(4), 479-487.

[172] Vredenburgh, J. J, Desjardins, A, et al. (2009). Experience with irinotecan for the treatment of malignant glioma." Neuro Oncol , 11(1), 80-91.

[173] Wakabayashi, T, Natsume, A, et al. (2008). A phase I clinical trial of interferon-beta gene therapy for high-grade glioma: novel findings from gene expression profiling and autopsy." J Gene Med , 10(4), 329-339.

[174] Wang, Y, Fei, D, et al. (2004). Biological activity of bevacizumab, a humanized anti-VEGF antibody in vitro." Angiogenesis , 7(4), 335-345.

[175] Wen, P. Y, & Kesari, S. (2008). Malignant gliomas in adults." N Engl J Med , 359(5), 492-507.

[176] Westphal, M, & Lamszus, K. (2011). The neurobiology of gliomas: from cell biology to the development of therapeutic approaches." Nat Rev Neurosci , 12(9), 495-508.

[177] Westphal, M, Yla-herttuala, S, et al. (2013). Adenovirus-mediated gene therapy with sitimagene ceradenovec followed by intravenous ganciclovir for patients with operable high-grade glioma (ASPECT): a randomised, open-label, phase 3 trial." Lancet Oncol , 14(9), 823-833.

[178] Wherry, E. J, Teichgraber, V, et al. (2003). Lineage relationship and protective immunity of memory CD8 T cell subsets." Nat Immunol , 4(3), 225-234.

[179] Wikstrand, C. J, & Bigner, D. D. (1980). Immunobiologic aspects of the brain and human gliomas. A review." Am J Pathol , 98(2), 517-568.

[180] Wobser, M, Keikavoussi, P, et al. (2006). Complete remission of liver metastasis of pancreatic cancer under vaccination with a HLA-A2 restricted peptide derived from the universal tumor antigen survivin." Cancer Immunol Immunother , 55(10), 1294-1298.

[181] Yamanaka, R, Homma, J, et al. (2005). Clinical evaluation of dendritic cell vaccination for patients with recurrent glioma: results of a clinical phase I/II trial." Clin Cancer Res , 11(11), 4160-4167.

[182] Yamanaka, R, Yajima, N, et al. (2003). Dendritic cell-based glioma immunotherapy (review)." Int J Oncol , 23(1), 5-15.

[183] Yang, I, Han, S. J, et al. (2010). The role of microglia in central nervous system immunity and glioma immunology." J Clin Neurosci , 17(1), 6-10.

[184] Yip, S, Miao, J, et al. (2009). MSH6 mutations arise in glioblastomas during temozolomide therapy and mediate temozolomide resistance." Clin Cancer Res , 15(14), 4622-4629.

[185] Yoshida, J, Mizuno, M, et al. (2004). Human gene therapy for malignant gliomas (glioblastoma multiforme and anaplastic astrocytoma) by in vivo transduction with human interferon beta gene using cationic liposomes." Hum Gene Ther , 15(1), 77-86.

[186] Zalutsky, M. R. (2004). Targeted radiotherapy of brain tumours." Br J Cancer , 90(8), 1469-1473.

[187] Zalutsky, M. R, Moseley, R. P, et al. (1989). Pharmacokinetics and tumor localization of 131I-labeled anti-tenascin monoclonal antibody 81C6 in patients with gliomas and other intracranial malignancies." Cancer Res , 49(10), 2807-2813.

[188] Zhang, J. G, Eguchi, J, et al. (2007). Antigenic profiling of glioma cells to generate allogeneic vaccines or dendritic cell-based therapeutics." Clin Cancer Res 13(2 Pt 1): 566-575.

[189] Zhu, J, Motejlek, K, et al. (2002). beta8 integrins are required for vascular morphogenesis in mouse embryos." Development , 129(12), 2891-2903.

Erlotinib in Glioblastoma – A Current Clinical Perspective

Georg Karpel-Massler and Marc-Eric Halatsch

Additional information is available at the end of the chapter

http://dx.doi.org/10.5772/58296

1. Introduction

Glioblastoma represents the most common primary brain tumor in adults. Despite improvements of multimodal therapy, the prognosis of this disease remains unfavorable. Thus, great efforts have been made to identify therapeutic agents directed against those specific molecular targets whose presence was shown to be associated with worse clinical outcomes. The epidermal growth factor receptor (HER1/EGFR) has been identified as one such target, and different compounds were developed to inhibit HER1/EGFR and/or its mutant form, EGFRvIII. However, clinical trials did not confirm the initial enthusiasm conveyed by promising results from experimental studies. Therefore, a therapeutic approach directed at inhibiting solely HER1/EGFR does not seem to translate into a clinical benefit. In this chapter we discuss the current therapeutic situation in the setting of glioblastoma while putting the spotlight on erlotinib, a HER1/EGFR-targeted small molecule tyrosine kinase inhibitor.

The epidermal growth factor receptor belongs to the HER family of receptors and consists of an extracellular ligand-binding site, a transmembraneous part and an intracellular tyrosine kinase (TK) domain (Wells, 1999). Docking of its ligands, *e.g.*, epidermal growth factor (EGF) or transforming growth factor-α (TGF-α), to the ligand-binding site activates the intrinsic TK. Subsequently, autophosphorylation of specific tyrosine residues within the cytoplasmic catalytic kinase domain of the receptor and initiation of cytoplasmic signaling cascades such as the ras-raf-mitogen-activated protein kinase (MAPK) pathway or the phosphatidylinositol 3-kinase (PI3-K)/Akt pathway occur (Arteaga, 2003; Scagliotti et al., 2004). As a consequence, diverse cellular functions such as proliferation or differentiation are regulated (Wells, 1999).

HER1/EGFR overexpression or ligand-independent activation was found in various epithelial malignancies (Earp et al., 2003). The causative relationship between dysregulation of the HER1/EGFR and neoplastic disorder is explained by the affection of downstream signal transduction which results in impaired apoptosis and/or stimulation of proliferation, tumori-

INTECH
open science | open minds

© 2014 The Author(s). Licensee InTech. This chapter is distributed under the terms of the Creative Commons Attribution License (http://creativecommons.org/licenses/by/3.0), which permits unrestricted use, distribution, and reproduction in any medium, provided the original work is properly cited.

genesis, angiogenesis and invasion (Halatsch et al., 2006). Dysregulated HER1/EGFR signaling may be caused by different mechanisms such as gene amplification resulting in HER1/EGFR overexpression as shown for 40-50% of glioblastoma (Salomon et al., 1995). Mutational changes of the intrinsic receptor structure constitute another mechanism that may lead to pathologically altered HER1/EGFR signaling. The so-called EGFRvIII accounts for approximately 60% of all HER1/EGFR mutants and is characterized by a constitutive activation (Frederick et al., 2000; Karpel-Massler et al., 2010). The expression of EGFRvIII was shown to confer cellular transformation and enhanced tumorigenicity (Nishikawa et al., 1994).

Despite recent improvements, the clinical efficacy of existing therapeutic modalities remains disappointing. Hence, in light of accumulating evidence for HER1/EGFR-mediated promotion of tumor growth and malignant transformation, substantial interest in the realization of HER1/EGFR-targeted therapeutic strategies developed. Small molecule tyrosine kinase inhibitors such as erlotinib (Tarceva®, Genentech Inc., San Francisco, CA, U.S.A.), a combined inhibitor of both, HER1/EGFR and EGFRvIII, are the clinically most advanced HER1/EGFR-targeted agents (Karpel-Massler et al., 2009). After promising results derived from experimental studies using erlotinib in a single agent approach were not confirmed by clinical trials, hopes now are set on the identification of other targeted agents enhancing the antineoplastic activity of erlotinib in a multi-targeted approach.

2. Current standard of care for patients with glioblastoma

Glioblastoma is the most frequently encountered astrocytic brain tumor in adults and accounts for more than 50% of all gliomas (Reardon, D.A. & Wen, 2006). The tumor rapidly infiltrates normal surrounding brain tissue. Patients with glioblastoma typically encounter tumor progression or recurrence, and median survival is only 14.6 months (Stupp et al., 2005). Neurologically safe, maximal surgical tumor resection is generally considered the first therapeutic measure for the treatment of newly diagnosed glioblastoma. However, localization of the tumor in or near eloquent brain areas will impose considerable restrictions on the radicality of the surgical procedure in order to avoid severe postoperative neurological deficits. Radiotherapy in combination with concomitant and adjuvant chemotherapy with temozolomide (Temodar®/Temodal®, Schering Corporation, Kenilworth, NJ, U.S.A.) is a viable postoperative treatment option. Whole brain irradiation (50-60 Gy) was shown by several randomized studies to increase survival by 14-36 weeks (Walker et al., 1980). While the chemotherapeutics that were initially used for the adjuvant treatment of glioblastoma were only of minor benefit, a randomized controlled trial in patients with newly diagnosed glioblastoma showed that administration of temozolomide concomitantly with and subsequently to radiation therapy significantly increased two-year survival from 10.4% to 26.5% and median survival from 12.1 to 14.6 months when compared to adjuvant radiation therapy alone (Stupp et al., 2005). With this study, a new therapeutic standard was established. Nevertheless, a progression-free survival and overall survival of only 6.9 and 14.6 months, respectively, strongly emphasize that further improvement of glioblastoma therapy is urgently needed.

Currently, a standard of care for the treatment of *recurrent* glioblastoma does not exist. In general, repeated gross tumor resection should be attempted. However, this strategy might not always be appropriate, especially when considering the fact that progressive tumor invasion may significantly increase the risk of provoking neurological deficits. Chemotherapeutics that were especially used before the temozolomide era upon tumor relapse include nitrosoureas such as carmustine (BCNU) or lomustine (CCNU) and alkylating agents such as procarbazine. However, the antineoplastic activity of these agents in clinical trials was shown to be rather modest (Rodriguez et al., 1989; Newton et al., 1990; Brandes et al., 2004). Irinotecan (Camptosar®, Pfizer Pharmaceuticals, New York, NY, U.S.A.), an inhibitor of topoisomerase I (Raymond et al., 2003; Reardon, DA et al., 2005), or bevacizumab (Avastin®, Genentech Inc., San Francisco, CA, U.S.A.), a humanized monoclonal antibody targeted to vascular endothelial growth factor (VEGF), represent two compounds that have been introduced more recently for the treatment of recurrent glioblastoma and that showed anti-glioblastoma activity (Stark-Vance, 2005).

3. Why interfering with HER1/EGFR or EGFRvIII-mediated signaling?

Given the poor therapeutic efficacy of current treatment measures for glioblastoma, the need for different therapeutic strategies is evident. HER1/EGFR is the most frequently amplified gene in glioblastoma, and its overexpression was found in more than half of these tumors which renders HER1/EGFR an outstanding therapeutic target (Salomon et al., 1995). Experimental studies show that HER1/EGFR stimulates tumor growth, invasion and migration (Lund-Johansen et al., 1990). In addition, data from clinical studies suggest that HER1/EGFR amplification is related to decreased overall survival and worse prognosis in patients with glioblastoma (Lund-Johansen et al., 1990; Shinojima et al., 2003).

EGFRvIII represents the most common mutant form of HER1/EGFR and is characterized by constitutive TK activity independent of ligand-binding (Batra et al., 1995; Frederick et al., 2000). Analysis of the expression of HER1/EGFR and EGFRvIII in bioptic glioblastoma specimens suggests concurrent overexpression of both EGFRvIII and HER1/EGFR in most of the tumors (Biernat et al., 2004). Moreover, in an experimental study using a murine model of human glioma xenografts, EGFRvIII expression was found to be related to increased proliferation, inhibition of apoptosis, and tumor formation (Nishikawa et al., 1994; Nagane et al., 1996). Other studies showed similar results and identified activation of the MAPK/ERK1/2 and PI3-K/Akt pathways as driving forces of cellular proliferation and tumor progression (Moscatello et al., 1998; Klingler-Hoffmann et al., 2001; Klingler-Hoffmann et al., 2003). In addition, in a murine orthotopic xenograft model of glioblastoma, administration of a monoclonal antibody targeting EGFRvIII (mAb 806) was shown to cause a significant decrease of tumor growth, increase of apoptosis and prolongation of survival (Mishima et al., 2001).

The tumor-specific properties of EGFRvIII have also lead to the development of EGFRvIII-targeted vaccines in order to provoke an immunologic response against EGFRvIII-bearing glioblastoma cells. Potential antitumor efficacy of EGFRvIII-targeted vaccines had been shown by experimental studies. Immunization of mice with transfected allogenic 300.19/EGFRvIII cells was reported to induce a major histocompatibility complex class I-restricted response against EGFRvIII-bearing syngeneic B16-F10 melanoma or 560 astrocytoma cells that were implanted intracranially (Ashley et al., 1997). In addition, vaccinated animals were shown to have a significantly longer median survival upon intracranial tumor challenge when compared to controls. Similar findings were reported for mice that were vaccinated with PEP-3-KLH (rindopepimut, CDX-110, Celldex Therapeutics, Needham, MA, U.S.A.), a conjugate of a peptide comprising the tumor-specific mutated segment of EGFRvIII (PEP-3) and keyhole limpet hemocyanin (KLH) (Heimberger et al., 2003). In this study, C3H mice received vaccination with 100 µg of PEP-3-KLH 8, 6 and 2 weeks prior to intracerebral administration of K1735 murine melanoma cells that were transfected with a murine homologue of the human EGFRvIII, and additional vaccination 4 days after intracranial implantation of the tumor cells. A more than 173% longer survival time was shown for mice vaccinated with PEP-3-KLH when compared to mice receiving only KLH. Moreover, mice with already established intracranial tumors that were treated with a single dose of the PEP-3-KLH vaccine 4 days after administration of the transfected K1735 cells had a 26% increase of median survival. Based on these promising preclinical data, several clinical trials were conducted. In two phase II trials, vaccination with PEP-3-KLH was examined in patients with EGFRvIII-expressing newly diagnosed glioblastoma. In the ACTIVATE trial, 18 patients underwent gross-total tumor resection prior to radiotherapy and concurrent chemotherapy with temozolomide followed by vaccination with PEP-3-KLH bi-weekly for 3 doses and continued monthly until progression (Sampson et al., 2010). The data were compared to a matched historical control group (n=17). The median progression-free survival and overall survival were 14.2 months and 26 months, respectively, versus 6.3 months and 15 months, respectively, in the control group. Notably, the patients who developed an EGFRvIII-specific antibody response had an overall survival of 47.7 months (n=6) compared to an overall survival of 22.2 months in patients lacking a specific antibody response (n=8). In the ACT II trial, 22 patients who met the same inclusion criteria as for the ACTIVATE trial received the same therapeutic regimen except for an additional treatment with temozolomide either at a dose of 200 mg/m^2 for 5 days of a 28-day cycle or at a dose of 100 mg/m^2 for 21 days of a 28-day cycle in conjunction with the vaccination therapy (Heimberger et al., 2009). Combination therapy of PEP-3-KLH and temozolomide was well tolerated, and a favorable median overall survival of 20.5 months was reported. An additional phase II study (ACT III) was conducted by Celldex Therapeutics. Sixty-five patients with newly diagnosed EGFRvIII-positive glioblastoma were enrolled in this single-arm multicenter study which was initially planned as a phase IIb/III randomized two-arm trial but had to be transformed into a single-arm design due to withdrawal of consent to participate in this study by 14 of the 16 patients that were randomized to the control group. In this study, a median overall survival of 21.8 months was reported which encouraged Celldex to launch two more studies: ACT IV, a randomized controlled phase III study in patients with newly diagnosed EGFRvIII-positive glioblastoma and ReACT, a phase II study in patients with EGFRvIII-positive recurrent glioblastoma. The final results of these studies are pending. However, what needs to be taken into account is the fact that only a part of the glioblastomas express EGFRvIII. For this subset of patients, however, vaccination with PEP-3-KLH might confer a significant clinical benefit.

4. Erlotinib for the treatment of glioblastoma

HER1/EGFR TK inhibitors such as erlotinib compete with adenosine triposphate and reversibly bind to the intracellular catalytic TK domain of HER1/EGFR or EGFRvIII thus inhibiting autophosphorylation of the receptor as well as further downstream signaling (Halatsch et al., 2006). In preclinical studies, erlotinib was shown to exert a variety of relevant antineoplastic effects in the setting of glioblastoma. Lal *et al.* showed that exposure of transformed D54-MG glioblastoma cells (D54-EGFRvIII) to 20 μM of erlotinib resulted in significant downregulation of certain genes encoding pro-invasive proteins and in significant inhibition of the invasiveness of D54-EGFRvIII cells (Lal et al., 2002). In a different study, erlotinib was shown to significantly reduce cellular viability of six human glioblastoma-derived tumor-initiating cell lines when given at a concentration of 5 μM (Griffero et al., 2003). This effect was shown to be in concordance with decreased EGF-induced phosphorylation of HER1/EGFR and subsequent inhibition of the MAPK signaling pathway by reduced phosphorylation of ERK1/2. Moreover, Halatsch *et al.* showed that the extent of erlotinib-mediated inhibition of anchorage-independent growth of glioblastoma-derived cell lines correlates inversely with the cellular capability to induce HER1/EGFR mRNA, emphasizing the important role of HER1/EGFR in the pathogenesis of glioblastoma (Halatsch et al., 2004).

Based on the positive findings reported by preclinical studies, much hope was set on the clinical application of erlotinib in glioblastoma patients. To date, several published studies have examined the effects of erlotinib on patients with recurrent or newly diagnosed glioblastoma. In phase I trials, erlotinib exhibited a reasonable safety profile and was generally well tolerated (Krishnan et al., 2006; Prados et al., 2006). In addition, EIAEDs were shown to accelerate drug metabolism of erlotinib which requires dose modification of erlotinib or a change in the antiepileptic drug regimen (Stupp et al., 2006). In terms of clinical efficacy, Raizer *et al.* examined the effects of erlotinib applied at a dose of 150 mg/d on 42 patients with recurrent glioblastoma and 43 patients with non-progressive glioblastoma following radiotherapy in a phase II trial (Raizer et al., 2010). For the patients with recurrent glioblastoma, median overall survival was reported as 6 months and median progression-free survival as only 2 months. Median overall survival and the 12-month overall survival were reported as 14 months and 57%, respectively, for the patients with non-progressive glioblastoma after radiotherapy. Thus, this study did not show a significant improvement of the clinical outcome attributable to the treatment with erlotinib in patients with recurrent glioblastoma or non-progressive glioblastoma after radiotherapy. However, Yung *et al.* showed that median overall survival and 6-month progression-free survival of 48 patients with recurrent glioblastoma who were treated with erlotinib reached or exceeded historical values for patients receiving chemotherapy for recurrent glioblastoma (Yung et al., 2010). Notably, this study was discontinued due to an insufficient number of responses after a planned interim analysis, and a control group was not included. Van den Bent *et al.* showed in a randomized controlled phase II trial that only 11.4%

of 54 patients with recurrent glioblastoma who were treated with erlotinib remained free of progression after 6 months compared to 24.1% of patients in the control group who received either temozolomide or BCNU (van den Bent et al., 2009). Moreover, median overall survival was shown to be similar across the treatment groups (7.7 months for the erlotinib group versus 7.3 months for the temozolomide/BCNU group).

Thus, taking erlotinib to clinical application in a monotherapeutic approach has so far fallen short of expectations. As a logical consequence, the question rose if erlotinib might provide a therapeutic benefit when combined with conventional radiochemotherapy. As outlined in detail in the following, the addition of erlotinib to a combined regimen of temozolomide and radiotherapy did not meet enthusiastic expectations and even raised the suspicion of inducing serious toxic side effects. In a phase I/II trial, Brown *et al.* studied the clinical efficacy of a combined treatment with erlotinib, temozolomide and radiotherapy in 89 patients with newly diagnosed glioblastoma (Brown et al., 2008). Erlotinib was administered at a dose of 150 mg/d starting 1 week prior to fractionated radiotherapy (60 Gy) and chemotherapy with temozolomide at a dose of 75 mg/m^2/d. After radiotherapy, treatment with erlotinib was continued and accompanied by up to six cycles of temozolomide at a dose of 200 mg/m^2/d for 5 days every 4 weeks. Median overall survival was reported as 15.7 months, and comparison to the "radiotherapy plus temozolomide arm" from the European Organisation for Research and Treatment of Cancer 26981/22981-National Cancer Institute of Canada trial revealed no significant difference (Mirimanoff et al., 2006). In contrast, Prados *et al.* showed in another phase II trial which included 65 patients with newly diagnosed glioblastoma or gliosarcoma receiving treatment with erlotinib and fractionated radiotherapy with concomitant and adjuvant temozolomide a marked improvement of median progression-free and overall survival (8.2 months and 19.3 months, respectively) when compared to a combined historical control (Prados et al., 2009). Rather disturbing results were reported from a phase II study published by Peereboom *et al.* (Peereboom et al., 2010). Twenty-seven patients with newly diagnosed glioblastoma were treated with a maximum dose of 150 mg/d erlotinib and radiotherapy (60 Gy in 30 fractions) with concurrent (75 mg/m^2/d for 42 days) and subsequent (12 four-week cycles comprising each 5 days of 150-200 mg/m^2/d) temozolomide. This trial was terminated preterm because of unacceptable toxicity and lack of efficacy. Median progression-free and overall survival were 2.8 months and 8.6 months, respectively. Twenty-two patients (67%) had progressive disease, and 4 patients (15%) had an adverse event. Three deaths occurred that were reported to be treatment-related. One patient died of pneumocystis carinii pneumonia despite treatment with pentamidine. Similarly, Brown *et al.* reported two cases of fatal pneumocystis carinii pneumonia (Brown et al., 2008). Again high expectations were disappointed.

5. Future perspectives

None of the therapeutic strategies evaluated so far involving erlotinib either alone or in combination with conventional adjuvant therapies represent a major success for the treatment of glioblastoma. Therefore, changing the general strategy towards a combined approach with

HER1/EGFR TK inhibitors and other targeted agents might provide a more pronounced clinical benefit for patients suffering from this disease.

In experimental studies, favorable effects were observed for the inhibition of downstream key regulators such as mammalian target of rapamycin (mTOR) and PI3-K in addition to the treatment with HER1/EGFR TK inhibitors. For example, phosphatase and tensin homolog deleted on chromosome 10 (PTEN)-deficient U87MG and SF295 glioblastoma cells that were subjected to a combined treatment with erlotinib and rapamycin, an mTOR inhibitor, showed significantly increased antiproliferative effects when compared to cells receiving erlotinib alone (reduction of proliferation by 38% versus 14%, respectively, in PTEN-deficient SF295 cells) (Wang et al., 2006). Another experimental study showed similar findings (Fan et al., 2007). In this study, additional inhibition of PI3-K using a dual mTOR/PI3-K inhibitor (PI-103) resulted in even more pronounced antiproliferative efficacy in PTEN-mutant glioma cells when combined with erlotinib in comparison to erlotinib combined with either mTOR or PI3-K inhibition. In a clinical pilot study including 22 patients with recurrent glioblastoma, Doherty *et al.* showed that patients treated with erlotinib or gefitinib in combination with sirolimus (rapamycine, Rapamune®, Wyeth Pharmaceuticals Inc., Ayerst, PA, U.S.A.) had a 6-month progression-free survival of 25% (Doherty et al., 2006). In addition, 32 patients with recurrent glioblastoma were treated with 150 mg/d (450 mg/d when on EIAEDs) of erlotinib and 5 mg/d (10 mg/d when on EIAEDs) of sirolimus in a phase II clinical trial (Reardon, DA et al., 2010). In this study, however, antitumor activity was negligible with no complete or partial responses and a median progression-free survival and a median overall survival of 6.9 weeks and 33.8 weeks, respectively.

Carboplatin was shown to have some antineoplastic activity in patients with recurrent glioblastoma and anaplastic astrocytoma (Prados et al., 1996). De Groot *et al.* examined the therapeutic efficacy of a combined regimen of the cytotoxic agent carboplatin and erlotinib in recurrent glioblastoma (de Groot et al., 2008). In this phase II study, 43 patients were treated with erlotinib at a dose of 150 mg/d that was escalated up to 200 mg/d as tolerated in combination with carboplatin administered once every 4 weeks at doses modified according to renal function. While this regimen was well tolerated, antineoplastic activity was modest. Median progression-free survival and overall survival were 9 weeks and 30 weeks, respectively, and only one partial response was achieved.

Tumor angiogenesis has been shown to be a crucial process for the growth and metastasis of solid tumors (Heath & Bicknell, 2009). The combined treatment with bevacizumab and HER1/EGFR-targeted agents has been evaluated by two recent phase II studies in the setting of recurrent high-grade glioma. Forty-three patients with recurrent glioblastoma were treated with 10 mg/kg bevacizumab, 125 or 340 mg/m^2 irinotecan (dose depending on EIAED comedication), and cetuximab, a monoclonal antibody targeted at HER1/EGFR (loading dose of 400 mg/m^2 followed by weekly administration of 250 mg/m^2) (Hasselbalch et al., 2010). Two complete responses (5%) and 9 partial responses (21%) were observed. Stable disease was achieved in 17 patients (40%). Median overall survival and progression-free survival were 30 weeks and 16 weeks, respectively. In the second phase II trial, twenty-five patients with recurrent primary glioblastoma were treated with 10 mg/kg bevacizumab every 2 weeks and concomitantly with 200 or 500 mg/d erlotinib (dose depending on EIAED comedication) (Sathornsumetee et al., 2010). Median overall survival and 6-month progression-free survival were reported as 42 weeks and 28%, respectively. Moreover, radiographic response was observed for 48% of the glioblastoma patients. Unfortunately, appropriate control groups were not included in this study. However, comparison to historical data of patients treated with bevacizumab only showed a similar progression-free survival and radiographic response. Thus, additional inhibition of HER1/EGFR does not appear to greatly increase the clinical efficacy when combined with bevacizumab in recurrent glioblastoma.

Overall, while promising results were reported by some early phase clinical trials evaluating the therapeutic efficacy of a combined treatment with HER1/EGFR TK inhibitors and other agents, further studies with a randomized controlled design and a larger patient population will be needed to make a final judgment.

Considering the fact that a multitude of different converging and diverging signaling pathways are involved in the maintenance and progression of glioblastoma, the failure of targeting of a single molecular determinant such as HER1/EGFR does not come as a surprise. Moreover, limiting the focus on therapeutic strategies targeted at already known oncogenic signaling pathways might impede further progress. Therefore, the search for novel targets is crucial in order to allow for a more efficient treatment of glioblastoma. A bioinformatic approach might help to identify molecules that are potentially relevant as tumor-driving forces. Halatsch *et al.* identified a panel of genes overexpressed in glioblastoma cells with an erlotinib-resistant phenotype by RNA microarray analysis of which some have been confirmed as promising co-targets *in vitro* (Halatsch et al., 2009; Karpel-Massler et al., 2013). Hopefully, in the future, broad molecular tumor screening will lead to the identification of individual molecular signatures amenable to successful multitargeting. Since these molecular signatures are likely to change during therapy, repeated therapeutic adjustments will be necessary based on updated molecular characteristics of the tumor (Cloughesy & Mischel, 2011). This kind of dynamic personalized therapy of glioblastoma will likely involve HER1/EGFR-targeted therapeutics such as erlotinib at one point.

Author details

Georg Karpel-Massler and Marc-Eric Halatsch

University of Ulm School of Medicine, Ulm, Germany

References

[1] Arteaga, C. (2003). HER1/EGFR: a molecular approach to cancer therapy. *Semin Oncol*, 30, 3-14.

[2] Ashley, D., Sampson, J., Archer, G., Batra, S., Bigner, D. & Hale, L. (1997). A genetically modified allogeneic cellular vaccine generates MHC class I-restricted cytotoxic responses against tumor-associated antigens and protects against CNS tumors in vivo. *J Neuroimmunol*, 78, 34-46.

[3] Batra, S., Castelino-Prabhu, S., Wikstrand, C., Zhu, X., Humphrey, P., Friedman, H. & Bigner, D. (1995). Epidermal growth factor ligand-independent, unregulated, cell-transforming potential of a naturally occurring human mutant EGFRvIII gene. *Cell Growth Differ*, 6, 1251-1259.

[4] Biernat, W., Huang, H., Yokoo, H., Kleihues, P. & Ohgaki, H. (2004). Predominant expression of mutant EGFR (EGFRvIII) is rare in primary glioblastomas. *Brain Pathol*, 14, 131-136.

[5] Brandes, A., Tosoni, A., Amista, P., Nicolardi, L., Grosso, D., Berti, F. & Ermani, M. (2004). How effective is BCNU in recurrent glioblastoma in the modern era? A phase II trial. *Neurology*, 63, 1281-1284.

[6] Brown, P., Krishnan, S., Sarkaria, J., Wu, W., Jaeckle, K., Uhm, J., Geoffroy, F., Arusell, R., Kitange, G., Jenkins, R., Kugler, J., Morton, R., Rowland, K., Mischel, P., Yong, W., Scheithauer, B., Schiff, D., Giannini, C. & Buckner, J. (2008). Phase I/II trial of erlotinib and temozolomide with radiation therapy in the treatment of newly diagnosed glioblastoma multiforme: north central cancer treatment group study N0177. *J Clin Oncol*, 26, 5603-5609.

[7] Cloughesy, T. & Mischel, P. (2011). New strategies in the molecular targeting of glioblastoma: how do you hit a moving target? *Clin Cancer Res*, 17, 6-11.

[8] de Groot, J., Gilbert, M., Aldape, K., Hess, K., Hanna, T., Ictech, S., Groves, M., Conrad, C., Colman, H., Puduvalli, V., Levin, V. & Yung, W. (2008). Phase II study of carboplatin and erlotinib (tarceva, OSI-774) in patients with recurrent glioblastoma. *J Neurooncol*, 90, 89-97.

[9] Doherty, L., Gigas, D., Kesari, S., Drappatz, J., Kim, R., Zimmermann, J., Ostrowsky, L. & Wen, P. (2006). Pilot study of the combination of EGFR and mTOR inhibitors in recurrent malignant gliomas. *Neurology*, 67, 156-158.

[10] Earp, H., Calvo, B. & Sartor, C. (2003). The EGF receptor family - multiple roles in proliferation, differentiation, and neoplasia with an emphasis on HER4. *Trans Am Clin Climatol Assoc*, 114, 315-333.

[11] Fan, Q.-W., Cheng, C., Nicolaides, T., Hackett, C., Knight, Z., Shokat, K. & Weiss, W. (2007). A dual phosphoinositide-3-kinase anti/mTOR inhibitor cooperates with blockade of epidermal growth factor receptor in PTEN-mutant glioma. *Cancer Res*, 67, 7960-7965.

[12] Frederick, L., Wang, X.-Y., Eley, G. & James, C. (2000). Diversity and frequency of epidermal growth factor receptor mutations in human glioblastomas. *Cancer Res*, 60, 1383-1387.

[13] Griffero, F., Daga, A., Marubbi, D., Capra, M., Melotti, A., Pattarozzi, A., Gatti, M., Bajetto, A., Porcile, C., Barbieri, F., Favoni, R., Lo Casto, M., Zona, G., Spaziante, R., Florio, T. & Corte, G. (2003). Different response of human glioma tumor-initiating cells to epidermal growth factor receptor kinase inhibitors. *J Biol Chem*, 284, 7138-7148.

[14] Halatsch, M.-E., Gehrke, E., Vougioukas, V., Bötefür, I., Efferth, T., Gebhardt, E., Domhof, S., Schmidt, U. & Buchfelder, M. (2004). Inverse correlation of *epidermal growth factor receptor* messenger RNA induction and suppression of anchorage-independent growth by OSI-774, an epidermal growth factor receptor tyrosine kinase inhibitor, in glioblastoma multiforme cell lines. *J Neurosurg*, 100, 523-533.

[15] Halatsch, M.-E., Löw, S., Mursch, K., Hielscher, T., Schmidt, U., Unterberg, A., Vougioukas, V. & Feuerhake, F. (2009). Candidate genes for sensitivity and resistance of human glioblastoma multiforme cell lines to erlotinib. *J Neurosurg*, 111, 211-218.

[16] Halatsch, M.-E., Schmidt, U., Behnke-Mursch, J., Unterberg, A. & Wirtz, C. (2006). Epidermal growth factor receptor inhibition for the treatment of glioblastoma multiforme and other malignant brain tumours. *Cancer Treat Rev*, 32, 74-89.

[17] Hasselbalch, B., Lassen, U., Hansen, S., Holmberg, M., Sorensen, M., Kosteljanetz, M., Broholm, H., Stockhausen, M.-T. & Poulsen, H. (2010). Cetuximab, bevacizumab, and irinotecan for patients with primary glioblastoma and progression after radiation therapy and temozolomide: a phase II trial. *Neurooncol*, 12, 508-516.

[18] Heath, V.L. & Bicknell, R. (2009). Anticancer strategies involving the vasculature. *Nat Rev Clin Oncol*, 6, 395-404.

[19] Heimberger, A., Archer, G., Mitchell, D., Bigner, D., Schmittling, R., Herndon II, J., Davis, T., Friedman, H., Keler, T., Reardon, D. & Sampson, J. (2009). Epidermal growth factor receptor variant III (EGFRvIII) vaccine (CDX-110) in GBM. *J Clin Oncol*, 27, No.15S, abs.2021.

[20] Heimberger, A., Crotty, L., Archer, G., Hess, K., Wikstrand, C., Friedman, A., Friedman, H., Bigner, D. & Sampson, J. (2003). Epidermal growth factor receptor VIII peptide vaccination is efficacious against established intracerebral tumors. *Clin Cancer Res*, 9, 4247-4254.

[21] Karpel-Massler, G., Schmidt, U., Unterberg, A. & Halatsch, M.-E. (2009). Therapeutic inhibition of the epidermal growth factor receptor in high-grade gliomas - where do we stand? *Mol Cancer Res*, 7, 1000-1012.

[22] Karpel-Massler, G., Wirtz, C. & Halatsch, M.-E. (2010). Ribozyme-mediated inhibition of 801-bp deletion-mutant *epidermal growth factor receptor* mRNA expression in glioblastoma multiforme *Molecules*, 15, 4670-4678.

[23] Karpel-Massler, G., Westhoff, M.-A., Zhou, S., Nonnenmacher, L., Dwucet, A., Kast, R.E., Bachem, M., Wirtz, C.R., Debatin, K.-M. & Halatsch, M.-E. (2013). Combined inhibition of HER1/EGFR and RAC1 results in a synergistic antiproliferative effect on established and primary cultured human glioblastoma cells. *Mol Cancer Ther*, 12, 1783-95.

[24] Klingler-Hoffmann, M., Bukczynska, P. & Tiganis, T. (2003). Inhibition of phosphatidylinositol 3-kinase signaling negates the growth advantage imparted by a mutant epidermal growth factor receptor on human glioblastoma cells. *Int J Cancer*, 105, 319-331.

[25] Klingler-Hoffmann, M., Fodero-Tavoletti, M., Mishima, K., Narita, Y., Cavenee, W., Furnari, F., Huang, H.-J.S. & Tiganis, T. (2001). The protein tyrosine phosphatase TCPTP suppresses the tumorigenicity of glioblastoma cells expressing a mutant epidermal growth factor receptor. *J Biol Chem*, 276, 46313-46318.

[26] Krishnan, S., Brown, P., Ballmann, K., Fiveash, J., Uhm, J., Giannini, C., Jaeckle, K., Geoffroy, F., Nabors, L. & Buckner, J. (2006). Phase I trial of erlotinib with radiation therapy in patients with glioblastoma multiforme: results of north central cancer treatment group protocol N0177. *Int J Radiat Oncol Biol Phys*, 65, 1192-1199.

[27] Lal, A., Glazer, C., Martinson, H., Friedman, H., Archer, G., Sampson, J. & Riggins, G. (2002). Mutant epidermal growth factor receptor up-regulates molecular effectors of tumor invasion. *Cancer Res*, 62, 3335-3339.

[28] Lund-Johansen, M., Bjerkvig, R., Humphrey, P., Bigner, S., Bigner, D. & Laerum, O. (1990). Effect of epidermal growth factor on glioma cell growth, migration, and invasion in vitro. *Cancer Res*, 50, 6039-6044.

[29] Mirimanoff, R., Gorlia, T., Mason, W., Van den Bent, M., Kortmann, R.-D., Fisher, B., Reni, M., Brandes, A., Curschmann, J., Villa, S., Cairncross, G., Allgeier, A., Lacombe, D. & Stupp, R. (2006). Radiotherapy and temozolomide for newly diagnosed glioblastoma: recursive partitioning analysis of the EORTC 26981/22981-NCIC CE3 phase III randomized trial. *J Clin Oncol*, 24, 2563-2569.

[30] Mishima, K., Johns, T., Luwor, R., Scott, A., Stockert, E., Jungbluth, A., Ji, X., Suvarna, P., Voland, J., Old, L., Huang, H. & Cavenee, W. (2001). Growth suppression of intracranial xenografted glioblastomas overexpressing mutant epidermal growth factor receptors by systemic administration of monoclonal antibody (mAb) 806, a novel monoclonal antibody directed to the receptor. *Cancer Res*, 61, 5349-5354.

[31] Moscatello, D., Holgado-Madruga, M., Emlet, D., Montgomery, R. & Wong, A. (1998). Constitutive activation of phosphatidylinositol 3-kinase by a naturally occurring mutant epidermal growth factor receptor. *J Biol Chem*, 273, 200-206.

[32] Nagane, M., Coufal, F., Lin, H., Bögler, O., Cavenee, W. & Huang, H. (1996). A common mutant epidermal growth factor receptor confers enhanced tumorigenicity on human glioblastoma cells by increasing proliferation and reducing apoptosis. *Cancer Res*, 56, 5079-5086.

[33] Newton, H., Junck, L., Bromberg, J., Page, M. & Greenberg, H. (1990). Procarbazine chemotherapy in the treatment of recurrent malignant astrocytomas after radiation and nitrosourea failure. *Neurology*, 40, 1743-1746.

[34] Nishikawa, R., Ji, X., Harmon, R., Lazar, C., Gill, G., Cavenee, W. & Huang, H. (1994). A mutant epidermal growth factor receptor common in human glioma confers enhanced tumorigenicity. *Proc Natl Acad Sci USA*, 91, 7727-7731.

[35] Peereboom, D., Shepard, D., Ahluwalia, M., Brewer, C., Agarwal, N., Stevens, G., Suh, J., Toms, S., Vogelbaum, M., Weil, R., Elson, P. & Barnett, G. (2010). Phase II trial of erlotinib with temozolomide and radiation in patients with newly diagnosed glioblastoma multiforme. *J Neurooncol*, 98, 93-99.

[36] Prados, M., Chang, S., Butowski, N., DeBoer, R., Parvataneni, R., Carliner, H., Kabuubi, P., Ayers-Ringler, J., Rabbitt, J., Page, M., Fedoroff, A., Sneed, P., Berger, M., McDermott, M., Parsa, A., Vandenberg, S., James, C., Lamborn, K., Stokoe, D. & Haas-Kogan, D. (2009). Phase II study of erlotinib plus temozolomide during and after radiation therapy in patients with newly diagnosed glioblastoma multiforme or gliosarcoma. *J Clin Oncol*, 27, 579-584.

[37] Prados, M., Lamborn, K., Chang, S., Burton, E., Butowski, N., Malec, M., Kapadia, A., Rabbitt, J., Page, M., Fedoroff, A., Xie, D. & Kelley, S. (2006). Phase I study of erlotinib HCl alone and combined with temozolomide in patients with stable or recurrent malignant glioma. *Neurooncol*, 8, 67-78.

[38] Prados, M., Warnick, R., Mack, E., Chandler, K., Rabbitt, J., Page, M. & Malec, M. (1996). Intravenous carboplatin for recurrent gliomas: a dose-escalating phase II trial. *Am J Clin Oncol*, 19, 609-612.

[39] Raizer, J., Abrey, L., Lassman, A., Chang, S., Lamborn, K., Kuhn, J., Yung, W., Gilbert, M., Aldape, K., Wen, P., Fine, H., Mehta, M., DeAngelis, L., Lieberman, F., Cloughesy, T., Robins, H., Dancey, J. & Prados, M. (2010). A phase II trial of erlotinib in patients with recurrent malignant gliomas and nonprogressive glioblastoma multiforme postradiation therapy. *Neurooncol*, 12, 95-103.

[40] Raymond, E., Fabbro, M., Boige, V., Rixe, O., Frenay, M., Vassal, G., Faivre, S., Sicard, E., Germa, C., Rodier, J., Vernillet, L. & Armand, J. (2003). Multicenter phase II study and pharmakokinetic analysis of irinotecan in chemotherapy-naive patients with glioblastoma. *Ann Oncol*, 14, 603-614.

[41] Reardon, D., Desjardins, A., Vredenburgh, J., Gururangan, S., Friedman, A., Herndon II, J., Marcello, J., Norfleet, J., McLendon, R., Sampson, J. & Friedman, H. (2010).

Phase II trial of erlotinib plus sirolimus in adults with recurrent glioblastoma. *J Neurooncol*, 96, 219-230.

[42] Reardon, D., Quinn, J., Vredenburgh, J., Rich, J., Gururangan, S., Badruddoja, M., Herndon, J.n., Dowell, J., Friedman, A. & Friedman, H. (2005). Phase II trial of irinotecan plus celecoxib in adults with recurrent malignant glioma. *Cancer*, 103, 329-338.

[43] Reardon, D.A. & Wen, P.Y. (2006). Therapeutic advances in the treatment of glioblastoma: rationale and potential role of targeted agents. *Oncologist*, 11, 152-164.

[44] Rodriguez, L., Prados, M., Silver, P. & Levin, V. (1989). Reevaluation of procarbazine for the treatment of recurrent malignant central nervous system tumors. *Cancer*, 64, 2420-2423.

[45] Salomon, D., Brandt, R., Ciardello, F. & Normanno, N. (1995). Epidermal growth factor-related peptides and their receptors in human malignancies. *Crit Rev Oncol Hematol*, 19, 183-232.

[46] Sampson, J., Heimberger, A., Archer, G., Aldape, K., Friedman, A., Friedman, H., Gilbert, M., Herndon II, J., McLendon, R., Mitchell, D., Reardon, D., Sawaya, R., Schmittling, R., Shi, W., Vredenburgh, J. & Bigner, D. (2010). Immunologic escape after prolonged progression-free survival with epidermal growth factor receptor variant III peptide vaccination in patients with newly diagnosed glioblastoma. *J Clin Oncol*, 28, 4722-4729.

[47] Sathornsumetee, S., Desjardins, A., Vredenburgh, J., McLendon, R., Marcello, J., Herndon II, J., Mathe, A., Hamilton, M., Rich Sr, J., Norfleet, J., Gururangan, S., Friedman, H. & Reardon, D. (2010). Phase II trial of bevacizumab and erlotinib in patients with recurrent malignant glioma. *Neurooncol*, 12, 1300-1310.

[48] Scagliotti, G., Selvaggi, G., Novello, S. & Hirsch, F. (2004). The biology of epidermal growth factor receptor in lung cancer. *Clin Cancer Res*, 10, 4227s-4232s.

[49] Shinojima, N., Tada, K., Shiraishi, S., Kamiryo, T., Kochi, M., Nakamura, H., Makino, K., Saya, H., Hirano, H., Kuratsu, J., Oka, K., Ishimaru, Y. & Ushio, Y. (2003). Prognostic value of epidermal growth factor receptor in patients with glioblastoma multiforme. *Cancer Res*, 63, 6962-6970.

[50] Stark-Vance, V. (2005). Bevacizumab and CPT-11 in the treatment of relapsed malignant glioma. *Neurooncol*, 7, 369.

[51] Stupp, R., Hegi, M., van den Bent, M., Mason, W., Weller, M., Mirimanoff, R. & Cairncross, J. (2006). Changing paradigms - An update on the multidisciplinary management of malignant glioma. *Oncologist*, 11, 165-180.

[52] Stupp, R., Mason, W., van den Bent, M., Weller, M., Fisher, B., Taphoom, M., Belanger, K., Brandes, A., Marosi, C., Bogdahn, U., Curschmann, J., Janzer, R., Ludwin, S., Gorlia, T., Allgeier, A., Lacombe, D., Cairncross, J., Eisenhauer, E. & Mirimanoff, R.

(2005). Radiotherapy plus concomitant and adjuvant temozolomide for glioblastoma. *N Engl J Med*, 352, 987-996.

[53] van den Bent, M., Brandes, A., Rampling, R., Kouwenhoven, M., Kros, J., Carpentier, A., Clement, P., Frenay, M., Campone, M., Baurain, J., Armand, J., Taphoorn, M., Tosoni, A., Kletzl, H., Klughammer, B., Lacombe, D. & Gorlia, T. (2009). Randomized phase II trial of erlotinib versus temozolomide or carmustine in recurrent glioblastoma: EORTC brain tumor group study 26034. *J Clin Oncol*, 27, 1268-1274.

[54] Walker, M., Green, S., Byar, D., Alexander, E.J., Batzdorf, U., Brooks, W., Hunt, W., MacCarty, C., Mahaley, M.J., Mealey, J.J., Owens, G., Ransohoff, J.n., Robertson, J., Shapiro, W., Smith, K.J., Wilson, C. & Strike, T. (1980). Randomized comparison of radiotherapy and nitrosoureas for the treatment of malignant glioma after surgery. *N Engl J Med*, 303, 1323-1329.

[55] Wang, M., Lu, K., Zhu, S., Dia, E., Vivanco, I., Shackleford, G., Cavenee, W., Mellinghoff, I., Cloughesy, T., Sawyers, C. & Mischel, P. (2006). Mammalian target of rapamycin inhibition promotes response to epidermal growth factor receptor kinase inhibitors in PTEN-deficient and PTEN-intact glioblastoma cells. *Cancer Res*, 66, 7864-7869.

[56] Wells, A. (1999). EGF receptor. *Int J Biochem Cell Biol*, 31, 637-643.

[57] Yung, W., Vredenburgh, J., Cloughesy, T., Nghiemphu, P., Klencke, B., Gilbert, M., Reardon, D. & Prados, M. (2010). Safety and efficacy of erlotinib in first-relapse glioblastoma: a phase II open-label study. Neurooncol, 12, 1061-1070.

Section 5

New Drugs for CNS Tumors – The Hope for the Future

Chapter 9

Comparative Preclinical Pharmacology and Toxicology for 4-demethyl-4-cholesteryloxycarbonylpenclomedine (DM-CHOC-PEN) — A Potential Neuro-Alkylating Agent for Glioblastoma (GBM) and Metastatic Cancers Involving the Central Nervous System

Lee Roy Morgan, Andrew H. Rodgers, Gerard Bastian, Edmund Benes, William S. Waud, Christopher Papagiannis, Dan Krietlow, Branko S. Jursic, Robert F. Struck, Gerald LaHoste, Melissa Thornton, Melody Luttrell, Edward Stevens and Rodger Thompson

Additional information is available at the end of the chapter

http://dx.doi.org/10.5772/58353

1. Introduction

4-Demethyl-4-cholesteryloxycarbonylpenclomedine (DM-CHOC-PEN), **1**, is a polychlorinated pyridine cholesteryl carbonate, (Fig. 1) that is a derivative of 4-demethylpenclomedine (DM-PEN, **2**) [1-4]. The latter is a non-neurotoxic metabolite of penclomedine (PEN, **3**, NSC 338720, 2-trichloromethyl-3,5-dichloro-4,6-dimethoxypyridine), that was identified during the NCI sponsored Phase I clinical trials with **3** [4-8]. **3** was found to be active *vs.* advanced cancers but possessed unacceptable neurotoxicity and discontinued from further study [5-10].

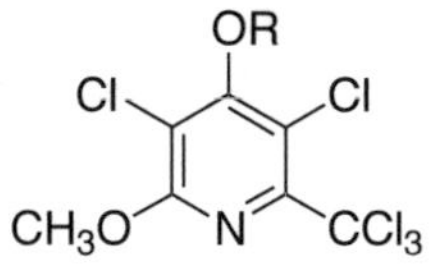

Where –**1**. DM-CHOC-PEN: R=CO_2-cholesteryl, **2**. DM-PEN: R=H, **3**. PEN: R=OCH_3

Figure 1. Penclomedine (PEN) and Analogs

INTECH
open science | open minds

© 2014 The Author(s). Licensee InTech. This chapter is distributed under the terms of the Creative Commons Attribution License (http://creativecommons.org/licenses/by/3.0), which permits unrestricted use, distribution, and reproduction in any medium, provided the original work is properly cited.

1 was synthesized at DEKK-TEC as part of a series of polychlorinated pyridine carbonates and carbamates that are lipophilic, non-neurotoxic alkylators of human xenograft brain and breast tumors implanted intracranially (IC) in mice [1-3].

Anticancer activity for **1** has been well documented *in vivo vs.* IC implanted human xenograft glioblastoma (U-251 and D-54) and breast cancer (MX-1) mouse models at doses lower or equivalent to its LD_{10} [1-3]. Over 25 carbonate and carbamate analogs of **2** have been synthesized and evaluated *in vivo* and **1** was the most active of the analogs *vs.* the above IC implanted human xenograft cancer models [1-3].

X-ray crystallography studies with **1** describe a perfectly linear configuration (Fig. 2) that includes a neutral heterocyclic ring linked through a stable carbonate group to a lipophilic cholesteryl moiety [2]. These basic characteristics plus the neutralizing effects (electrophilic) of the polyhalogenated substitutions on the pyridine ring probably contribute to **1**'s ability to form micelle particles that penetrate the blood brain barrier, and accumulate in CNS tumor tissues [1, 11].

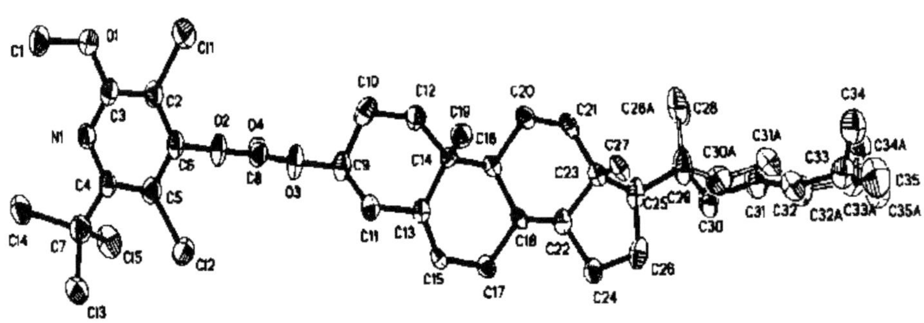

Figure 2. Structural characteristics of **1**

A mechanism of action has been proposed for **1** that involves cross-linking across the trichloromethyl group with tumor DNA in the major groove *via* N^7-guanine cross linking in a G-X-C sequence [1]. This mechanism of action would allow **1** to be administered in combination with many of the clinically significant DNA major groove-alkylating drugs, that include methylating agents [*e.g.* dacarbazine and temozolomide (Temodar^R)] and chloroethylating agents [*e.g.* bis(chloroethyl)-nitrosourea (BCNU) and clomesone] – all of which form carbonium ion-mediated adducts *via* O^6-guanine in *contrast* to binding with N^7-guanine, as does **1** [12].

The pharmacokinetics, metabolic fate and toxicology of **1** in three animal species (mice, rats and dogs) are reviewed here.

Cognitive/behavioral studies have been conducted in rats and dogs and are reviewed in depth.

2. Materials and methods

2.1. Drug formulation and chemicals

1 and **2** were synthesized by DEKK-TEC, Inc., using GLP/GMP guidelines, as previously described [1]. **1** is very stable in the solid state under ambient temperature and was administered in various vehicle media for the animal studies. For the rat studies, **1** was formulated as a buffered emulsion of soybean oil (20%), egg yolk lecithin (10%), glycerin (3%), histidine (3.1%) and water emulsion (containing 2-7 mg/mL of **1**) [IND 86,876]. For the mouse and dog IV studies, **1** was formulated as a 0.3% Klucel+0.3-3.3% Tween® 80, saline suspension and for the oral mouse study an emulsion of **1** in a 8% Tween-80®/Neobee®-1053 (Squibb) solution was used.

2.2. High pressure liquid chromatography (HPLC) analysis of 1 and a metabolite, 2

HPLC analysis was performed using an Agilent Technologies (New Castle, DE) 1200 model HPLC fitted with a diode array UV detector set at a wavelength of 244 nm (λ_{max} for **1**). A Rheodyne Model 7725 injection port (Cotati, CA, USA) with a 20μL sample loop was used to inject the samples. Chromatograms were recorded with an Agilent Technologies integrator. Samples were chromatographed using an Alltech 150 x 4.6 mμ column that contains *Luna* C8 (2) 100A packing (diameter of particles=5 mμ).

The mobile phase for **1** consisted of 80% THF: 20% water and for **2**, was 45% THF: 47% water, which was degassed, filtered through a 0.45 μm Rainin filter (Woburn, MA, USA) and delivered at a flow rate of 1.0 mL/min.

Plasma and erythrocyte samples were stored at-74°C until analyzed. Standard solutions were prepared by dissolving 6 mg of **1** or **2** in 20 mL THF. Internal standards were 20 mg of cholesteryl benzoate (**ChB**, Sigma Aldrich Co) or phenol (**P**, Sigma Aldrich Co) each in 20 mL THF. All solutions were stable for at least 2 months at 5° C. Standard assays for **1** and **2** consisted of 0.25 mL of plasma, 25 μL of **1** or **2** and internal standard (**ChB** or **P** – 2 μL) and 2 mL dichloromethane. The samples were vortexed for 10 min and frozen to separate the layers. The bottom organic layer was removed with a 25 gauge needle and glass syringe, filtered through a 0.45 mm Acrodisc syringe filter and evaporated to dryness under vacuum, reconstituted with 100 μL of THF and analyzed as below.

Control dog and rat whole blood and plasma samples were spiked with **1** in the concentration range 5-1000 ng/mL, plus 20 μL of the above **ChB**. Similar controls were prepared for **2** (ng/mL) and its int. std. – **P**. Peak-area ratios of **1/ChB** or (**2/P**) *vs*. the concentration of **1** or **2** (ng/mL) were subjected to linear regression analysis. Retention times for **1** and **ChB** were 6.41 and 4.63 min., respectively and for **2** and **P** were 6.6 and 18.5 min., respectively.

Verification of the HPLC assays included calibration curves derived from the assay of five (5) erythrocyte and eleven (11) plasma standards in duplicate prepared each with **1** and **2** (0.5 ng/mL-600 μg/mL). Plasma and erythrocyte samples were obtained from healthy rats and dogs and spiked with **1** or **2** and their respective internal standards. Drug concentrations in all samples were calculated using the results of linear regression analysis. Reproducibility was higher than 85%. Limit of quantitation for **1** and **2** was 0.2 ng/mL.

2.3. P-glycoprotein (P-gp) transport studies

Cell lines-three (3) human cancer cell lines-A549: *lung*; MCF7: *breast*; and HeLa: *ovarian* were obtained from ATCC, Manassas, MD, and maintained in culture in a temperature controlled (36 °C), 5% carbon dioxide, and humidity controlled incubator system. All culture transfers were in a laminar flow hood under sterile conditions. Tissue culture medium used was RPMI 1640 containing 10% FBS and penicillin/streptomycin/fungizone (1%) – all purchased from InVitrogen.

Material preparation-Rho was prepared in distilled water as a stock solution (1 mg/mL), stored frozen at-22° C. Rho (0.2μg/mL) was added to the culture medium in the presence or absence of Vpml and/or **1**. Vpml (2-23 μg/10 mL) was prepared in PBS solution and **1** (0.5-73 μg/10 mL) in PBS+5% DMSO.

A typical assay-contained: **1**-7.3 μg/mL, Vpml-2.5 μg/mL and Rho-0.2 μg/mL. Cells per test system were 0.8-1.2 x 10^6/mL. Incubations occurred in the above incubator conditions for the times and schedules discussed below. Experiments were conducted in triplicate and at times as specified in the Results. Reaction incubations were 15-60 minutes in length as discussed in the Results section.

Post incubation-After treatment, cells were rapidly trypsinized (~2 min), washed with cold PBS and kept on ice until analyzed. Assay conducted with a Becton-Dickinson FACS-ARIA II flow cytometer with CELLQUEST software. The Rho fluorescence was measured at laser excitation 488 nm with emission at 530 nm and is expressed in arbitrary units compared to control cells (untreated). Measurements were conducted on 10,000 cells per assay.

2.4. Animals

Adult Sprague-Dawley mice [Crl: CD1(ICR) BR] (males 20-25 g and female 18-25 g) and rats [Crl: CD1(ICR) BR] (males 300-350 g and female 225-250 g) were obtained from Harlan Industries (Indianapolis, IN), housed in groups of three-five per cage in light-controlled (12 h/day) and temperature-controlled (24°C) animal isolators with filtered vents and exhausts. They were fed a diet of Purina Laboratory Chow (Purina Feed) and received tap water *ad libitum*. The rats were fasted and 3-4 mL of blood was drawn *via* the jugular vein. The order of bleeding was alternated (one animal from each dose group, then repeating) to reduce handling and time biases.

Adult male and female beagle dogs (6.5-7.5 mo. of age, 6.5-9.49 kg) were raised and maintained at MPI Research (Mattawan, MI). They were fed a diet of Purina Dog Chow (Purina Feed), received tap water *ad libitum* and exercised per IACUC protocol. Mouse, rat and dog were euthanized with phenobarbital/ketamine anesthesia and/or carbon dioxide inhalation. The chest cavities were exposed to insure death. Institutional animal care and use committees (IACUC) reviewed and approved all the studies.

All mice, rat and dog studies were conducted at MPI Research (Mattawan, MI) under GLP regulations as described in the Guide for the Care and Use of Laboratory Animals, Office for Laboratory Animal Welfare, NIH, Bethesda, MD.

For mouse toxicity studies, **1** was administered IV bolus *via* the tail vein or per oral gavage; for the dog studies, **1** was administered as an IV bolus *via* the femoral vein and for rats, administration was during a 3 h IV infusion via indwelling femoral vein catheters. The observation period for all studies was 14-days – followed with euthanasia. For the rat and dog studies, complete necropsies with complete blood pharmacokinetic parameters, hematology, coagulation profiles, clinical chemistry and urine analyses were performed. For the mouse studies physical/gross necropsy examinations were conducted.

For the acute behavioral studies, rats received drugs and controls to identify/verify gross behavioral patterns employing a Morris modified water maze (4′ x 3′ x 1.5′) with a single layer of white polyethylene peanuts that floated (in 6″ of water) and covered a single mounting stage [13, 14]. Adult female rats (Hsd:SD, 175-225 g.) were grouped 3-6 animals per drug arm. The test agents were dissolved in or suspended in 5% aqueous Tween^{R} 80-hydroxypropyl cellulose in 5% saline and administered intraperitoneally (IP). Controls received the vehicle only. Swimming trials began – 1, 2, 3 and 20 hours post-dosing. For each time period post-dosing, the rats were challenged on six (6)-back-to-back swim trial events to find the platform. The daily swimming times and ranges were compared to vehicle controls *vs*. chemotherapeutics alone in rats. The data (latency to find the platform) was analyzed by variance (ANOVA). Body weights and water temperature-prior to each dosing and during each FOB assessment were monitored.

2.5. Pharmacokinetic studies

Groups of rats (5/sex) were administered 100, 200, or 300 mg/kg of **1** as a 3 h timed infusion and samples of blood collected (in EDTA tubes) at various time points IPEOI:-15,+10,+45 min, 1.5, 3, 6, 8, 12, 24 h and 14-days. Each animal possessed an indwelling femoral catheter for ease of the study. The catheters were flushed after each blood draw. The plasma and erythrocytes were separated and stored separately at -74°C until analyzed.

Adult beagle dogs (8 M) were administered **1** as a slow bolus injection once through a femoral vein in doses of 10, 20, and 30 mg/kg. A 20-gauge venous catheter was inserted into a saphenous vein for bleeding and samples were withdrawn at 0, 5, 15, and 30 min. and 1, 1.5, 2, 4, 8, 12 and 24 h into EDTA containing tubes. Plasma was separated and stored at-70° C until assayed. Animals were anesthetized with ketamine.

2.6. Animal pharmacokinetic data analysis

Model parameters were estimated using Micropharm software and nonlinear least squares regression was performed using Simplex and Gauss Newton algorithms []. An open two-compartment model provided the best fit. Clearance, volume of distribution and half-lives were derived from estimates of the model parameters.

2.7. Data analysis

Data analysis was performed on all plasma and *in vitro* studies and analyzed via non-linear regression using a non-weighed quasi-Newtonian/simplex fitting algorithm (Statistical software available from Stat soft, Tulsa, OK).

3. Results

3.1. Stability studies

Bulk drug product, **1**, as crystals, has been observed to remain stable for > four (4) years under ambient conditions [1]. The final clinical product (2 mg/mL) was stored at refrigerator temperatures (4-8° C) for 1.5 years without deterioration [15].

To further document product stability a 50:50 mixture of **1** (as the clinical product) with 10% Intralipid[R] (Fresenius Pharmaceuticals) was infused at room temperature over 8 h into a sterile container. Aliquots were withdrawn at 0, 0.5, 1, 2, 3, 4 h and analyzed by HPLC as described above. Decomposition of **1** during an 8-hour infusion at room temperature was 6% (mean for 4-runs). The breakdown product, **2**, could not be identified during this extended simulated infusion study [11].

3.2. Toxicity

Acute oral and IV toxicity study results for **1** in mice, rats and dogs are presented in Table 1 which presents median lethal dose values observed. The oral study with mice failed to produce toxicity at maximal administered doses of 0.8-2 g/kg. Volume restrictions prevented higher escalations. The drug (oral) was not active in the xenograft models, thus additional oral administration route studies were terminated. Two separate single IV mouse-dosing studies calculated a $LD_{10/50}$ of 136/385 mg/kg (for both sexes; with 95% confidence limits) – Table 1. Specific lethal/sublethal values and details are discussed in Table 1.

Clinical signs generally reflecting the deteriorating state of both mice and rats post dosing were observed in both sexes for **1** in a dose-dependent manner and included body surface staining, decreased activity, lethargy, loss of appetite, decreased defecation, tremors, and/or whole-body edema. The lethal experiences were sedation followed by respiratory arrest. No seizures or loss of coordination was observed for the survivors.

3.3. Acute single dose intravenous studies in mice

Adult male and female mice, 10 animals per sex per dose level, were intravenously dosed with 50, 100, 200, 400 and 600 mg/kg. No animals died at 0 or 100 mg/kg, 1 animal died at both 50 and 200 mg/kg doses, 7 of 10 animals died at 400 mg/kg and 8 of 10 animals died at 600 mg/kg (Table 1). Various clinical signs reflecting treatment-related effects were noted in both sexes, oftentimes in a generally dose-dependent manner. These clinical signs included decreased activity, rapid/difficult/slow/shallow breathing, limbs splayed, tremors and skin

http://dx.doi.org/10.5772/58353

cold to touch. No seizures or loss of coordination was noted. The deaths at 400 and 600 were of a very immediate nature, occurring within minutes or less post-dose, with no clinical signs exhibited prior to death. While transient incidences of rapid breathing were also noted in a couple of control animals, a definitive relationship to the vehicle was unclear. No definitively clear treatment-related body effects were noted in those mice surviving the 14-day observation period when compared with controls. No macroscopic findings were noted in any animal at necropsy.

Neither aplastic bone marrow nor splenic depletion of lymphocytes was noted.

Species	No/ Sex	Doses (mg/kg)	Method	$LD_{10/50}$ (mg/kg)	Time* (Days)	Comments
Mice	36 M	50-600	IV	132/385	2-14 days	Deaths were erratic
	36 F		Bolus	($LD_{10/50}$)		
Mice	30 M	800-2000	Oral –	0.8 – 2.0 g/d x	21 days	
	30 F		Gavage	5d – no deaths		No deaths
Rat	73 M		IV	100		1-Rat died @ 100 mg/kg; cholesterol – elevated, but acceptable
	73 F	50-300	Infusion	(LD_{10})	15 days	
Dog	8 M		IV			
	8 F	10-30	Bolus	>30.0	10 days	No deaths
Dog	4 M		IV			
	4 F	10-30	Bolus	>30.0	10 days	No deaths

*The time of the last death.

Table 1. Medial dose summary for **1**

Based on the conditions and findings of this study, the intravenous LD_{10} for **1** was calculated to be 136 mg/kg (95% confidence limits could not be calculated) in mice (combined sexes), while the intravenous LD_{50} was calculated to be 385 mg/kg (95% confidence limits).

3.4. Sub-chronic oral mouse toxicity (Table 1)

A study was conducted in groups of 10 male/10 female mice per dose. The study evaluated **1** administered daily for five days at doses of 0, 800, 1000, 1200, 1500 and 2000 mg/kg per gavage to mice. Only one death occurred at 800 mg/kg on day 2 after dosing. All animals demonstrated some degree of lethargy and unkempt appearance. Similar body appearances were noted with the controls. No seizures were noted.

3.5. Acute single dose intravenous studies in rats (Table 1)

A rat study was conducted with the objectives to evaluate and characterize acute toxicity, maximum tolerated dose (MTD), and evaluate pharmacology (including pharmacokinetic parameters) of **1** when intravenously (IV) administered over 3-hours, as an emulsion to rats. The same formulation that is being administered to patients via IV infusion in clinical trials was used for the rats (see Materials). A detailed clinical examination of each animal was performed daily and included evaluations of the skin, fur, eyes, ears, nose, oral cavity, thorax, abdomen, external genitalia, limbs and feet, respiratory and circulatory effects, autonomic effects such as salivation, nervous system effects, including tremors, convulsions, reactivity to handling, and psychological behavior.

Initially, a dose range finding (DRF) study was conducted that consisted of four (4) treatment groups – each group included 3-M/3-F that were single dosed IV infusions and monitored – no deaths were observed. The IV doses of **1** administered were – 50, 100, 150 and 200 mg/kg/dose.

The main study phase consisted of a control group (10-M/10-F) that each received the vehicle only and three groups (10-M/10-F) that each received a single IV infusion of **1** at dose levels of 100, 200 or 300 mg/kg. One male (1) rat in the 100 mg/kg group became moribund and was euthanized. No animals died in the 200 or 300 mg/kg dosed groups. No external related body effects were noted in the rats surviving the 14-day observation period. Both liver and spleens were target organs noted to be enlarged and evaluated in detail as discussed below.

The rats were divided into 2-groups that were euthanized either on Day-2 or Day-15. Complete macroscopic/microscopic examinations and complete clinical chemistry, hematology, coagulation studies and urinalysis were completed on all animals.

There were no meaningful hematological effects noted. On Day-2, erythrocytes, hemoglobin, and hematocrit tended to be higher in the 300 mg/kg/dosed group. These changes were most likely a result of fluid imbalances relative to reduced water intake. Monocytes were increased in both sexes at 200 and 300 mg/kg/dose and lymphocytes were decreased in males at 300 mg/kg/dose. Neutrophils were elevated in all groups on Days-2 and 15 and were attributed to stress and/or route of administration. All other changes were resolved by Day-15 and all values returned to normal pre-drug limits.

There were no test article-related effects on coagulation parameters or on urine analysis values.

The most significant findings were **1**'s related effects on the clinical chemistry analytes in the lipid profile studies (Table 2). Both alterations in the cholesterol and triglyceride profiles were significantly affected post dosing with **1**. Cholesterol and **2** are formed following the metabolism of **1** by the liver and/or peripherally (Scheme 1). The total cholesterol levels significantly increased in all groups *vs.* the control vehicle group. Increased levels of LDL-cholesterol were the pre-dominant variant observed on Day-2. However, by Day-15 the total cholesterol levels had returned to within normal limits and the total cholesterol was predominantly accounted for as a HDL-variant.

http://dx.doi.org/10.5772/58353

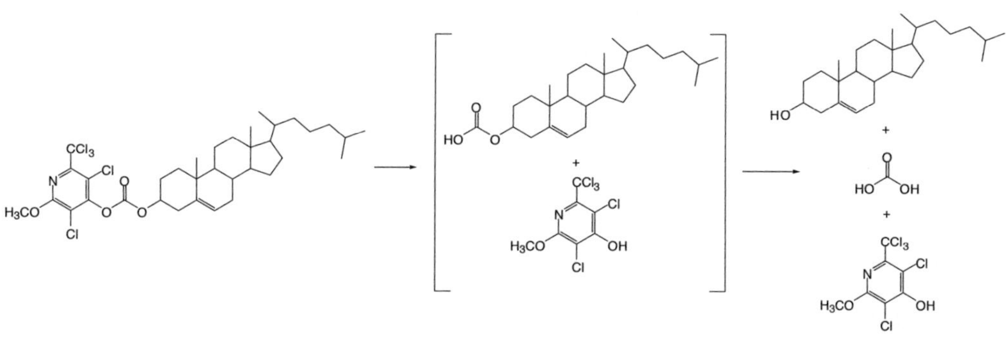

Scheme 1. Metabolism of **1**

Parameter	Day	Vehicle	100 mg/kg	200 mg/kg	300 mg/kg
(mg/dL)		**(M/F)**	**(M/F)**	**(M/F)**	**(M/F)**
Cholesterol	2	50/ 49.4	106.4[a]/77.8	206.4[b]/157.4[b]	188[b]/165.6[b]
(Total)	15	36.8/63.6	45.5/63.6	49.6[a]/48.8	51.8[a]/61.4
HDL-variant	2	27.4/34.4	33.6/36.8	25.2/30.8	25.6/28.8
	15	26.6/51.8	32.3/51.2	35.6[a]/40	37.8[b]/49.6
LDL-variant	2	134/5.4	66.0/31.3	210.2/142.6	183.6/156
	15	6.6/4.4	7.5/5.6	7.2/4.4	6.8/4.4
Triglycerides	2	38.8/29	54.8/40	109.8[a]/45.8	81/110.6
	15	36.6/43.8	37.3/34.4	33.8/28.4	46.2/30.8

No of animals in each group – 5; [a]Significantly different from control ($p<0.05$); [b]Significantly different from control ($p<0.01$).

Table 2. Summary of lipid profiles in rats dosed with 1 as an IV infusion (Day 1)

The triglycerides also increased in the 200 and 300 mg/kg groups on Day-2 post-dosing, which resolved by Day 15. The females demonstrated the most significant elevations in both triglycerides and LDL-cholesterol. On Day 15 the profiles for both total cholesterol and triglycerides had returned to WNL. Table 2 reviews cholesterol and triglyceride trends.

Alanine aminotransferase (ALT) in males, and γ-glutamyl transferase (GGT), and alkaline phosphatase in females were minimally to mildly elevated at the 300 mg/kg/dose on Day 2. All of the findings noted on Day-2 had resolved by Day-15.

Various clinical signs reflecting treatment-related effects were noted, mostly lethargy that cleared. No behavioral alterations were noted.

Macroscopic/microscopic examinations revealed increased sizes of the livers and spleens. On Day-2, the 200 and 300 mg/kg groups possessed vacuolated macrophages in the liver (Kupffer cells) and spleen. By Day-15 the macrophages contained smaller oil aggregates and clusters within hepatic sinusoids. The findings in both the spleen and the liver showed trends toward resolution by Day-15 with both biliary hyperplasia in the liver and splenic focal necrosis resolving; vacuoles were smaller and cell cytoplasm had a more eosinophilic tint seen in both livers and spleens, albeit the vacuoles still expanded the cytoplasm of the cells. The latter changes are artifacts resulting from the extraction of drug/lipids/cholesterol from hepatic/splenic macrophages during fixation/preparation of tissues for microscopic examination. The changes seen on Day-2 in the spleens and the livers trended towards resolution by Day-15. Controls (vehicle alone) did not demonstrate the above changes.

Transitory changes in the hepatic profile are considered 2° to stasis of **1** in hepatic sinusoids with biliary congestion that results in cysts and shunting of blood to the spleen resulting in splenic cysts and fatty deposits.

Although the above findings resolved by Day-15, they must be considered adverse – based on the degree of elevation in triglycerides (3-fold) and LDL-cholesterol (30-fold in females) seen in some groups. The control group received the vehicle alone – soybean oil and egg yolk lecithin – both rich in triglycerides and did not demonstrate abnormal lipid profiles or the liver/spleen changes.

Based on the conditions and findings of this study, the intravenous LD_{10} of **1** in rats was calculated to be 100 mg/kg (95% confidence limits could not be calculated) – Table 1.

3.6. Acute dog IV toxicity (Tables 1, 3)

A single IV dose study was performed in adult Beagle dogs, which consisted of **1** administered once as an IV bolus. Sixteen (16) adult beagle dogs (8 male and 8 female) divided into three groups received a single intravenous injection of **1**. The experimental design and results are presented in Table 3.

No treatment related effects on survival, hematology, urinalysis, or macroscopic and microscopic evaluations were noted during the study. Numerous clinical signs reflecting treatment-related effects were noted in both sexes of all groups, including the control group, and exhibited no dose-dependent pattern, clearly suggesting that the effects were attributable to the 0.3% Klucel+1.92% Tween 80 vehicle rather than **1**. Pertinent clinical signs noted included decreased activity, emesis, impaired righting reflex, limb function impaired, breathing slow/shallow, red skin discoloration (entire body, ears, or face), swelling (face and/or nose/muzzle), skin cold to touch, eyes swollen, slow gum capillary refill time, feces-mucoid/soft/discolored/watery, lacrimation, salivation, sclera injected, vocalization, tremors, and urination decreased. The effects were of immediate onset (within one hour post dose), with most of the signs clearing by Day 2 of the study. However, decreased activity persisted for Days 2, 3, or 4 in some of the animals and through the remainder of the study. No clear treatment-related body weight effects were noted during the study when comparing treated groups *vs.* controls. Slight body weight losses were noted in some animals which were non-dose related. The latter observations were in all probability attributable to the vehicle.

Route/Schedule	Dose (mg/kg)	Number and Sex		Observations
IV once	0	2M	2 F	No deaths
	10	2 M	2 F	No deaths
	20	2 M	2 F	No deaths
	30	2 M	2 F	No deaths

Table 3. Acute IV toxicity in the dog

There were marked elevations of alanine aminotransferase (ALT), and sorbitol dehydrogenase (SDH) in males in both controls and all treated animals on Day 2. Increased aspartate aminotransferase (AST) was observed in one (1) male with remarkably increased values for AST, ALT and SDH. The other male in this group exhibited only mildly increased values on Day 2 for these parameters. Similar trends were noted in females. ALT and SDH were highest on Day 2 for all dose levels, including controls. This acute and transient effect on liver enzymes exhibited no dose-dependent pattern and attributable to the vehicle. The latter finding was not observed to this extent in the rat study which used a different vehicle. The above was verified in a second group of 4M/4F.

The dog hematological studies confirmed that the 10-30 mg/kg doses do not produce myelosuppression, thrombocytopenia or anemia.

Treatment-related neurotoxicity was not observed following the single IV bolus administration of **1** to dogs. A second opinion review was obtained (RT), who conducted silver stains and confirmed MPI's observation that there were no microscopic pathological CNS changes present in the brains of dogs treated with **1** (FDA IND – 68,876) [14].

3.7. Summary Median Lethal Dose (Single Dose)

Table 1 summarizes the toxic effects of single IV dose administrations of **1** in mice, rats and dogs. Three intravenous studies were conducted under FDA GLP guidelines. The summary of the median lethal single dose (LD_{50}) values were calculated by combining the data from the acute single dose studies according to species and are available only for mice and dogs.

3.8. Acute rat behavioral studies

Rats in groups (5-females) received **1**, **2**, or **3** in a dose range finding (DRF) screen to identify and verify gross behavioral patterns (Table 4). Documentation of drug cognitive/learning abilities were conducted in a Morris modified water maze with adult female rats (Hsd:SD, 175-225 g.) which were grouped 3-6 animals per drug arm (Table 5).

Impaired learning behavior has not been observed for **1** or **2** in contrast to observed data for **3** during the first 1-3 h and at 20 h periods post-dosing (Table 5). A vehicle and a 5-FU control were included for comparison. The observations noted for **3** and 5-FU support the literature reports that both drugs impair memory in patients receiving the drug [16-18]. The described

Drug	Dose (mg/kg) IP	1 - 4 Hours	5th Hour	7th Hour
Vehicle (Controls)	0.5 mL	Alert; normal behavior	Alert; normal behavior	Alert; normal behavior
Mk-801 (control)	0.05 once	Lethargic	Lethargic	Lethargic
5-FU (Chemo Control)	78	Lethargy, eyes closed	More alert	Normal behavior
3	400-800 once	Eyes closed; spastic; lethargy	Less lethargy; spastic	Normal behavior
2	350-600 once	No acute toxicity; no spasms	Normal behavior	Normal behavior
1	100 & 300 once	No acute toxicity; no spasms	Normal behavior	Normal behavior

Table 4. Rats - gross behavior patterns (5 female rats per group, 160-168 g)

assay is a simple, reproducible quantitative assessment of impaired visuospatial cerebellar-learning/memory and performance functions *via* swimming and navigating a water maze. The treated and control rats were timed to navigate to find a hidden platform – Figures 3 and 4.

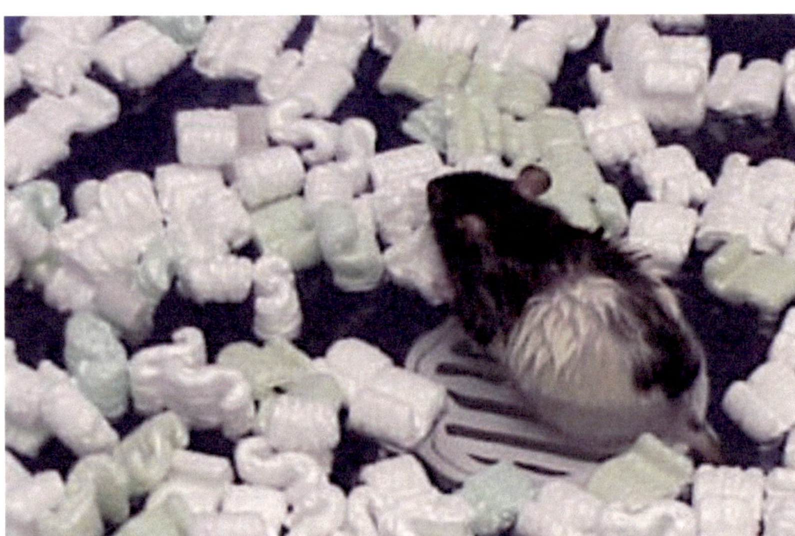

Figure 3. A rat on the water maze platform.

A control memory impairment agent, MK-801, is included to demonstrate complete impalement. In contrast, **1** and **2** had little or no influence on learning/memory, while **3** produced long lasting impairment.

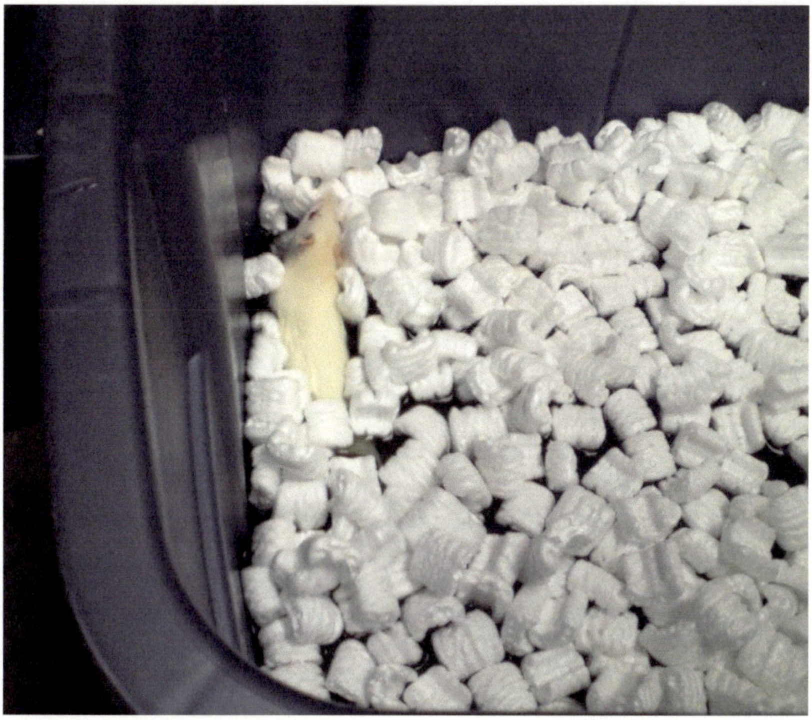

Figure 4. A rat swimming through the peanuts.

3.9. Brain/tumor penetration

Adult male mice (athymic NCr-nu/nu – NCI-Frederick Production Area, NCI) were sedated and intracerebrally (IC) implanted with U251 glioma cells (10^6) from tissue culture. The mice were divided into 5-control and 5-treated with **1**. The latter group was administered **1** (135 mg/kg/day) IP daily for two consecutive days (q1d x 2) beginning 4-days post inoculation of cells. Four hours after the second treatment the animals were sacrificed and the brains removed intact (cerebellum included), flash frozen in liquid nitrogen and stored at -77 °C until assayed.

The intact frozen brains (~1.3 g) were coronal sliced into three sections in a mouse brain blocker (Kopf). The encapsulated gliomas were easily identified and separated readily from normal brain tissue with a scalpel and using microscopic 'touch finger printing' – separation verified. The tumor tissues were weighed, pooled and homogenized in 10 mL saline at 5°C. This process was repeated for the normal brain tissue. The cold homogenates were separately extracted with 10 mL dichloromethane, the organic layer separated and evaporated to dryness.

The residues were dissolved in dichloromethane and underwent preparative TLC on silica gel plates (Sigma-Aldrich, Milwaukee, WI) with a mobile phase – hexane/dichloromethane:10/30. The respective spots for **1** and **2** were extracted with dichloromethane, concentrated and analyzed by HPLC (for procedure, see-Methods). **1** and **2** were present in the gliomas extracts -62 and 11 ng/g, resp. (avg.) were present in the gliomas, but none in the normal brain tissue.

TREATMENTS				LEARNING - IMPROVEMENT (MEAN) *[DIFFERENCE BETWEEN 1st AND 6th TEST – SAME TIME PERIOD]				MEMORY – IMPROVEMENT/IMPAIRMENT [Differences Between 1 – 20 hrs]				
								1Hr→	2Hr→	3Hr→		
Agent	Dose (mg/kg/ dose	#Rats	Schedule	1 Hr	2 Hr	3 Hr	20 Hr	2 Hr	3 Hr	20 Hr	1 Hr → 20 Hr (Overall)	
				Fold↑	Fold↑	Fold↑	Fold↑	Fold↑	Fold↑	Fold↑	Fold ↑	Time (sec)
Control	Saline	24	_	3.2	1.3	2.1	2.0	3.0	0.7	1.6	3.5	35.1
MK-801	0.05	3	QD X 1	0**	0**	0**	0**	0	0	0	0	0
5-FU	78	6	QD X 1	1.7	1.3	1.7	8.2	1.0	0.6	1.3	0.7	-13.5
3	400	6	QD X 1	0.8	1.3	0.6	1.2	1.4	1.7	0.6	1.0	-1.2
2	135	6	QD X 1	6.7	1.5	1.7	2.4	4.0	1.0	1.0	3.5	42.1
1	100	6	QD X 1	3.2	1.3	1.8	3.8	3.2	0.6	1.5	2.4	23.6

*Rats were tested – six (6) separate trials – 1, 2, 3 and 20 hrs post dosing. The rats are timed to swim to the stage. The fold improvements are recorded in the table. For hours 1, 2, 3, and 20 post dosing, two values are given for each drug. The first number (X) for each hour is the difference (in seconds) between the initial and final attempts (first – sixth run). A negative number indicates complete lack of learning throughout six runs – taking a longer amount of time on the sixth try than the first. The next value (indicated with *) is X fold performance improvement. This is calculated by initial/ final time. <1 indicates complete lack of improvement (taking longer on the last try than the first). Doses used were the therapeutic values as determined from the tumor models.

**MK-801-is a NMDA (N-methyl-D-aspartate) inhibitor that produced a solemn effect that prevented the rats from swimming and learning. After 3-days the rats were equivalent *vs.* control. 5-FU has been associated with memory loss in patients treated with chemotherapy (17).

Table 5. Evaluation of the behavioral activity of penclomedine analogs in female rats

Five (5) control mice bearing IC implanted U251 cells (non-treated) were used as the dissection and extraction controls. No chemicals were identified in the above extraction assays or in the brains from the control tumor/normal mice.

3.10. Normal brain penetration

Adult male rats [Crl: CD1(ICR) BR] (325-350 g wt) in groups of 5 animals were dosed intraperitoneally with 50 mg/kg of DM-CHOC-PEN in 0.3% Klucel/Tween80/saline daily x 2 days. On the 3rd day the rats were sacrificed and the intact brains removed (~1.9 g) and each homogenized in 10 mL saline at 5°C. To the cold homogenates, 20 mL dichloromethane was added and shaken for 30 minutes. The organic layer was removed and evaporated to dryness under vacuum at room temperature. The residues were dissolved in 1 mL of tetrahydrofuran and 100 μL chromatographed on silica gel plates with hexane:dichloromethane (1:1) as solvent. DM-CHOC-PEN was identified at R_f 0.74 with an additional spot – R_f 0.51. All spots were cut out, extracted with THF and analyzed by HPLC. DM-CHOC-PEN and a polar metabolite were identified by HPLC (see below).

DM-CHOC-PEN was calculated to be present-100 ng/g (avg.) of whole brain. The more polar peak (R_f 0.51) was not DM-PEN and present at 20 ng/g of whole brain. ^{1}H-NMR of the latter fraction identified a pair of peaks at δ 5.68 & δ 5.75-consistent with loss of a methylene chlorine and binding to an NH-group, possible adduct. The material possessed a cholesteryl carbonate moiety. Normal brain tissue was used as a control.

3.11. Pharmacokinetic studies in rats and dogs (Table 5)

Plasma concentration-time profiles for **1** in adult rats post a 3-hour single dose IV infusion of 100, 200 and 300 mg/kg are presented in Fig. 5. Mean pharmacokinetic parameters for rats summarized in Table 6, Figs. 5 and 6 were – $T_{1/2\alpha}$ 15+/-7 h, $T_{1/2\beta}$ 19.1+/-1.3 h and CL 22.2+/-6.5 L/h for **1**, which could be detected 24 h post infusion. As mentioned previously and outlined in Scheme 1, **1** is metabolized to 2 and cholesterol, which are compared in Fig. 6 for the 100 mg/kg dose. The levels of 2 and cholesterol paralleled each other, as expected.

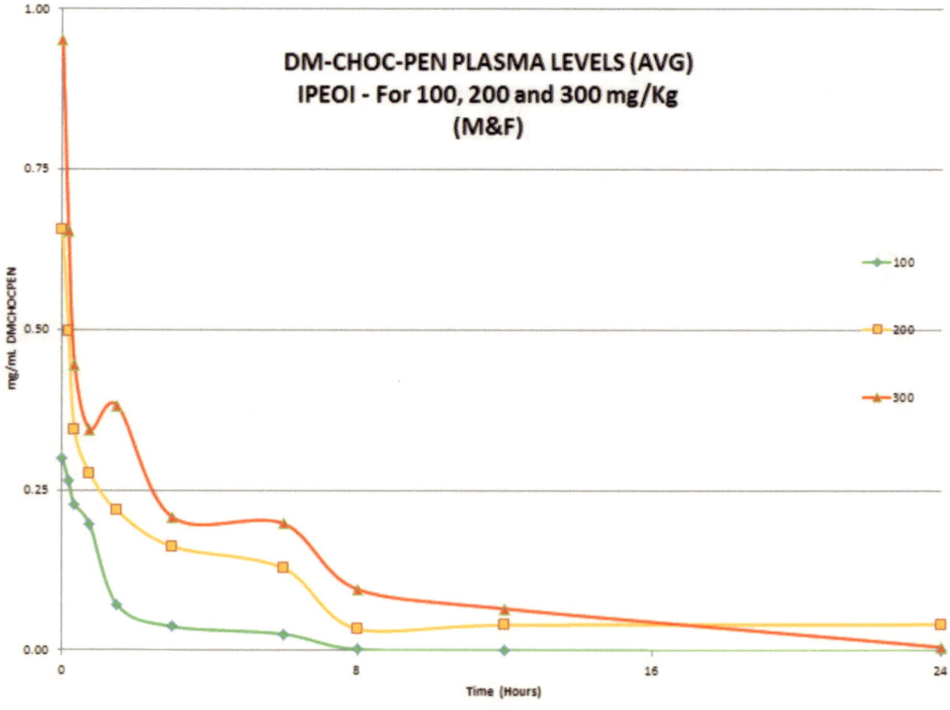

Figure 5. Mean plasma levels for **1** IPEOI – 4-rats per group.

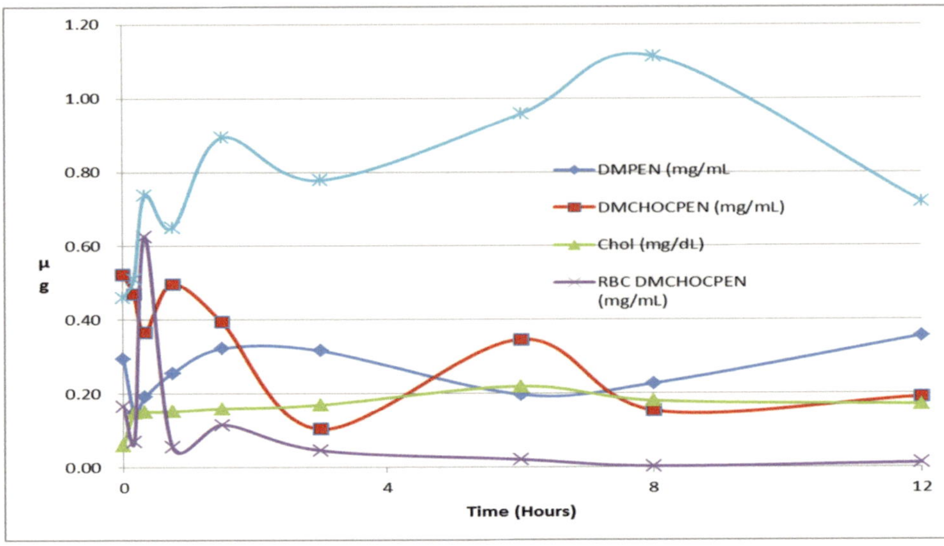

Figure 6. Mean plasma and rbc levels for **1, 2** and cholesterol, IPEOI for **1** after IV infusion (200 mg/kg) – 4-rats per group.

The shifts noted in the bioavailability for **1** *vs.* **2** are suggestive of an enzyme overload – a Michaelis Menten effect (Fig. 6). For rats, the AUC and C_{max} values *vs.* doses of **1** administered were linear – Figs. 7 & 8. Dog pharmacokinetics for **1** are compared to the rat values in Table. For dogs, plasma clearance was constant between 10 and 30 mg/kg. The plasma clearance is 328.8 L/h *vs.* 346.8 L/h; demonstrating the PK linearity of **1**. Differences seen between rats and dogs are due to the fact that rats received **1** during a 3-hr IV infusion and dogs *via* an IV bolus injection – thus not comparable.

Dose	Specie (N)	$T_{1/2}\alpha$ (h)	$T_{1/2\beta}$ (h)	AUC (mg*h/L)	Cl (L/h)
10 mg/kg	Dog (4)	1.23 (Mean)	21.6 (Mean)	0.42 (Mean)	328.8 (Mean)
		0.53 (SD)	16.00 (SD)	0.17 (SD)	221.2 (SD)
30 mg/kg	Dog (4)	0.63 (Mean)	18.7 (Mean)	1.12 (Mean)	346,8 (Mean)
		0.09 (SD)	10.7 (SD)	0.09 (SD)	54.5 (SD)
100 mg/kg	Rat (5)	0.51 (Mean)	2.48 (Mean)	1.05 (Mean)	30.4 (Mean9.99
		0.05 (SD)	0.8 (SD)	0.53 (SD)	(SD)
200 mg/kg	Rat (5)	0.25 (Mean)	6.94 (Mean)	3.46 (Mean)	16.9 (Mean)
		0.1 (SD)	2.1 (SD)	0.46 (SD)	4.04 (SD)
300 mg/kg	Rat (5)	0.12 (Mean)	4.0 (Mean)	5.17 (Mean)	19.40 (Mean)
		0.06 (SD)	1.2 (SD)	1.74 (SD)	9.13 (SD)

(Males & females combined)

Table 6. Comparative PK parameters of **1** in rats and dogs

http://dx.doi.org/10.5772/58353

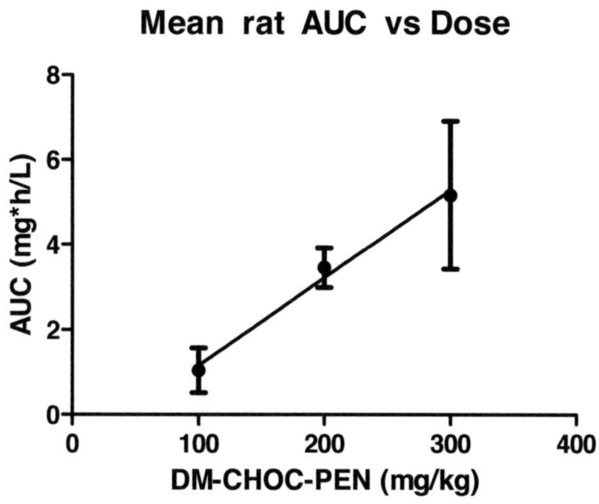

Figure 7. AUC *vs.* dose for **1**

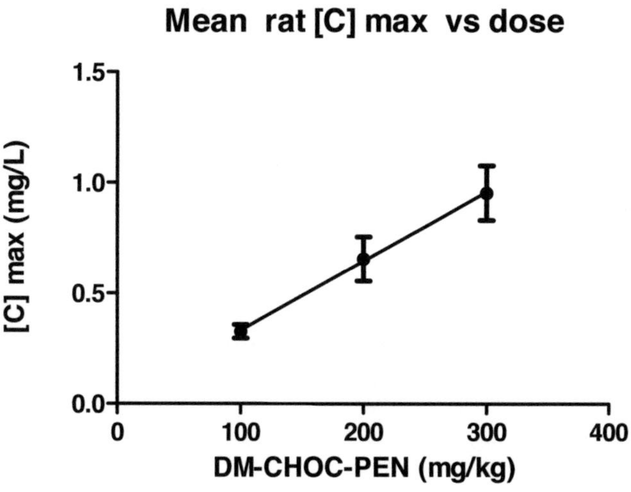

Figure 8. $[C]_{max}$ *vs*. dose for **1**

3.12. P-glycoprotein (P-gp) transport (Table 6)

The results of incubating Rho in the presence or absence of Vpml and/or **1** are summarized in Table 7.

Six reaction conditions (**1-6**) are reviewed, where:

1 – is the result from incubating cell lines with Rho for 15 minutes.

2 – is the result from incubating cell lines with Vpml for 1 hour and then adding Rho during the last 15 minutes of incubation.

3 – is the result from incubating the cell lines with Vpml for 15 minutes, adding **1** after an incubation time of 30 minutes and then adding Rho during the last 15 minutes – total incubation time, 60 minutes.

4 – is the result from treating the cell lines simultaneously with Vpml and **1** for 45 minutes and then adding Rho and continuing the incubations for an additional 15 minutes – total incubation time – 60 minutes.

5 – is the result from incubating the cell lines with **1** for 15 minutes and then adding Vpml for additional 45 minute incubation. Rho is added during the last 15 minutes of the incubation.

Finally, **6** is the result of incubating each of the cell lines for 1 hour with **1** alone and then adding Rho during the last 15 minutes of incubation.

The results summarized in Table 7 for the 3 sensitive cell lines are coherent: The rate of incorporation of Rho is lower when cells are treated by the mixture of Vpml and DM-CHOC-PEN or Vpml alone but not when the cells are treated with DM-CHOC-PEN alone (mean fluorescence intensity of 6 roughly the same for control cells). This is interpreted as meaning that DM-CHOC-PEN has no effect on the function of P-gp transport.

Cell Line	Mean Fluorescence Intensity for Total Cells (Mean) (x 10^3)*					
	Rho	Vpml + Rho	Vpml → DM + Rho	Vpml + DM +Rho	DM + Vpml + Rho	DM + Rho
	1	2	3	4	5	6
HeLa	19.3**	15.0	15.6	18.2	16.0	17.6
A549	23.2	20.8	16.4	13.2	17.9	21.8
MCF-7	10.5	6.5	5.9	6.2	7.4	8.9

*Cell concentration per each assay. Average of triplicate assays.

Table 7. P-glycoprotein transport of **1**

4. Discussion

The rationale for the pre-clinical development of **1**, a polychlorinated pyridine cholesteryl carbonate, was based on observed antitumor activity *vs.* IC implanted human xenografts growing in mice, in comparison with standard therapy [1,2]. **1** was synthesized during an attempt to design and develop polychlorinated pyridine carbonates that could penetrate the BBB, with cytotoxic activity *vs.* intracranially growing brain tumors and without neurotoxicity [1,2].

We report here the results of acute toxicity and pharmacology studies with single intravenous injections of **1** in groups of rodents and dogs. The end-point of all the studies was to identify drug toxicity and an acceptable starting dose for a Phase I clinical trial in humans with advanced cancer.

The IV LD_{10} single-dose value for mice (sexes combined) was calculated as 139 mg/m^2. The mouse study generally displayed a typical dose-response effect (with the exception of one death at 50 mg/kg), with **1** being slightly more toxic in males than in females at the two highest doses.

A sub-chronic oral mouse toxicity study was conducted at MPI Research, Mattawan, MI, under GLP conditions in male/female mice. The study evaluated **1** in an emulsion administered per oral gavage daily for five days at doses of 0, 800, 1000, 1200, 1500 and 2000 mg/kg per gavage to mice. Only one death occurred at 800 mg/kg on day 2 after dosing. All animals demonstrated some degree of lethargy and unkempt appearance, but no seizures. Similar body appearances were noted with the controls.

Adult rats were treated once with single IV infusions of **1** in doses of 50, 100, 150, 200, and 300 mg/kg. One (1) death occurred at the 100 mg/mL dose level. No deaths occurred in the treated vehicle group. There were no meaningful effects on hematology parameters. On Day-2 erythrocytes, hemoglobin, and hematocrit tended to be higher at the 300 mg/kg/dose. These changes were most likely a result of fluid imbalance. Monocytes were increased in both sexes at 200 and 300 mg/kg/dose and lymphocytes were slightly decreased in males at 300 mg/kg/dose level. Neutrophils were elevated relative to expected ranges in all groups on Days-2 and 15 and were attributed to stress and/or route of administration. All other changes were resolved by Day 15 and all values returned to normal pre-drug limits. There were no test article-related effects on either coagulation or on urinalysis parameters.

The most significant abnormal findings were the statistically increased plasma values for cholesterol and triglycerides in the 200 and 300 mg/kg treated groups. LDL-cholesterol was significantly elevated in females – increased from 5.4 to 142 and 156 mg/dL for the 200 and 300 mg/kg groups, resp. This elevation is significant and considered a SLT (CTEP.v4). The triglycerides were increased by 4-fold in the 300 mg/kg group females, however, they return to normal values by Day-15. Hepatic and splenic deposits of fats were also noted on gross and microscopic examinations which cleared by Day-15.

Cholesterol is released during metabolism of **1** (Table 2 & Scheme 1). The early formation of LDL-cholesterol is not a surprise since the formation of the LDL-variant is the initial natural method to 'initially encase cholesterol molecules'. The cholesterol is cleared through the liver as the HDL-variant. Triglycerides were elevated secondary to increased cholesterol and the lipid character of the emulsion vehicle, which also rapidly reversed [3].

Although the above cholesterol and triglyceride findings resolved by Day-15, they must be considered adverse – triglycerides (3-fold) and LDL-cholesterol (30-fold in females). The control group received the vehicle alone – soybean oil and egg yolk lecithin – both rich in triglycerides and did not demonstrate abnormal lipid profiles.

Alanine aminotransferase (ALT) in males, and γ-glutamyl transferase (GGT), and alkaline phosphatase in females were minimally to mildly elevated in the 300 mg/kg group on Day-2. All of these findings on Day-2 resolved by Day-15. Transient elevations in transaminases were considered to be 2° to hepatic clearance of the drug. Neither gross nor microscopic evidence of toxicity (other than hepatic cysts) was noted at autopsies, including CNS. Table 7 compares calculated starting therapeutic doses for humans [19].

A single IV dose administration study was performed in adult beagle dogs employing single doses (10 – 30 mg/kg) of **1**. No treatment related fatalities occurred. Numerous clinical signs reflecting treatment-related effects were noted in both sexes of all groups. Pertinent clinical signs noted included decreased activity, autonomic hyperactivity – vomiting, decreased urination, salivation, and lacrimation. The effects were of immediate onset (within one hour post dose), with most of the signs clearing by Day-2 of the study. However, decreased activity persisted for Days 2, 3, and 4 in some of the animals and through the remainder of the study. Slight body weight losses noted in some animals were not dose-dependent and it could have been attributable to the clinical signs (and associated stress) caused by the vehicle. There were marked elevations of aspartate aminotransferase (AST), alanine aminotransferase (ALT), and sorbitol dehydrogenase (SDH) noted in controls and all treated groups and apparently attributable to the vehicle – a Klugel/Tween mixture that will not be used in the clinical studies. All liver functions reversed by Day-15. This acute and transient effect on liver enzymes exhibited no dose-dependent pattern and was also apparently attributable to the vehicle. The latter finding was not observed in the rat study.

No hematological deficiencies were noted in any group. Drug-related neurotoxicity was not observed. This was confirmed by second opinion (RT), who conducted silver stains and confirmed MPI's observation that there were no microscopic pathological CNS changes present in the brains of dogs treated with **1** [19].

Based on the conditions and findings of this study, a single bolus intravenous injection of **1** to groups of beagle dogs at dose levels of 10, 20 and 30 mg/kg produced no effects that were directly related to the test article; instead they were probably attributable to the 0.3% Klucel +1.92% Tween® 80 vehicle used.

Pharmacokinetic studies were conducted in two species – rats and dogs. Parameters were obtained from Gauss Newton algorithm modeling [3]. The values are compared in Table 6. No statistical differences between male and female rats were noticed. The differences in half life can be explained in reference to administration routes – dog-IV bolus *vs*. rat – IV infusion over 3 hrs. Similarly, the clearance is higher in the bolus studies as expected with a surge of drug being filtered.

In the learning/cognitive screening study, rats treated with **3** took a longer period of time to find the pedestal *vs*. **1**, **2** and the controls. Despite normal gross appearance of the rats after 7 hr (Table 4), the **3** treated animals demonstrated impaired learning (Table 5). There were no signs of learning impairment noted in the rats treated with **1** or **2**, as was seen for **3**. **2** is a polychlorinated 4-hydroxypyridine (Fig. 1) and exists as a zwitterion that is too polar to cross the BBB. This behavior has been observed for other 4-hydroxypyridines [20]. The water

http://dx.doi.org/10.5772/58353

swimming maze assesses impaired visual spatial processing, as well as memory. The observations for 5-FU (drug control) confirmed literature reports of learning/memory impairment post dosing in humans [16].

The drug penetrated human glioblastoma tumor tissue growing IC in mice, with none detectable in the normal tissue. This only reinforced our interest in using the drug to treat patients with cancers involving the CNS.

1 does not have effects on the P-gp transport system. In the current study, Rho was selected as an indicator of **1**'s interaction/inhibition with the P-gp protein transport system in three (3) human cancer cell lines-A549: *lung*; MCF7: *breast*; and HeLa: *ovarian*. Verapamil (Vpml) is a known inhibitor of the P-gp pathway and was included as a positive control, providing additional support that **1** is not a substrate for the P-gp transmitter system and not rejected *via* the high energy ATP-binding cassette (ABC) transport systems [11].

Both **1** and **2** bind to erythrocytes and could penetrate the blood brain barrier (BBB) and IC growing cancers attached to rbcs *via* breaks in the BBB (penetration routes of metastatic cancers) or sites of neo-angiogenic networks. However, as previously published, **2** alone is not active *vs*. IC implanted human breast and glioma tumors implanted in a mouse model; the presence of **2** in the IC implanted tumors (see Results-*Brain/tumor penetration*) must be due to IC steroid esterase hydrolysis of **1** [21].

Thus, preclinical studies, conducted under GLP guidelines are presented as support for **1** to enter Phase I clinical trials as treatment for advanced cancer with CNS involvement. Table 8 reviews calculated starting doses and data satisfied the FDA's requirements for an IND (IND 68,876), which has completed a Phase I clinical trial – DTI-021 [19]. The phase I clinical trial is nearing completion with acceptable toxicities and responses noted in patients with advanced cancer involving the CNS system [15].

Drug	Species	Acute IV LD_{10}	Comparable Human IV Dosage*
DM-CHOC-PEN	Mouse	136 mg/kg/d	39 $mg/m^2/d$ (10% of LD_{10})
DM-CHOC-PEN	Rat	100 mg/kg/d	60 mg/m^2 (10% of LD_{10})
DM-CHOC-PEN	Dog	>30 mg/kg/d	>100 $mg/m^2/d$** (1/6th HNSTD)

* Standard conversion **Based on the highest dose – 30 mg/kg used in the dog studies

The initial level of dosing in the Phase I clinical trial has been established as 39 mg/m^2 (IND 86,876) (19).

Table 8. Estimated comparable human intravenous dosages

Acknowledgements

Supported by NCI/SBIR grants – 5R44CA85021 and 1R43CA132257

Author details

Lee Roy Morgan[1], Andrew H. Rodgers[1], Gerard Bastian[4], Edmund Benes[1], William S. Waud[6], Christopher Papagiannis[7], Dan Krietlow[7], Branko S. Jursic[2], Robert F. Struck[5], Gerald LaHoste[3], Melissa Thornton[1], Melody Luttrell[1], Edward Stevens[2] and Rodger Thompson[8]

1 DEKK-TEC, Inc., New Orleans, LA, USA

2 Department of Chemistry, University of New Orleans, Lakefront, New Orleans, LA, USA

3 Department of Psychology, University of New Orleans, Lakefront, New Orleans, LA, USA

4 Service de Pharmacologie, CHU Pitie'-Salpetriere, Paris, France

5 Cancermedica, LLC, Birmingham, AL, USA

6 Southern Research Institute, Birmingham, AL, USA

7 MPI Research, Mattawan, MI, USA

8 Veterinary Neuropathology, Birmingham, AL, USA

References

[1] Morgan LR, Struck RF, Waud WR, LeBlanc B, Rodgers AH, Jursic BS. Carbonate and carbamate derivatives of 4-demethylpenclomedine as novel anticancer agents. Cancer Chemotherapy and Pharmacology, 64: 829-836, 2009.

[2] Morgan LR, Struck RF, Waud WR, Jursic BS, Serota D, Papagiannis C, Rodgers AH. Carbonate and carbamate derivatives of 4-demethylpenclomedine as novel anticancer agents. Molecular Targets and Cancer Therapeutics, 23, 231, 2007.

[3] Morgan LR, Struck RF, Rodgers AH, Serota DG. Preclinical Toxicity of 4-Demethyl-4-cholesteryloxylcarbonylpenclomedine (DM-CHOC-PEN). Proc. Amer. Assoc. Res., 48: abst. 5614, 2007.

[4] Waud WR, Tiwari A, Schmid SM, Shih T-W, Strong JM, Hartman NR, O'Reilly S,

[5] Struck RF. 4-Demethylpenclomedine, an antitumor-active, potentially non-neurotoxic metabolite of penclomedine. Cancer Res, 57:815-817, 1997.

[6] Berlin J, Stewart JA, Storer B, Tutsch KD, Arzoomanian RZ, Alberti D, Feierabend C, Simon K, Wilding G (1998) Phase I clinical and pharmacokinetic trial of penclomedine using a novel, two stage trial design for patients with advanced malignancy. J Clin Oncol, 16:1142-1149.

[7] O'Reilly S, Grochow L, Donehower RC, Bowling K, Chen TL, Hartman N, Struck R, Rowinsky EK. Phase I and pharmacologic studies of penclomedine, a novel alkylating agent in patients with solid tumors. J Clin Oncol, 15: 1974-1984, 1997.

[8] Jodrell DI, Bowman A, Stewart M, Dunlop N, French R, MacLellan A, Cummings J, Smyth JF. Dose-limiting neurotoxicity in a phase I study of penclomedine (NSC 388720, CRC 88-04), a synthetic alpha-picoline derivative, administered intravenously. Brit J Cancer, 77: 808-811, 1998.

[9] Berlin J, Wahamaki A, Tutsch KD, Alberti D, Feierabend C, Binger, K, Arzoomanian, RZ, Volkman, J, Karca J, Mornocha, R, Stewart J, Wilding G. Phase I, pharmacokinetic and bioavailability study of oral penclomedine administered daily x 5 every four weeks. Proc. Amer. Assoc. Cancer Res, 40: 92, 1999.

[10] O'Reilly S, O'Hearn E, Rowinsky EK, Struck RF, Molliver ME. Neuroanatomic studies of the cerebellar effects of penclomedine. Proc. Amer. Assoc. Cancer Res, 37:

[11] 374-375, 1996.

[12] O'Reilly S, O' Hearn E, Struck RF, Rowinsky EK, Molliver ME. The alkylating agent penclomedine induces degeneration of purkinje cells in the rat cerebellum. Invest New Drugs, 21:269, 2003.

[13] Morgan LR, Struck RF, Waud W, Jursic BS, Serota DG, Papagiannis C, Rodgers AH, Thornton, ME, GS LaHoste. Comparative pharmacokinetics and intermediary metabolism of 4-demethyl-4-cholesteryl-oxycarbonylpenclomedine (DM-CHOC-PEN), EORTC/ AACR/NCI (Berlin), Abst 871, 2010.

[14] Pletsas D, Wheelhouse RT, Pletsa V, Nicolaou A, Jenkins TC, Bibby MC. Kytopoulas SA. Polar, functionalized guanine-O^6 derivatives resistant to repair by O^6-alkylguanine-DNA alkyltransferase: implications for the design of DNA-modifying drugs. Eur. J. Med Chem., 11: 1-10, 2006.

[15] Morris, R. Development of water-maze procedure for studying spatial learning in the rat. J. Neuroscience Methods, 11: 47-60, 1984.

[16] Saab, BJ, Saab, AMP, Roder, JC. Statistical and theoretical considerations for the platform re-location water maze. J. Neurosci. Meth. 198:44-52, 2011.

[17] Weiner RS, Friedlander P, Gordon C, Mahmood T, Ware ML, Bastian G, Rodgers AH, Urien S, Morgan, LR. A first-in-humans: phase I clinical for 4-Demethyl-4-cholesteryl-oxycarbonylpenclomedine (DM-CHOC-PEN). Proc Amer. Assoc. Cancer Res., 54, 1173, 2013.

[18] Dietrich J, Han R, Yang Y, Mayer-Proschel M, Noble M. CNS progenitor cells and oligodendrocytes are targets of chemotherapeutics *in vitro* and *in vivo*. J Biol. 5:22-32, 2006.

[19] Konat GW, Kraszpulski M, James I, Zhang HT, Abraham J. Cognitive dysfunction induced by chronic administration of common cancer chemotherapeutics in rats. Metabolic Brain Diseases, 23:325–333, 2008.

[20] Common chemo drug can cause memory problems. In: the Times-Picayune News Paper, New Orleans, LA, B-3, pg 3, 2008 and ref cited.

[21] Morgan LR. A Phase I Trial: Safety and tolerance of 4-demethyl-4-cholesteryloxy-carbonylpenclomedine (DM-CHOC-PEN)-a potential neuro-alkylating agent for glioblastoma and metastatic cancers of the central nervous system, FDA IND 68,876, 2010.

[22] Morgan LR, Rodgers AH, Bastian G, Benes E, Waud WR, Jursic BS, Struck RF, LaHoste G, Thornton M, Luttrell M, Stevens E, Thompson R. Comparative preclinical pharmacology and toxicology for 4-demethyl-4-cholesteryloxycarbonylpenclomedine (DM-CHOC-PEN): A potential neuro-alkylating agent for glioblastoma and metastatic cancers of the central nervous system. ECCO in European J Cancer, Abst. 57, 2011.

[23] Lund-Pero, M, Jeppson, B, Arneko-Nobin, B, Sjogren, HO, Holmgren, K, Pero, RVV. Non-specific steroidal esterase activity and distribution in human and other mammalian tissue. Clin. Chim Acta, 224: 9-20, 1994.